16/
μx/osc

DISEASES OF THE NERVOUS SYSTEM

Diseases of
The Nervous System

DESCRIBED FOR
PRACTITIONERS AND STUDENTS

by
F. M. R. WALSHE
M.D., D.Sc., F.R.C.P.(Lond.); F.R.S.,
D.Sc.(Hon.), Nat. Univ. Ireland

PHYSICIAN IN CHARGE OF THE NEUROLOGICAL DEPARTMENT, UNIVERSITY COLLEGE HOSPITAL, LONDON;
PHYSICIAN TO THE NATIONAL HOSPITAL FOR NERVOUS DISEASES, QUEEN SQUARE;
FELLOW OF UNIVERSITY COLLEGE, LONDON

FIFTH EDITION
(REPRINT)

EDINBURGH
E. & S. LIVINGSTONE LTD.
16 & 17 TEVIOT PLACE
1947

First Edition	.	September 1940
Second Edition	.	August 1941
Reprinted	.	. May 1942
Third Edition	.	March 1943
Reprinted	.	January 1944
Fourth Edition	.	April 1945
Reprinted	.	January 1946
Fifth Edition	.	January 1947
Reprinted	.	September 1947

Printed in Great Britain

Preface to Fifth Edition

THE continued favour shown to this text-book by readers and reviewers has made necessary the preparation of a fresh edition; the fifth in six years. I have taken the opportunity to recast in part the chapters dealing with intracranial tumour and with cerebral vascular disease, and to make such minor additions and changes as the advance of knowledge, the flux of opinion and the valuable suggestions of correspondents have shown to be expedient. To all who by their kind interest have helped me in this way I am most grateful: in particular to Mr. Wylie McKissock in connection with Chapter III, and to Dr. Maurice Mitman in respect of the treatment of acute meningitis. To my old friend and colleague, Dr. Greenfield, I am indebted for the photographs that supplement the diagrams of spinal cord lesions.

To Mr. Charles Macmillan of Messrs. Livingstone I wish especially to express my gratitude for his constant sympathetic interest and help. To him I owe it that this book emerges in more pleasing form from the "battledress" that it has worn for the past five years.

F. M. R. WALSHE.

1946.

Preface to First Edition

THE writing of a simple text-book adapted to the needs of the student and the practitioner has been the avowed aim of more authors than have achieved it, and it is not difficult to discover how many works so designed have failed of their purpose. The task of selection, of emphasis and—in particular—of omission that necessarily goes to the writing of a book intended to give this circle of readers all they need and no more than this in the simplest form is one of difficulty.

It is more often true of affections of the nervous system than of those of other systems that they tend to pass for their final investigation and interpretation into the hands of the specialist. The methods—clinical, laboratory, and radiological—that may be needed in this process do not come in question while the case is still in the hands of the court of first instance: the general practitioner. It is, therefore, idle to burden the exposition by describing signs and procedures that in the nature of things he will never be called upon to employ. Yet few writers of the designedly simple text-book are found able to resist the temptation to mention, however briefly and uselessly, something of everything, and few are willing to face the imagined reproach that they have left out something new, rare, or ingenious.

Further, there is a growing tendency in neurological writings to employ a complex and redundant terminology that is fast rendering them unintelligible to all but professed neurologists, and to multiply the enumeration and description of those eponymous signs and syndromes by means of which enterprising clinicians stake out their claims, as it were, upon the human body. All this is a very tyranny of words and stifles thought in terminology.

It is, then, in a neglect of the essential simplicity of presentation and economy of information that the writer of the simple text-book so easily loses sight of his purpose and produces a work that, whatever its merits as a précis of information upon its subject, is not what it set out to be: a practical guide to the student and the general practitioner.

It is often said, and not without truth, that clinical neurology is largely a study in the applied anatomy and physiology of the nervous system. While the aphorism expresses what may usefully be the outlook of the professed neurologist, and has characteristically been his outlook in this country, it has been disastrous in its effects upon those not specially interested in this branch of medicine, for it has invested the subject with a legend of unsurmountable difficulty and complexity. The specialization of function within the nervous system and the apparently innumerable masses of grey matter and pathways, and the many symptom-complexes of lesions involving them, lead many students during the period of their clinical training to abandon the attempt to grapple with a body of knowledge, perhaps the most lucid in medicine, that they hope and try to persuade themselves will be of no practical importance to them in the general practice of medicine.

Some twenty years in the teaching of neurology have convinced me that both students and practitioners tend too easily to accept defeat in this way before a case of nervous disease and to evade—or to pass to the pathologist or the radiologist, not rarely in vain—diagnostic problems the solution of which is easily within reach of simple clinical observation were they but methodically and confidently tackled.

Therefore in the following pages I have tried to deal only with what is possible in general practice in the matter of diagnostic methods and of treatment, to strip the subject of unnecessary complexities and to confine myself to what I have seen and believe to be true. Hence the reader will hear but little, for example, of the ventriculogram or of the electro-encephalogram. He will have no occasion to make or to interpret either. He need not look in this book for lists or descriptions of the host of eponymous signs and syndromes, nor for the plague of polysyllabic words of classical derivation in too common use to describe disorders of function and pathological changes that can be discussed in plain English. He will find no more anatomy or physiology than the relatively few elementary facts necessary to the recognition and localization of nervous diseases.

In treating of neurological diagnosis there is a tendency to cast this almost wholly in an anatomical mould, and, in consequence, written descriptions of nervous disease are too often little more than dull catalogues of localizing signs, with brief commentaries upon their features and frequency.

The subject thus becomes purely a matter of memorizing and the reader is given no pictures for his mind. Yet what the clinical observer sees when he confronts his patient is a state of disordered function, one of a continuous series of such states that began with the onset of the illness and will continue to its end. The illness is not a simple matter of a lesion to be localized, but is *a sequence of events. It is something with an existence in time as well as in space.* Diagnosis must, therefore, concern itself as much with the life/history of the illness as with the anatomical seat of the disease process.

It is equally essential that text-book accounts of disease should be based upon this notion of an illness as a process, the story of which is to be told. To write a narrative, therefore, and not a mere "*catalogue raisonné"* should be the aim of the medical author, as it was of the writers of the outstanding text-books of the late nineteenth century, such as Gowers, Murchison, Byrom Bramwell and others.

This book is planned in two sections. In the first is attempted a general statement of the principles of neurological diagnosis with summary descriptions of the characteristic symptom-complexes of disease of the nervous system. In the second are given accounts of the commoner nervous diseases. The degree of detail given will be found to vary from malady to malady according to the relative importance of each in the general practice of medicine. The unevenness of treatment thus enforced is deliberate.

A number of the rarer affections of the nervous system find no mention in these pages. The brief summaries which commonly do service for their description in most simple text-books do not suffice for their recognition at the hands of those who are not professed neurologists, and thus serve no good purpose. Their omission here allows of a fuller and more adequate account of those diseases which it is reasonable to expect every doctor to recognize.

In the present state of knowledge no consistent method of grouping of nervous diseases is practicable. The pathogenesis of some of the most familiar of them remains obscure, and from the practical point of view an ætiological classification even when it is possible may separate quite artificially syndromes that have to be considered together when the task of clinical diagnosis is undertaken. Thus, a case presenting muscular wasting as its prominent feature may belong to any one of an ætiologically diverse collection of neuromuscular affections, yet for practical purposes all varieties of muscular atrophy are best grouped together. Hence, consistency of plan has not been attempted. The grouping of diseases, or their treatment in separate chapters, has been adopted on what have seemed to me the grounds best suited to the clinical approach.

A brief account of the common psychoneuroses has been included. It may appear unduly sanguine to hope to give within the compass of a single chapter a useful account of this very important aspect of medicine when we recall what a vast literature has grown up around it within the present century. However, much of this is concerned with hypothesis, and the essential task of diagnosis—the clinician's first task —has usually been a Cinderella at this carnival of literary expansiveness. It is, therefore, with diagnosis that the chapter on the psychoneuroses has been mainly concerned, save for a digression upon the pathogenesis of the so-called "traumatic" neurosis, a subject upon which a candid statement is long overdue.

In conclusion I wish to express my grateful thanks, for their criticism and advice, to my teacher, colleague and friend, Professor T. R. Elliott,

F.R.S., and to the late Dr. T. A. Ross. For what in the way of omissions, defects and errors may have survived their kindly criticism I am wholly responsible. To the publishers, Messrs. E. and S. Livingstone, my warmest thanks are due for their help and for the trouble they have taken to meet my wishes.

F. M. R. WALSHE.

1940.

Contents

PART I

GENERAL PRINCIPLES OF NEUROLOGICAL DIAGNOSIS

x

PART II

DESCRIPTIVE ACCOUNT OF THE MORE COMMON DISEASES OF THE NERVOUS SYSTEM

Illustrations

PART I

GENERAL PRINCIPLES OF NEUROLOGICAL DIAGNOSIS

A

CHAPTER I

Introduction : Non-Anatomical Factors in Diagnosis

WHAT clinical examination reveals to us in the patient is a state of disordered function, one of a continuous series of such states that began with the onset of his illness and will continue to its end. Diagnosis, therefore, consists not merely in the simple localization of a lesion or disease process within the nervous system, but also in the interpretation of the entire sequence of events that have made up the illness. This illness, then, has to be thought of as something having an existence in time as well as in space, and no conception of nervous disease is adequate or real that does not embody this idea of an active process. Here, then, we have a non-anatomical or time factor that must be taken into account.

A simple example will make this clear. If in the course of a physical examination of a young adult we find spastic weakness of the legs, increased tendon jerks and clonus, loss of abdominal reflexes and extensor plantar responses, we may correctly infer that there is a lesion of the lateral columns of the spinal cord involving the pyramidal tracts. Further than this examination does not take us, and to ascertain the nature of the lesion and its probable future behaviour we must know the sequence of states of disordered function that have preceded and led up to the state found on examination. If, for example, we learn that the illness has been characterized by marked remissions or fluctuations in the severity of the symptoms over a period of time, we shall have acquired information suggesting the possibility that we are dealing with the pathological process known as disseminated sclerosis, one of the commonest organic nervous affections in young adults. It is well known that this affection may present remarkable clinical variations from week to week, or month to month, as well as from case to case; and for this reason those not specially familiar with it are prone to regard it as a malady of which no clear image can readily be formed, and as one to be safely diagnosed only by a tedious process of exclusion. Yet this is so only if we think of it purely in terms of physical signs. If we look upon it as a whole, that is, as a series of states of disordered function, then it is seen to possess a most striking individuality, a unity in diversity shown by few other forms of illness. In a word, physical examination can be fully interpreted only in its context of history. Careful history-taking and assessment are, therefore, of the very essence of diagnosis, and provide a task not less difficult, and perhaps even more beset with pitfalls, than physical examination.

These pitfalls are of two kinds. In the first place, the patient does not always know what is and what is not relevant to his medical history. For example, let us return to the case of disseminated sclerosis. A significant item in the patient's past history is often the occurrence of a temporary blurring of vision in one eye—the expression of that retrobulbar neuritis with which the clinical course of the malady so frequently opens. This episode may have occurred years before the development of the symptoms for which the patient is now seeking advice. It bears no obvious relation to those symptoms; it may not even be recalled by the patient. In either case it is not mentioned by him, and unless questions directly designed to elicit information on this point are put nothing will be heard of it. The examiner must, therefore, know what to ask for and how to ask for it without putting the answer in the patient's mouth. He can do this only if he looks at illness from the point of view here emphasized.

A second difficulty arises from the almost universal tendency of the layman to describe his symptoms, not directly but in terms of what he thinks them due to. A history of past trauma is the red herring most commonly drawn across the trail of relevant fact in this connection, but there are others. For example, the patient who is slowly developing a weakness of his legs, finds them tire easily and ache when they are tired, or he may be enduring the lightning pains which commonly usher in the clinical course of tabes dorsalis. He thereupon says that he has "neuritis" or "rheumatism," and only careful questioning may discover *the facts* upon which he bases this interpretation. Yet it is facts rather than amateur interpretations that are needed in diagnosis. The frequency with which, in cases of slowly developing organic nervous disease, this "diagnosis" of the patient is accepted and made the basis of what must almost certainly be futile or inadequate treatment shows clearly that the clinician is not always sufficiently on his guard against this common source of error and misunderstanding. He must, therefore, be an active and informed partner in this process of eliciting the story of an illness.

THE MODES OF DISTURBANCE OF NERVOUS FUNCTION

We have seen that there are two factors in neurological diagnosis, the behaviour from time to time of the pathological lesion, and its localization. We have now to consider how such a lesion may disturb the functions of the nervous system and thus produce symptoms.

The nervous system is inaccessible to such direct methods of examination as are possible in the case of the thoracic and abdominal viscera. Save for the optic nerve head which is visible in the fundus of the eye the central nervous system is enclosed within the bony framework of the skull and vertebral column and is wholly removed from observation. In the first instance, then, diagnosis depends upon the investigation and interpretation of disorders of function in tissues innervated by the nervous system. These disorders which make up the subjective symptoms and objective signs of nervous disease are themselves the outward indication of disturbances of function in the nervous tissues, and we may now state the general principles which seem to govern the disturbance of nervous function.

These are most easily understood if we take an illustrative case: that of the common cerebral hæmorrhage into the substance of the brain from rupture of a central branch of the middle cerebral artery. This hæmorrhage produces a sudden gross local destruction of cerebral tissue. At the moment that the blood pours from the ruptured vessel into the region of the corpus striatum the subject has what is called apoplexy, that is, he becomes suddenly unconscious. The cerebral hemispheres cease to function, "the organism ceases to be aware of its surroundings and only the lower nuclei go on functioning without the control of those at higher levels." Should the victim survive, he regains consciousness and is then found to have hemiplegia. Indeed, the presence of this can be detected even while he is comatose. At first hemiplegia is flaccid, that is, the muscles are lax; the affected limbs drop inertly if lifted and the tendon reflexes may be diminished. In the course of the ensuing few weeks this flaccid hemiplegia changes its characters. The muscles of the affected limbs become hypertonic, *i.e.* spastic, and the tendon jerks undergo a marked increase. Other features, such as associated movements, also develop.

This sequence of events illustrates three of the modes of disorder of nervous function. Let us take them in order.

The apoplexy, or coma, which passes off in a few days, cannot be due to the direct destruction of tissue by the hæmorrhage, since, while this destruction is necessarily permanent, the coma is transient. The coma, therefore, is no more than *a temporary cessation of function in the parts of the cerebral hemispheres left intact by the lesion,* and able later to resume activity. This temporary abrogation of function in response to a sudden destruction of a small part of the cerebral hemispheres is spoken of as "cerebral shock." We learn from it that although there is a complicated differentiation of function within the brain, yet this organ normally acts as a whole and tends to respond as a whole to damage of one part. We have, therefore, in the sudden coma of cerebral hæmorrhage an example of the shock symptom. It consists of a temporary paralysis of function.

The hemiplegia, on the other hand, is a direct result of destruction of tissue, that is, of the pyramidal fibres in the substance of the hemisphere. It is, in consequence, relatively permanent. *It is a paralysis of function in tissues destroyed by the lesion.*

When we come to the final stage, that of *spastic* residual hemiplegia, we find that, in addition to the paralysis of function produced as above described, there are now certain symptoms that clearly betray excess of function or overaction. These are the abnormally increased muscle tone and tendon jerks and the involuntary associated movements. These cannot be a direct result of destruction of tissue, but are *due to the uncontrolled action of intact mechanisms in the brain released from higher control.* Symptoms of this order we speak of as "release symptoms."

From their nature it will be clear that release symptoms may persist indefinitely. They play a very important part in the clinical pictures of many chronic nervous affections, and may even dominate this picture; for example, the tremor and muscular rigidity of paralysis agitans and the writhing movements of athetosis are in the category of release symptoms.

A fourth category of symptoms remains for description. A local lesion or some general abnormal state may stimulate nerve cells to excessive activity. If nerve cells of the cerebral motor cortex are rendered hyperexcitable, as they may be, by a certain grade of oxygen deprivation, the result is *an excessive discharge of activity which produces a convulsion.* This muscular spasm may then be spoken of as an excitation or irritation symptom.

To summarize: the functions of any given portion of the nervous system may be directly paralysed by its destruction; such paralysis is apt to be permanent. Nervous functions may be temporarily paralysed by shock when a lesion involves some other part of the nervous system.

The functions of part of the nervous system may be released from control and overact when some higher level of the system is destroyed, or they may be increased by direct stimulation or, as it is often called, by irritation.

Symptoms resulting from destruction and release tend to be permanent, while those due to shock and to irritation are transient. In respect of irritation some qualification of this generalization is necessary. The persisting pain that may follow certain injuries to peripheral nerves and goes by the name of causalgia (see pages 37, 280, 287) is an example of an enduring irritation. Facial hemispasm (see page 266) may be so regarded, while some believe that the spontaneous pain of the thalamic syndrome is an irritative and not a release symptom.

It may be stated in conclusion that the entire range of signs and symptoms in nervous disease are the expression of these four modes of disturbance of nervous function.

A final law governs the production of disordered function in disease of the nervous system. When any given function normally under the control of the nervous system is undergoing dissolution as the result of disease, its most recently acquired and most complex features are the first to go. In the case of the motor functions of the hand and arm, skilled movements are the first to be lost and the most severely impaired. Thus the movements involved in playing a musical instrument, or in some other skilled occupation, may be impaired at a time when simpler movements of the hand, such as grasping, are unimpaired. In the case of the speech function the same considerations hold, and the power of expressing thought or emotion in a foreign tongue may be lost when the power of such expression in the individual's native tongue is preserved. Further, these most vulnerable functions return last and least completely during a recovery process.

THE TIME FACTOR IN SYMPTOM PRODUCTION

We have seen that the clinical characters of an affection of the nervous system depend not alone on the localization of the lesion but also upon its behaviour in time, and we have seen the four ways in which a lesion may disturb the functions of the nervous system. It remains to consider the influence of the time factor in determining the degree and kind of disturbance of function; that is, in producing the symptomatology of nervous diseases.

In general it may be stated that a pathological process or lesion of sudden development tends to produce maximal disturbance of function, while a slowly developing lesion leads to less disturbance and may even be well established before its presence is revealed by any disorder of function. For example, the sudden hemiplegia of cerebral hæmorrhage is accompanied by the shock phenomenon of coma, whereas the gradually developing hemiplegia caused by a new growth is not so accompanied. Again, a gunshot wound of the cerebellum will give rise to the grossest cerebellar ataxy, while a tumour within that structure may cause much destruction of tissue without giving rise to a full-fledged syndrome of cerebellar disease.

An even more striking illustration of the role of the time factor in determining symptomatology is afforded by compression of the spinal cord. Thus a sudden crushing of the cord in the thoracic region is followed at once by total flaccid paraplegia, loss of knee and ankle jerks, retention of urine and total sensory loss. A very different picture is produced by gradual compression of the spinal cord, as, for example, by a tumour. We see now the progressive development of a spastic paraplegia, with greatly increased muscle tone in the extensor muscles of the limb, the tendon jerks are exaggerated and there is clonus, and instead of retention of urine we probably see precipitancy of urine followed by incontinence.

Here, as in a previous example, it is the phenomenon of shock resulting from a sudden damage to the cord which is responsible for the picture of sudden total transection of the cord. When this shock passes off, reflex activity returns in the isolated portion of the cord.

It follows, from what has been said, that the time factor is determined in the main by the nature of the pathological process, though in the case of gradual and sudden compression of the cord this process is in essentials the same, time alone being the factor decisive in determining the resulting state of disordered function.

SOME GENERAL CONSIDERATIONS ON ÆTIOLOGY

In those succeeding chapters which describe particular affections of the nervous system, the term "ætiology" is used in the somewhat restricted sense common in clinical medicine, as implying the specific cause: e.g. a micro-organism or a trauma, of the illness, but it is important that the wider implications of the term should be remembered. The former tendency to think of illness as simply due to defect or disorder in some component of a human machine has given place to the notion of illness as a vital reaction of the organism as a whole, or in other words, as a form of behaviour in response to adverse factors. These factors are invariably multiple, even in the case of an infection, and for purposes of discussion may be divided into environmental and internal. Environmental factors include injury, heat, cold, chemical agencies, nutritional factors, infections, and psychological factors of some diversity. Environmental factors and internal factors are closely interrelated; for example, the individual may be susceptible to an infection only when environmental factors have lowered his resistance. Amongst internal factors (characteristics of the individual) some are inherited, some acquired. Age and sex are amongst internal factors determining in part the response of the individual to external factors. When we speak of "cause" in respect of illness, therefore, we see that there are aspects of cause in the environment and aspects of cause in the individual. In other words, ætiology is necessarily and invariably a complex of factors. In conclusion, we may say that there are three fields of observation in the determination of ætiology: the field of the person (his anatomical, physiological, and psychological characteristics); the field of the environment; and the field of structure or mechanism, that is, what part of the organism is the seat of the primary and essential disease reaction.

A factor which is found to be of significance in the causation of illness is the psychological factor, in the sense that adverse psychological influences may set up physiological disturbances which in turn may lead to structural lesions. Examples of this sequence of events are perhaps not so well ascertained in the case of neurology as in general medicine, and the time has not come for any final assessment of a primary psychological factor in what is commonly spoken of as organic nervous disease. The subject is referred to again on page 313.

These observations, then, are of general import, but the following special points bearing on nervous diseases may be further discussed.

THE INFLUENCE OF AGE, SEX, AND HEREDITY

These factors also are not without their importance in diagnosis.

Age.—Experience shows that certain affections of the nervous system have age periods of predilection for their appearance. Thus epilepsy commonly makes its appearance before adult life is reached, and it follows that if a child gives a history of recurrent epileptic fits and is found to be otherwise healthy, we may safely make a diagnosis of epilepsy. But if an apparently healthy middle-aged adult begins to be liable to fits of the same order, we should, in view of the known behaviour of epilepsy, hesitate to make this diagnosis, suspecting rather that we were dealing with a "symptomatic" epilepsy, the fits being the expression of some gross cerebral disease, in all probability a new growth, since this is the common basis of generalized fits appearing for the first time in middle age in a subject presenting no other indications of disease. Other examples of this order will readily occur to the mind, and they indicate that among the factors that go to the making of diagnosis the age of the subject may on occasion be a most important one.

Sex.—This is not a factor of wide importance in neurological diagnosis. It is true, perhaps, that certain maladies are more commonly seen in one sex than in the other, but statistical considerations are of comparatively little value in the assessment of the individual case. It may be admitted that the pseudo-hypertrophic form of muscular dystrophy is found almost exclusively in males, but comparable examples are rare.

Heredity.—It is not proposed to summarize the Mendelian laws of inheritance, but it may be said that there are a number of forms of heredo-familial degeneration of the neuro-muscular system that, with some variations, obey these laws. Therefore, the history of the appearance of a malady in ascendants or siblings tends to narrow very appreciably the field of differential diagnosis.

On the other hand there are several affections of the nervous system that on inconclusive grounds have been alleged to show heritable qualities, but cannot be brought within the scope of any known laws of inheritance. Idiopathic epilepsy is such a malady.

Migraine is another paroxysmal disorder of nervous function commonly regarded as heritable, and here, as in the case of epilepsy, there is no evidence of inheritance according to any known laws, and no knowledge of what precisely it is that may be inherited.

Apart, then, from the recognized heredo-degenerations of the nervous and muscular systems, the role of heredity in nervous diseases is rather a matter of speculation than one of knowledge. A different aspect of inheritance, the importance of which in connection with the nervous system it is not yet possible to assess, arises in connection with hæmolytic diseases of the new-born.

In some 90 per cent. of these the mother is Rh. negative: *i.e.* her red cells do not contain the Rh. factor. Icterus gravis neonatorum is such a hæmolytic disease, it may be accompanied by severe bile staining of the corpus striatum, and followed in those children that survive by gross disturbances of nervous function of the order of double athetosis.

CHAPTER II

Anatomical or Localizing Factors in Diagnosis

WHEN all due consideration has been given to the non-anatomical factors in neurological diagnosis, it has to be admitted that the main clinical features of nervous disease, especially of its more chronic varieties, are chiefly determined by the localization of the disease process within the nervous system. Indeed, this is what we might anticipate from what we know of the structure and organization of the system.

Fortunately for the routine diagnosis of all but the more uncommon forms of nervous disease, the main subjective symptoms and objective signs fall into relatively few groups, and if these be known the problems of localizing diagnosis do not present the great difficulties commonly supposed to attach to them.

On the whole, it may be said that the most reliable and most easily assessed disorders are those of movement and of the reflexes. In the early stages of many common nervous diseases, such, for example, as disseminated sclerosis, abnormal reflexes may be the only unequivocal indications of organic disease. Sensory changes, on the other hand, rarely exist apart from associated motor and reflex abnormalities; they are more difficult to assess than these and less reliable in many cases.

THE ORGANIZATION OF THE MOTOR SYSTEM

From both the anatomical and physiological points of view it is usual to consider the motor system as comprising four components: (1) the upper motor (pyramidal) neurone, (2) an extrapyramidal system of neurones, (3) the cerebellar system, and (4) the lower motor neurone. This grouping will be followed here, and the following brief summary of the organization of the motor system will make its significance clearer.

There is evidence that in the spinal cord there are reflex mechanisms that subserve a variety of movements, locomotor and defensive, but the maintenance of posture which is necessary for these movements to be effective is a function of reflex arcs that have their centres in the pons and medulla. But even these two systems do not provide all that is necessary to stance and movement, and other reflex mechanisms centred in the midbrain are essential. When all these are normally operative, in such an animal as the decorticated cat, the animal can stand, walk, run, and jump more or less normally—but purely reflexly and only upon adequate stimulation. In other words the mechanism for co-ordination of movement is situated in the segmental nervous system, and the cerebellum and basal ganglia play no discoverable part in it. Superimposed upon this mechanism are the various nuclei figured in Fig. 2. What their precise role in the regulation of movement and of posture may be is far from fully known, but with the segmental mechanisms already referred to they form the entire motor system of lowlier forms of animal life and are thus sometimes referred to as the "old motor system." Set over this basic mechanism are the upper motor neurone (pyramidal system) and the cerebellar system. The former is regarded as the sole channel by which the subordinate motor mechanisms are activated in the performance of voluntary motor acts. It breaks up the large movements reflexly co-ordinated by the subordinate mechanisms into elementary components and builds these up into the innumerable combinations and permutations of movement that are the repertoire of voluntary movements characteristic of the intact organism. In performing this analytic and synthetic function, the upper motor neurone utilizes the cerebellar system, and if this be put out of action voluntary movement (unlike reflex movements) becomes grossly disordered (cerebellar ataxy). It is probably in the harmonious combination of movement and posture that the cerebellum has its role.

There is, however, a still higher level of motor function not included in the four categories already mentioned. This has its anatomical seat in the frontal cortex immediately anterior to the so-called "motor cortex" in which the pyramidal system arises. Its functions are known as eupraxic, and in it are finally represented the skilled movements and movement-complexes that we learn during life. The eupraxic centres play upon the motor cortex and set it in action to initiate voluntary motor activities.

It follows from this brief summary that a loss of function of eupraxic centres does not cause a true paralysis of movement, but an inability to initiate movements *at will*—though these may still be performed spontaneously, as it were, when attention is not directed to their performance. This defect, which will be later described, is known as motor apraxia. Loss of function of the upper motor neurone leads to impairment or loss of voluntary movement, to a true paralysis of movements. Disorders of function of the extrapyramidal system on the other hand, do not lead to paralysis or loss of movements but to disorders of posture, muscle tone, and co-ordination, while, finally, loss of function of the lower motor neurone (ventral horn cell and its axone) cuts off the skeletal musculature from the nervous system and leads to a total loss of all muscular activity, reflex and voluntary, with other consequences to be described.

We may now proceed to consider briefly *the anatomy* of these components of the motor system.

The upper motor neurone consists of the pyramidal tract and the cells in the cerebral cortex from which it arises. Formerly thought to arise solely from the so-called giant cells of Betz, it is now clear that the pyramidal fibres in fact arise from pyramidal cells of a wide range of sizes in the fifth layer of the grey matter of the ascending frontal convolution and immediately adjacent parts of the cortex anterior to this. Of these pyramidal cells a small proportion, lying mainly at the upper end of the convolution, are large and possess coarse Nissl-staining granules in the cytoplasm. These are the Betz cells. From them arise some of the long pyramidal fibres that go to the lumbar enlargement of the cord, but by far the greater proportion of pyramidal fibres, which outnumber the Betz cells by about 40 to 1, arise from pyramidal cells that are generally of smaller size and contain fewer and smaller granules. The Betz cell does not constitute either a morphological nor a physiological category apart from other pyramidal cells in the same cortical layer and region. The suggested division of all this cortical region into two distinct physiological mechanisms, the "motor" and the "premotor" cortex, each having distinct functions, has no validity, though it seems likely that from the anterior part of this region there arise corticopontine fibres that play a part in the regulation of muscle tone (see page 15). The pyramidal fibres pass deep from their origin and, gathering together, enter the posterior limb of the internal capsule, traverse the brain stem and, reaching the lower end of the medulla, decussate and come to lie in the lateral column of the spinal cord as the pyramidal tract (see Fig. 2). Finally, the fibres enter the grey matter of the ventral horn and end round the motor cells therein.

The extrapyramidal system of neurones (the old motor system) is a more complex and less completely elucidated component. It comprises the corpus striatum (caudate nucleus, putamen, globus pallidus), the substantia nigra, corpus subthalamicum, red nucleus and vestibular nucleus, as well as other masses of grey matter (reticular nuclei) in the brain stem. Short tracts connect these masses of grey matter with each other and with other parts of the brain, and there are also certain long descending paths, namely, the (small) rubrospinal tract, the vestibulospinal, and reticulospinal tracts. Like the pyramidal neurone all these impinge upon the ventral horn cells in the spinal cord. Their situations are indicated in Fig. 2.

The cerebellar system comprises the cerebellum and its afferent and efferent paths, not all of which are represented in Fig. 2.

Finally, there is *the lower motor neurone*, the final channel of access to the muscles, hence its name "the final common path" conferred upon it by Sherrington.

Physiologically considered, the pyramidal or upper motor neurone may be accepted as the main executive organ in the initiation of voluntary movements. In the "motor cortex" are represented all the movements of which the individual is capable.

Since there are many more such movements than there are muscles, a muscle takes part in many different movements. These movements range in complexity from such a simple matter as the flexion of a finger to the movements of writing or those involved in the playing of a

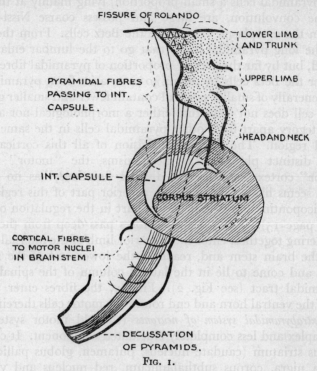

FISSURE OF ROLANDO

LOWER LIMB AND TRUNK

UPPER LIMB

PYRAMIDAL FIBRES PASSING TO INT. CAPSULE.

HEAD AND NECK

INT. CAPSULE

CORPUS STRIATUM

CORTICAL FIBRES TO MOTOR NUCLEI IN BRAIN STEM

DECUSSATION OF PYRAMIDS.

Fig. 1.

ORIGIN AND COURSE OF PYRAMIDAL TRACT.

Diagram representing the origin and course of the pyramidal fibres (upper motor neurone). The stippled area indicates the cortical field of origin of these fibres immediately anterior to the fissure of Rolando. At the upper part of this field are represented the giant cells of Betz from which a very small proportion of the pyramidal fibres arise. The majority arise from other pyramidal cells over an area the anterior limits of which have not yet been accurately delimited, but which corresponds to the "motor cortex" of Sherrington.

The "giant cells" are represented by triangles, the smaller cells by dots. The course of the fibres through the internal capsule and brain-stem is represented. In the latter the fibres destined for motor nuclei in the brain-stem turn dorsalwards from the pyramid.

musical instrument. Much the same muscles take part in all of these, and it is *these movements and not the individual muscles which carry them out that are represented in the motor cortex. Hence it follows that a lesion of this mechanism causes a paralysis of movements and not a paralysis of individual muscles.* Thus, a muscle may take part in two movements, one of which becomes paralysed while the other is left. This may be easily verified in many cases of residual hemiplegia. In such a case the patient commonly cannot extend the wrist, but is able to clench the fist. If, when he attempts to do the latter, we place a finger on the extensor tendons at the wrist we shall feel them tighten, fixing the hand in the mid-position while the fingers flex. If now we ask the patient to extend the wrist and digits fully, we shall find no contraction of these extensors, for the movement in which they are now a component is paralysed. This state of affairs shows quite clearly that the cerebral motor cortex is concerned with movements and knows nothing of muscles.

We have seen that the upper motor neurone impinges upon the lower motor neurone. The latter innervates muscles as such, and when it is out of action we see paralysis of individual muscles.

The essential difference between these two modes of innervation may be seen if we consider again the voluntary clenching of the fist already cited. In this movement three groups of muscles are concerned: (1) the flexors of the fingers which contract. We speak of these as the *agonists* in this movement. (2) The extensors of the fingers which are inhibited and relax. We speak of these as the *antagonists* in this movement. (3) The extensors of the wrist which contract to fix the hand in the mid-position. We speak of them as the *synergists* in this movement. Therefore, the motor cortex when active innervates a co-ordinated movement involving several muscles. The lower motor neurone innervates muscles but does not achieve co-ordinated action between different muscles.

As has already been stated, our knowledge of the functions of the extrapyramidal system is very imperfect. It is not directly concerned with the initiation of voluntary movements, but probably with the regulation of posture. The cerebellum, as we have seen, functions under the direct control of the upper motor neurone and it also is concerned with the regulation of posture in the performance of voluntary movements.

Muscle Tone.—During the following account of disorders of the motor system the terms "muscle tone," "hypertonus," "spasticity," "hypotonus," and "atonia" will frequently recur and some definition of the governing term "tone" must be given. The sense given to it by the physiologist is a complex one and often seems to have little or no relation to the clinician's use of it. The following summarizes the physiologist's conception in the barest outline. When a muscle with normal innervation is passively stretched its fibres actively resist the stretch and enter into an active state of increased and sustained tension. This response is a reflex reaction evoked by the stimulation of sensory end-organs in the fleshy part of the muscle (stretch receptors), and is known as a stretch reflex. Even the apparently relaxed normal muscle, attached at each extremity, is in a constant slight degree of tension thus induced. If such a muscle be further stretched by gravity, by manipulation, or by the elicitation of its tendon jerks, it responds by an additional development of tension. To short-lived stretch the response is equally short-lived, as we see in the tendon jerk, but to sustained stretch the response is maintained, or tonic. The degree of tension thus produced is called the normal tone of the muscle. In certain conditions of experimental production, or of disease of the nervous system, this tone is changed, either in the direction of increase (hypertonus) or of decrease (hypotonus or atonia). Various factors influence the degree of tone in the normal subject besides stretch of the reacting muscle. Thus stretch of other remote muscles and stimuli arising in the otolith organs of the ear are all capable of causing variations in tone, and these variations are outwardly expressed in changes of attitude.

In other words, muscle tone provides the background of posture upon which active movements occur, and is an important element in the co-ordination of movement.

It is this "stretch reflex" with which the clinician is concerned and which he calls tone, but his methods of detecting its presence and of determining its departures from the normal are widely different from the methods adopted in its experimental study. The clinician commonly estimates tone by the manipulation of the limbs and this gives him a sense of the degree of tension in the muscle. In short, to the clinician the word "tone" means the active elastic tension he feels when he passively stretches a muscle. Palpation of the belly of a muscle gives no reliable indication of this tone.

Experience gives him the knowledge of what is the normal degree of elastic resistance in the muscle when he passively stretches it in this

---

(Reference to Fig. 2.)

A. The cortico-spinal or pyramidal tract arises in the cerebral cortex of the ascending frontal convolution and the region immediately anterior to it, and, traversing the internal capsule and brain-stem, decussates in the medulla. It then runs in the lateral column (see B.) of the spinal cord to terminate in the grey matter of the ventral horn around the motor cells. The various nuclei which are included in the extrapyramidal system are indicated by stippling. The paths which arise in them include the vestibulo-spinal tract, originating in the vestibular nucleus, and running down in the ventral column of the cord. The small rubro-spinal tract which, arising in the red nucleus, immediately decussates and comes to take position in the cord ventral to the pyramidal tract. The reticulo-spinal tract which, arising in scattered nuclear masses in the pons and medulla, also runs down in the lateral column of the cord ventral to the rubro-spinal tract. The fibres of all these paths ultimately turn into the grey matter and form synaptic junctions with the ventral horn cells.

The short tracts between the various components of the extrapyramidal system are also indicated. C.N., caudate nucleus. D.N., dentate nucleus. C.S., corpus subthalamicum. G.P., globus pallidus. I.C., internal capsule. Put., putamen. S.N., substantia nigra.

The extrapyramidal system is sometimes spoken of as "the old motor system" in contradistinction to the "new motor system" which comprises the cortico-spinal system.

B. Transverse section of the cord, showing the relative positions occupied by the various motor tracts.

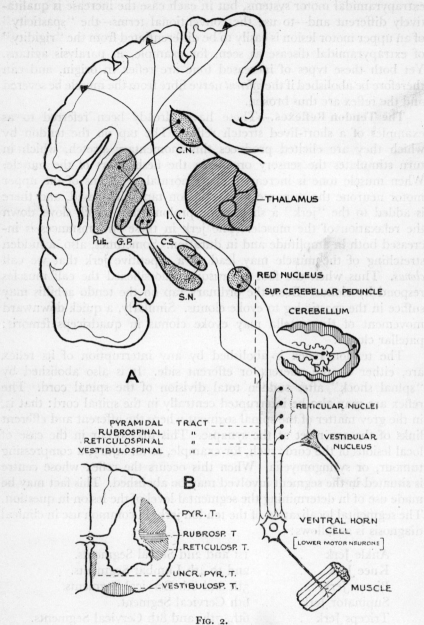

C.N.

THALAMUS

I.C.

Pul.   G.P.   C.S.

RED NUCLEUS

SUP. CEREBELLAR PEDUNCLE

CEREBELLUM

S.N.

D.N.

A

RETICULAR NUCLEI

PYRAMIDAL   TRACT
RUBROSPINAL   "
RETICULOSPINAL   "
VESTIBULOSPINAL   "

VESTIBULAR
NUCLEUS

B

PYR. T.

RUBROSP. T.
RETICULOSP. T.

UNCR. PYR. T.
VESTIBULOSP. T.

VENTRAL HORN
CELL
[LOWER MOTOR NEURONE]

MUSCLE

FIG. 2.
A AND B. THE MOTOR SYSTEM.

B

way. He finds it increased in disease both of the pyramidal and of the extrapyramidal motor systems, but in each case the increase is qualitatively different and—to use the conventional terms—the "spasticity" of an upper motor lesion is easily to be differentiated from the "rigidity" of extrapyramidal disease as seen, for example, in paralysis agitans. Yet both these types of increased tone are reflex in origin, and can therefore be abolished if the *afferent* nerve fibre from the muscle be severed and the reflex arc thus broken.

The Tendon Reflexes.—These have already been referred to as examples of a short-lived stretch reflex. The tap on the tendon by which they are elicited produces this momentary stretch, which in turn stimulates the sensory organs in the fleshy part of the muscle. When muscle tone is increased above normal in lesions of the upper motor neurone the response to the tendon tap is increased, and there is added to the "jerk" a short tonic prolongation which slows down the relaxation of the muscle. The jerk in these circumstances is increased both in amplitude and in duration. Sometimes, also, a sudden stretching of the muscle may lead to a repetitive jerk that we call *clonus*. Thus when the foot is brusquely dorsiflexed the calf muscles respond by clonus. Even the ordinary tap on the tendo achillis may suffice in the spastic leg to evoke clonus. Similarly, a quick downward movement of the patella may evoke clonus in quadriceps femoris; patellar clonus.

The tendon reflex is abolished by any interruption of its reflex arc, either on the afferent or efferent side. It is also abolished by "spinal shock" after sudden total division of the spinal cord. The reflex arc may also be interrupted centrally in the spinal cord: that is, in the grey matter of the spinal segment where the afferent and efferent links of the arc meet at the synapse. This may occur in the case of local lesions of the cord: such, for example, as an injury, a compressing tumour, or syringomyelia. When this occurs the reflex whose centre is situated in the segment involved may be abolished. This fact may be made use of in determining the segmental level of the lesion in question. The segmental localization of the tendon jerks in common use in clinical diagnosis is as follows:

Ankle Jerk	. .	1st and 2nd Sacral Segments.
Knee Jerk	. .	2nd to 4th Lumbar Segments.
Biceps Jerk	. .	5th and 6th Cervical Segments.
Supinator Jerk	.	6th Cervical Segment.
Triceps Jerk	. .	6th, 7th, and 8th Cervical Segments.

Sometimes the abolition of a tendon jerk by a lesion in its appropriate spinal cord segment is associated with the appearance of an alternative response: as, for example, when lesions involving the grey matter of the 5th and 6th cervical segments lead to the appearance of flexion of the fingers when the lower end of the radius is tapped with a view to eliciting the supinator jerk. This phenomenon is spoken of as "inversion" of the reflex. This form of inversion is frequently seen in injuries of the cervical cord associated with damage to the 5th and 6th cervical vertebræ, a common site of injury.

There is no absolute standard as to what constitutes a normal degree of briskness in a tendon jerk. In persons free from any organic affection of the nervous system it is apt to vary from time to time, and from individual to individual. In the organically sound individual, however, there is a *uniform* degree of briskness of all tendon jerks. Differences of briskness between the tendon reflexes in a limb, or between one side and the other, betray the presence of organic disease.

Anything which leads to a general increase in muscle tone will increase the amplitude of the tendon jerks. When the individual's attention is deeply occupied, or his emotions of any kind aroused, such a slight general increase of tone ensues, and in these circumstances the tendon jerks are found to be increased. This fact is made use of in the procedure of "reinforcement" when there is difficulty in eliciting the tendon jerks. The patient is asked to make some strong muscular effort, such as clenching his fists, setting his jaw, or interlocking the bent fingers of his hands and then pulling them away from each other.

In the healthy subject the knee and ankle jerks are always present, and the arm jerks (biceps, triceps, and supinator) also. This statement, however, calls for this reservation, that in children below the age of about eighteen months the arm jerks and the ankle jerks may be difficult if not impossible of elicitation, and that in aged persons the ankle jerks may be diminished or lost.

Clonus has been mentioned as indicative of an upper motor neurone lesion, but it should be remembered that a form of clonus may be present in association with a general exaggeration of tendon jerks in unstable or debilitated persons apart from organic disease of the nervous system. Such a clonus may be distinguished from that of organic disease. The latter commonly develops most easily and is longest maintained when the foot is in a degree of plantarflexion, it is increased in force as the examiner's hand presses the foot up in the direction of dorsiflexion, and it is not easy to stop the clonus when it is well-developed except by letting the foot drop. The clonus not associated with organic disease usually occurs with the foot not plantarflexed and can readily be stopped by pressing this further towards dorsiflexion. It is also commonly less regular in rate and amplitude than the true clonus of the spastic limb.

The Cutaneous Reflexes.—When certain regions of the skin are lightly stroked or scratched, muscles innervated from the spinal segment corresponding to the sensory innervation of the stimulated area of skin respond by a brisk, short-lived contraction. This is the so-called cutaneous reflex. Thus, stroking the skin of the abdominal wall leads to quick brief contraction of the underlying abdominal muscle: the abdominal reflex. It is usual to divide the abdominal wall into four quadrants, two upper and two lower, in the examination of this reflex. The four abdominal reflexes thus obtainable are present in the majority of normal persons even when the abdominal wall is obese, and this latter condition should rarely be accepted as an adequate explanation of the absence of the abdominal reflexes. Sometimes the lax abdominal musculature of the multiparous woman may fail to give the reflex responses. *The normal plantar reflex* (flexor plantar response) is another cutaneous reflex of clinical importance. Stroking or scratching of the sole should evoke a plantarflexion of the great and little toes and usually of the entire foot, with an associated contraction of tensor fascia femoris and of quadriceps: an accompaniment not found with an extensor plantar response. In lesions of the upper motor neurone this is replaced by a totally different reflex, the extensor, or Babinski, type of plantar response.

GENERAL REMARKS ON DISORDERS OF THE MOTOR SYSTEM

From what has been stated of the composition of the motor system it follows that co-ordinated movement results from the combined and harmonious activity of the various components of a complex structure, and it will be understood that the character of disorders of movement and of posture will vary according to the particular component that is not acting normally, or is out of action. The notions of loss and of release of function have already been briefly mentioned, but it should be borne in mind that the disordered movements (weak, ataxic, or tremulous, etc.) that we observe in the subjects of disease of the motor system result from the combined activity of those components of this system that are left in action. Thus, the ataxy of cerebellar disease is due to voluntary attempts to compensate for the loss of normal cerebellar participation in movement; that is to say, this ataxy is produced by what is left of the motor mechanism. We have, therefore, four main categories of motor disorder; that produced when the pyramidal system is acting defectively or not at all, that resulting from loss or impairment of the extrapyramidal mechanisms, that resulting from cerebellar lesions, and that seen when the lower motor neurone, the last and only link between muscles and nervous system, is involved. There are thus four main syndromes of motor disorder. Since disease does not invariably respect anatomical or physiological unities, we may

4 syndromes of motor disorder
  a. upper motor
  b. lower motor
  c. cerebellar
  d. x-tra pyramidal

ANATOMICAL OR LOCALIZING FACTORS IN DIAGNOSIS   21

expect to see syndromes of motor disorder that embrace more than one of the components of the motor system. Yet despite the complexities that may from time to time be thus produced in the clinical pictures we observe, the existence of four main and characteristic syndromes is clear.

THE SYMPTOMATOLOGY OF LESIONS OF THE UPPER MOTOR NEURONE

The symptoms fall into two distinct groups: those due to loss of function in the upper motor neurone, and those due to overaction (release) in subordinate extrapyramidal neurones. When the lesion is suddenly produced the phenomenon of "shock," as already described, ensues and it is not until this has passed off that the release symptoms make their appearance. With a gradually progressive lesion, however, both paralysis and release symptoms develop simultaneously.

Throughout this account, spasticity, increased tendon reflexes, clonus, and the extensor type of plantar response are spoken of as "release" symptoms due to loss of control when the upper motor neurone, that is, the pyramidal system, is out of action. Yet there are indications, both clinical and experimental, that a pure and uncomplicated lesion of this system produces *loss of movements only, and that some other cortical efferent path must also be put out of action before this group of release symptoms can occur.* Actually, this system, whatever its anatomical identity, must lie in such close juxtaposition to the pyramidal neurone that in states of disease in man both are commonly involved together, hence the almost invariable association of this group of release symptoms with the loss of movements characteristic of a pyramidal lesion. Therefore, *for clinical purposes* it is unnecessary to take this possible double origin of the syndrome of spastic paralysis into consideration.

Taken together the symptoms are as follows:—

(1) Loss of voluntary movements.
(2) Increase of muscle tone: spasticity.
(3) Increase of tendon jerks and clonus.
(4) Loss of cutaneous reflexes.
(5) Extensor (Babinski) type of plantar response.
(6) Associated movements.

(1) *Loss of voluntary movements.*—The movements of the limbs suffer more severely than those of head, neck, and trunk. In the limbs movements are affected in order of severity as follows: Upper Limb— isolated movements of the fingers and all skilled movements of the hands, extension of wrist and fingers, extension at the elbow, clenching of the fist, flexion at the elbow, and—least affected—elevation and

adduction at the shoulder. Lower Limb—dorsiflexion of toes and foot, eversion of the foot, flexion at knee and hip, plantarflexion of foot and toes, and, least severely, extension at knee and hip and inversion of the foot.

In the face, movements of the lower face are more severely impaired than those of the upper part of the face. Deglutition is unaffected, but articulation may be transiently disordered. Bilateral movements of the trunk are little if at all affected.

(2) *Increase of muscle tone.*—Clinically this increase is noteworthy in the limb musculature only. We have seen that the loss of voluntary movement is in a measure selective, some movements being more severely affected than others. Similarly, the incidence of increased tone, or of spasticity as it is often called, is also selective, In the upper limbs it is most marked in the flexor muscles of forearm and arm and in the adductors of the shoulder. In the lower limbs it is characteristically most marked in plantarflexor and extensor muscles. Its presence is readily detected by passive stretching of the muscles, when a clearly increased resistance can be felt. This has the following qualities, most easily elicited in the knee extensors. If the thigh rests upon the examiner's left forearm, placed under it as the patient lies in bed, and the right hand grasps the leg just above the ankle, on flexing the leg at the knee a few degrees of movement are easily carried out without marked resistance, but once this range is passed an active resistance is felt to develop quickly in quadriceps, and more force is needed—considerable force in some cases—to continue the flexion. After another thirty degrees of flexion this resistance melts quickly, and the rest of the movement is relatively easily carried out. This sudden waxing and then waning of tone in the hypertonic limb has been spoken of as " clasp-knife rigidity." In the upper limb passive extension at the elbow will reveal a similar state. In some cases of spastic paraplegia this hypertonus may be extreme and may defeat the attempt to flex the leg passively as described above. In others, again, it may be only just appreciable to the careful observer, and in these circumstances is found in the finger flexors of the upper and in the plantarflexors, and perhaps also the knee extensors, of the lower limb.

(3) *Increase of tendon jerks and clonus.*—These features have already been described (page 15).

(4) *Loss of cutaneous reflexes.*—A characteristic, yet not invariable feature of upper motor neurone lesions is the loss of cutaneous reflexes. The abdominal reflexes commonly disappear when the upper motor neurone is the seat of disordered function, but this is not quite invariably so. Thus, in infantile hemiplegia and in very long-standing hemiplegia in adults, originally lost abdominal reflexes may return. In disseminated sclerosis an early bilateral disappearance of abdominal

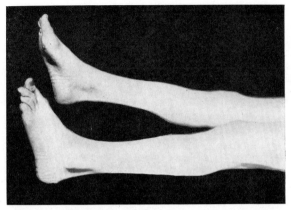

A

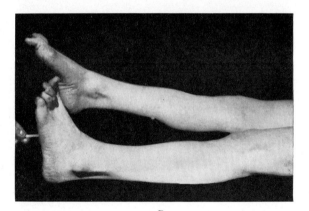

B

Fig. 3.

THE EXTENSOR AND CROSSED EXTENSOR PLANTAR
RESPONSES.

These photographs illustrate the Babinski and the crossed
plantar responses in a case of spastic paraplegia. A shows the
resting position of the limbs. B shows plantar stimulation of the
left sole giving a Babinski response. The foot and great toe of the
opposite side are seen to have gone into marked plantarflexion
(crossed plantar response).

To face page 22.

reflexes is almost the rule, but in amyotrophic lateral sclerosis they may be preserved in the presence of other signs of gross disorder of the upper motor neurone. The normal flexor plantar response is abolished and is replaced by a reflex response of a different character as well as of different form, namely, the extensor or Babinski type of plantar response.

(5) *The extensor (Babinski) type of plantar response.*—There is perhaps no more important single physical sign in clinical neurology. It consists of an upgoing (dorsiflexion) movement of the great toe when the sole of the foot is stroked or scratched. In many instances, however, it may be obtained from a very much wider receptive field, both cutaneous and deep. Thus, pinching the skin of the foot or leg—occasionally as high as the thigh in certain cases of spastic paraplegia—pressure over bony points round the ankle, a stroking pressure over the shin, and other devices may elicit the response.* The region most sensitive is the lateral half of the sole of the foot, and the reflex may be obtainable here alone in cases where the interference with pyramidal function is but slight. It should, therefore, always be elicited from here and not from the mesial border of the sole. It is usually accompanied by dorsiflexion of the foot and often by flexion at hip and knee. These wider movements are an integral part of the total response to stimulation of the sole, and this response is in fact a limb flexion or withdrawal. It corresponds to the flexion reflex of the spinal animal. Sometimes in cases of paraplegia-in-extension (see page 25) the eliciting of this reflex may be accompanied by plantarflexion of the foot and great toe of the opposite side, the so-called crossed plantar response which corresponds to the crossed extension reflex of the spinal animal (see Fig. 3).

(6) *Associated movements.*—The phenomena commonly so-called are in fact changes in posture rather than movements. When the hemiplegic patient yawns or stretches, the affected arm tends to extend involuntarily at the elbow, wrist, and fingers, remaining rigidly in this new attitude until the yawn passes off, when the original resting posture is resumed. Simultaneously the leg goes into rigid extension with the foot plantarflexed. A comparable reaction of the limbs of the hemiplegic side accompanies any forceful or sustained movement of the normal limbs, though in this case the arm usually goes into increased

---

* Despite what has been said in the preface concerning eponymous signs, the name of Babinski has become too firmly attached to the extensor plantar response to be detached now. Further, the alternative title "extensor plantar response" is incorrect in that the response is one of dorsiflexion and not one of extension. It should be remembered also that the receptive field of the response may be a very much wider one than the sole of the foot, and, therefore, we may reasonably object to the perpetuation of such titles as Oppenheim's, Gordon's, and Chaddock's reflexes, which are no more than the "extensor plantar response" elicited from different parts of its wide receptive field. Protest may here be made against the growing and objectionable practice of recording the state of the plantar response by the expressions "Babinski positive" and "Babinski negative." The first is tautological, the second erroneous, for there is only one Babinski response.

flexion at all joints. These reactions are in the nature of tonic reflexes and are seen only when a marked degree of spasticity is present.

Hemiplegia.—This is the most familiar picture of upper motor lesion. (1) *Of acute onset and in the initial stage.* The patient is commonly unconscious. There may be conjugate deviation of head and eyes away from the side of the lesion, and slight ptosis on this side may be present. The check on the paralysed half of the face may flap in and out with each breath, particularly when breathing is stertorous. While the entire musculature is flaccid, that of the paralysed limbs is most so, so that the thigh muscles spread out as the patient lies supine and gives this part of the limb a broader appearance than its fellow. For a week or more the temperature of the hemiplegic half of the body may be from 1·5° to 2° F. higher than on the opposite half. Sometimes acute trophic lesions develop; œdema of hand and foot with blistering, and bedsores. The abdominal reflexes are abolished on the paralysed side. Only in the most deeply comatose cases are the tendon jerks abolished. The plantar response is extensor on the affected foot.

(2) *Spastic residual hemiplegia.*—As shock passes off the patient regains consciousness, the presence of hemiplegia becomes more fully apparent and release symptoms begin to make their appearance. The active deviation of the head and eyes away from the side of the hemiplegia passes off, but for a week or more there may remain some defect in conjugate deviation of the eyes towards the hemiplegic side. At first, also, the tongue may be thrust out towards the hemiplegic side (impelled thereto by the genioglossus muscle of the normal side), but this passes off except in cases that remain severely paralysed. The base of the tongue often lies higher on the paralysed side.

There is relatively slight weakness of the upper part of the face, but more severe paresis of the lower face. The facial weakness is more marked on voluntary than on emotional movement (*e.g.* smiling). It may at first be impossible to "wink" the eye of the affected side without closing the opposite eye. The loss of voluntary movement is most severe in the arm, and both here and in the leg it shows the distribution already mentioned (page 21). There is some weakness of trunk muscles, as seen in the striking inability of the patient to sit up in bed, or—later—in a chair, without falling towards the paralysed side. He also finds it difficult to turn over in bed.

As spasticity gradually develops it takes the distribution described on a previous page (page 22). The arm tends to adopt an attitude of general flexion and adduction, and although perhaps severely paralysed is found to return to this position persistently unless it is fixed in extension by the side. From the onset the leg is extended and rotated out, with the foot plantarflexed, and it so remains except in cases of long-standing hemiplegia in demented and bedridden patients. These tend to lie on one side and this leads to flexion of the legs, which finally come to be fixed in this attitude.

The changes in tendon reflexes and in the plantar responses are those characteristic of upper motor neurone lesions.

Recovery of movement develops in the face and leg, and later, and much less perfectly, in the upper limb. The hand may never regain any movements other than simple flexion of all the fingers simultaneously. In most cases of hemiplegia the extensor (Babinski) plantar response on the paralysed side remains freely elicitable only from the sole of the foot, but the other devices already mentioned may evoke it from the leg below the knee. When the patient yawns the paralysed arm goes into very rigid spasm and half extends while the wrist and fingers also extend. The limb returns to its resting position as the yawn passes off. A little more has to be said before the description of hemiplegia is complete. Vascular lesions in the region of the internal capsule are the commonest cause of hemiplegia, and they do not respect anatomical arrangements of nerve fibres. Hence it is that when the posterior limb of the internal capsule is extensively destroyed the sensory radiations which lie caudal to the pyramidal fibres, and the optic radiations which are placed still further caudally may be involved, so that a hemi-anæsthesia, with or without a crossed homonymous hemianopia (see page 45), may in these circumstances accompany the hemiplegia.

Paraplegia.—There are two clinical forms of spastic paraplegia, paraplegia-in-extension and paraplegia-in-flexion. The former represents a paraplegia of pure upper motor neurone type, the latter is due to the interruption in the spinal cord of extrapyramidal motor paths in addition to that of the pyramidal tract. It is generally seen in the later stages of spinal cord compression and in any severe paraplegia from an extensive lesion.

(1) *Paraplegia-in-extension.*—All paraplegias of gradual onset from lesions involving the upper motor neurone belong to this type at their onset. Such a paraplegia develops the following sequence of signs. The first movement to be weakened is that of dorsiflexion of the foot, so that this tends to drag when the patient tires. In this way the toe of the shoe is worn down rapidly and the foot is apt to catch when on uneven ground. Next, flexion of the limb as a whole weakens and the leg tends to shuffle in walking. At the same time the tendon jerks increase in briskness and spasticity slowly develops in the extensor and plantarflexor muscles. The normal plantar response changes to the extensor type at a very early stage in this process, sometimes before appreciable weakness can be detected on clinical examination. Finally, the legs come to be rigidly extended and show more or less severe

adductor spasm. They may go into spontaneous clonus from time to time, or into sudden single extension spasms.

In lesions involving only the pyramidal system this form of paraplegia is retained (as, for example, in amyotrophic lateral sclerosis), but if other pathways in the cord are involved it changes gradually to the second type, that of paraplegia-in-flexion.

(2) *Paraplegia-in-flexion.*—Except in a single circumstance to be mentioned, this state follows and never precedes paraplegia-in-extension. It indicates a more complete interruption of conduction of descending impulses in the cord and an approach to separation of the cord below the level of the lesion from higher levels of the nervous system.

Involuntary flexor spasms make their appearance, they gain in force and frequency, and finally the legs come to lie fully flexed, with the knees pressed tightly against the abdominal wall. Voluntary power wanes rapidly when this flexion develops, flexion and dorsiflexion are completely lost and extension is feeble. It may require great force to pull the legs into the extended position, and once extended they rapidly resume flexion. The extensor type of plantar response now becomes very easy of elicitation and is accompanied by forceful flexion of the entire limb. In addition, this response may be obtained from an increasingly wide field, which sometimes includes the distal two-thirds of the entire limb. Below the middle of the thigh, pinching or pricking the skin, or deep stroking over bones and muscles all elicit it in a forceful and complete form. The knee jerks, and later the ankle jerks, may diminish and become difficult if not impossible to obtain. This picture is the final stage of an unrelieved compression of the spinal cord and of many cases of disseminated sclerosis. Sensory loss and loss of sphincter control usually accompany it.

(3) *Sudden Total Transection of the Cord.*—Such a lesion produces immediately total flaccid paralysis of the limbs, total sensory loss, loss of tendon jerks, retention of urine, and sometimes transient absence of all plantar response. The sudden interruption of descending impulses from the brain produces a condition of "spinal shock" which may last permanently if—as is frequently the case—death ensues within a few weeks. But if life is preserved, and the patient does not suffer from infected bedsores or cystitis, spinal shock begins to pass off in a few weeks. The knee and ankle jerks may return, the type of plantar response described under paraplegia-in-flexion is found and this form of paraplegia may develop. Sometimes the stroking of the sole produces not only the extensor response with limb flexion, but also the involuntary passage of some (but not all) of the urine in the bladder.

(4) *Combined Lesions of the Dorsal and Lateral Columns of the Cord.*— It may be useful to mention here the influence which a lesion of the afferent fibres of the dorsal columns has upon the clinical picture of

an upper motor neurone lesion in the cord. Such a state of affairs is seen in Friedreich's ataxy and in most cases of subacute combined degeneration of the cord. The tendon jerks are abolished and there is no hypertonus, but the abdominal reflexes are commonly lost and the plantar responses are of the extensor type. To the weakness ensuing upon the lateral column (pyramidal) lesion there is added some degree of sensory ataxy from impairment or loss of postural sensibility.

THE SYMPTOMATOLOGY OF LESIONS OF THE EXTRAPYRAMIDAL SYSTEM

With one rare exception (that of a vascular lesion involving the nucleus subthalamicus) diseases involving this system are chronic affections of gradual onset. There is no true paralysis of voluntary movements, but some of the release symptoms which predominate in these circumstances hamper voluntary movement in different ways, make it exhausting to the subject and thus lead to the appearance of some weakness. The essential clinical components of the different symptom-complexes of extrapyramidal motor system disease are:—

(1) Disorders of muscle tone.
(2) Involuntary movements.

There are three main symptom-complexes:—

(a) The tremor-rigidity syndrome of paralysis agitans.
(b) Athetosis.
(c) The choreiform syndrome.

Since, as we have seen (page 13), the normal functions of the structures composing the extrapyramidal system are very incompletely known, it is not surprising that attempts to correlate these three symptom-complexes with lesions in different components of the system have not been very satisfactory or conclusive. We are not at present in a position to differentiate syndromes of the putamen, or globus pallidus one from another, and hypotheses on the subject are not within the scope of the present work.

(a) This will be more fully described under the heading of paralysis agitans, but some general features may be mentioned. The muscular hypertonus differs qualitatively from that seen in lesions of the upper motor neurone, although like this it is a reflex rigidity arising from stretch. It is uniform throughout the entire range of passive or active movement of the muscle. Hence it has been described as a "lead pipe" rigidity. It feels to the examining hands much like the sensation of bending a soft lead pipe. If tremor is also present, and sometimes

even when this is not visible, a curious tremor in the muscle is to be
felt as the muscle is stretched. This gives a sensation somewhat as
though the extending muscle were "giving" over a cog, hence the
term "cogwheel" rigidity sometimes used. This rigidity invades the
entire skeletal musculature except that of the external muscles of the
eyes. It "damps down" the range of movement, so that the play of
facial expression dwindles and finally disappears, giving the patient
a mask-like expression. Only strong emotional stimuli break up this
fixity, and then a slow smile waxes and wanes over the patient's face.
In walking the arms cease to swing, and the legs move slowly and in
short steps. This rigidity maintains a fairly constant level. The tremor
is a rhythmical movement of a rate of about four per second. It is not
constantly maintained, often ceasing when the patient is at rest,
always when he is asleep, and increasing with stress of emotion or in
fatigue. It may cease while the limb is in active movement through
space, returning again when some fixed attitude is taken up. The
tendon jerks may be increased, but clonus is not seen. The abdominal
reflexes remain brisk and the plantar responses of normal type. In
this syndrome, tremor is occasionally entirely absent. In other cases
it predominates. When tremor is coarse rigidity tends to be minimal,
but is never wholly absent.

(*b*) *Athetosis.*—The characters of this are aptly expressed by the
term "mobile spasm" applied to athetosis by Gowers. It seems to
consist in irregular accesses of hypertonus into the musculature which
give rise to slow writhing movements and curious postures of the
limbs and hands. The fingers are often hyperextended at the metacarpo-
phalangeal joints. These movements are always aggravated in force
and amplitude when voluntary movement is attempted and under the
influence of emotion. No signs of upper motor neurone lesion may be
found, but in some instances (*e.g.* in infantile hemiplegia) these signs
may co-exist with athetosis. There is a congenital form of bilateral
athetosis in which the movements of the face, tongue, and of articulation
are disordered. As in the tremor-rigidity syndrome eye movements
escape.

(*c*) *The Choreiform Syndrome.*—The involuntary movements that
come in this category are commonly superimposed upon voluntary
movements, but when well-developed may occur also when the patient
is at rest. They are jerky inco-ordinate movements of the limb, trunk,
and facial muscles, ocular movements commonly escaping. It may be
considered doubtful, however, whether the involuntary movements of
rheumatic chorea really belong either to the group of release symptoms
or to that of extrapyramidal disorders. In severe cases of chorea, *e.g.*
chorea gravidarum, they are incessant, of great violence, and are
accompanied by delirium or great excitement. It is probable, therefore,

that these movements come in the category of excitation or "irritation" symptoms, the seat of the disturbance being cortical.

There is, however, a rare form of progressive chorea seen in middle-aged and elderly persons, sometimes associated with mental disorder (Huntington's chorea) in which the involuntary movements are probably release manifestations associated with disease in the basal ganglia. In these circumstances, the movements occupy—in appearance—a position intermediate between those of athetosis and those of rheumatic chorea. Choreiform movements commonly occur on a background of diminished tone.

THE SYMPTOMATOLOGY OF CEREBELLAR LESIONS

Cerebellar ataxy is the general term applied to the sum of disorders of voluntary movement that follow loss of cerebellar function. Very many components have been described as together making up this ataxy, but in truth very few of these are true components, *they are merely the particular form the ataxy takes according to the clinical test employed to demonstrate it, and according also to the particular movements being examined.** Thus it is obvious that if in a case of cerebellar disease we test eye movements we shall see something different from what we may expect if we test the very complex movements of the hand and arm, and because we call the disorder of the former nystagmus and that of the latter intention tremor there is no reason whatever for supposing, as is commonly done, that we are looking at two distinct modes of inco-ordination. We are in fact seeing the same disorder in different circumstances. If this is borne in mind the complexity and obscurity which invest descriptions of cerebellar ataxy are largely disposed of.

The essence of cerebellar ataxy is a disturbance of postural fixation not only of parts actually in movement but of parts which should be maintaining the necessary background of attitude in the rest of the musculature. Another aspect of this defect is seen in acute cerebellar lesions as a marked flaccidity or atonia of the muscles. This is perhaps no more than an extreme expression of the defect in postural fixation, or tone, already mentioned.

Clinically, and employing the customary tests, this defect shows itself in the following ways:—

(1) *Eye movements.*—On conjugate deviation to the side the eyes show a series of regular horizontal jerks known as nystagmus. On

---

* The reader will note that the complex terminology usually employed in describing cerebellar ataxy is omitted from this account. The omission is deliberate, for this terminology does not analyse the clinically observed phenomena into physiological components. On the contrary it renders any account of cerebellar ataxy almost unintelligible, and obscures the real nature of the disorder of movement in question.

deviation to the right, for example, the eyes move briskly in the desired direction but the deviation is not sustained and the eye more slowly recedes towards the mid-position, only to be brought back to the deviated position by a quick jerk. This is plainly the expression of a defect of postural fixation, corrected by voluntary efforts to maintain deviation. It is, in fact, a form of intention or action tremor of the eye muscles. In unilateral lesions of the cerebellum, the nystagmus is slower and its range wider when the eyes are moved towards the side of the cerebellar lesion than when they turn away from the side of the lesion. In cases of cerebellar abscess and of auditory nerve fibroma this difference may be very striking.

(2) *Articulatory movements.*—These are so affected as to produce what is called "scanning" or "staccato" speech. Each component syllable in a word is pronounced deliberately and slowly as though it were a separate word, and is not run together with its fellow syllables as in normal speech. In severe cases, the disorder may render speech almost unintelligible.

(3) *Movements of the hands and arms.*—When the limbs move through space, as, for example, when the patient is asked to touch index finger-tip to nose, the limb starts on its course and soon begins to develop a coarse, irregular, to-and-fro jerky movement which increases in coarseness as the finger approaches its objective. This it finally reaches and may then shake on the nose. In addition, these jerks, which seem due to voluntary efforts to correct a tendency of the limb to fall away, are apt to be forceful and to cause the hand to overshoot the mark when the patient is trying to pick up some object or to carry out some such movement as the doing up of buttons.

Further, if the patient be asked to perform alternating movements, such as alternate pronation-supination of the wrist, this inherent defect—intention tremor—becomes aggravated. The movements are irregular in rate and amplitude—generally excessive in range—and are thus slower than normal. In addition, the rest of the arm, postural fixation being defective, may enter into the movement and this renders the latter still more ataxic.

(4) *Movements of the legs.*—The same disorders appear here, rendering the gait irregular and staggering. In walking the postural steadiness of the head and trunk musculature is also defective, and thus the maintenance of stance may be grossly disordered. The trunk sways irregularly and the patient may be unable either to stand or to walk.

In unilateral lesions of the cerebellum these disorders are confined to the same side as that of the cerebellar lesion. The tendon jerks are swinging in character, but remain of normal briskness. Cutaneous and plantar reflexes are normal. There is no loss of any form of sensation in a pure cerebellar lesion.

THE SYMPTOMATOLOGY OF LESIONS OF THE LOWER MOTOR NEURONE

When the motor nerve supply to a muscle is cut off the muscle is completely paralysed, becomes flaccid, its tendon reflex is abolished, and it proceeds to waste. Finally, fibrous changes take place in its structure, it shortens and is said to undergo contracture. During the active process of wasting, in cases where the interruption of nerve supply is incomplete or slowly progressive, small groups of muscle fibres show irregular twitchings known as fibrillation. The degenerating muscle wholly, or even partly, cut off from the nervous system by a lesion of the lower motor neurone is usually extremely tender to pressure, may be painful and subject to cramps.

During this phase of degeneration in the muscle it may show what is known as *the reaction of degeneration*. Healthy muscle in normal connection with the nervous system responds by a tetanic contraction when its motor nerve is stimulated by a faradic current. The muscle itself does not respond to this form of stimulation, but only to the continuous or galvanic current. It then does so by a short-lived contraction when the current is made and broken. Once the axis cylinders of the motor nerve are degenerated (Wallerian degeneration) this nerve cannot any longer conduct the faradic stimulus and hence there is no response to faradism. The denervated and degenerating muscle fibres themselves show an altered response to direct stimulation by the galvanic current. This response may be greater than normal, but is slower in waxing and in passing off, and it may spread along the muscle in a slow wave. These altered reactions are the reaction of degeneration. This is not a full statement of the qualitative changes that may be seen, but it contains the essential and important items, and to it may usefully be added this proviso: that electrical testing of muscular reactions is rarely of value unless carried out by someone with experience, and that it is comparatively rare for this testing to provide diagnostic information that cannot more easily and reliably be obtained by other means. During the third week of a total Bell's palsy the retention by the paralysed muscles of normal electrical reactions enables us to say that quick and perfect recovery will take place, while the presence of the reaction of degeneration at this time indicates that recovery will be delayed for many months. This, perhaps, is the commonest important indication for the use of electrical testing of muscles, and, therefore, in general this testing is of little importance in neurological diagnosis.

THE ORGANIZATION OF THE AFFERENT NERVOUS SYSTEM

The afferent components of the nervous system may be said to determine and govern the activity of the entire nervous system. There are two such components, sensory and non-sensory. The impulses which pass upwards in the sensory pathways enter consciousness and form the basis of sensation in all its forms, while those which traverse the non-sensory afferent pathways never enter consciousness at all but subserve important reflex functions which are essential to the mainten-ance and regulation of muscle tone and thus of posture. The afferent links of certain reflex arcs which pass through the spinal cord also belong to the latter system.

THE SENSORY SYSTEM

ANATOMICAL.—The sensory pathway, like the motor, consists of a relay of neurones passing between periphery and brain. Arising in the various end-organs in skin and deeper skeletal tissues, it ascends the

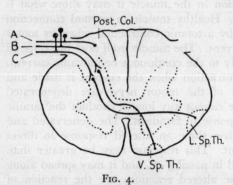

FIG. 4.
REARRANGEMENT OF SENSORY FIBRES ON ENTERING THE CORD.

A diagram of a transverse section of the spinal cord representing an entering dorsal root. A indicates the fibres which turn upwards in the dorsal column of the side of entry to sub-serve tactile, postural, and vibratory modes of sensibility. B represents a fibre subserving tactile sensibility which, crossing the midline, turns upwards in the ventral spino-thalamic tract. C represents the fibres which subserve thermal and painful sensibility. These cross the midline and turn upwards in the lateral spino-thalamic tract.

peripheral nerve and traverses the dorsal root to enter the dorsal column of the spinal cord in what is called the root entry zone.

In its peripheral course this pathway conveys the impulses underlying all modes of sensi-bility, but on its entry into the cord it undergoes a rearrange-ment in which the various im-pulses are grouped according to quality: *i.e.* physiologically. Impulses underlying tactile, pressure, postural and vibra-tory sensibility travel upwards in the dorsal columns in the primary neurone, forming the *uncrossed sensory path* (Fig. 4). On reaching the dorsal column nuclei at the lower end of the medulla the primary neurone ends in a synapse with the cell of the secondary neurone, which at once decussates (decussation of the fillet) and having crossed the middle line turns upwards next to the median raphe as the mesial fillet. This neurone traverses pons and midbrain and ends in the lateral nucleus of the thalamus. Here the third neurone arises and continues the path to the sensory cerebral cortex, where the impulses which it carries reach consciousness.

The impulses underlying painful (superficial and deep) and thermal sensibility are conducted by the primary neurone to the grey matter of dorsal horn. Here the neurone ends and the secondary neurone arises. This crosses in the neighbourhood of the grey commissure of the cord to reach the lateral column of the opposite half of the cord, where it turns up as the *crossed sensory path*, or, in anatomical terms, the lateral spino-thalamic tract. This runs upwards in the lateral region of the medulla and pons, approaches the fillet in the midbrain and ends with it in the thalamus. It is thought that the impulses carried by this path may reach consciousness in the thalamus. The path does not continue on to the cerebral cortex.

Tactile sensibility, as well as travelling by the uncrossed sensory path has a crossed pathway (ventral spino-thalamic tract) in the ventral column of the cord on the side opposite to the entry of the conducting fibres.

This rearrangement of the sensory pathway is shown diagrammatically in Fig. 4.

PHYSIOLOGICAL.—The modes of sensibility may be divided into superficial (cutaneous) and deep. Of *cutaneous sensibility* there are four primary modes: light touch, cold, warmth, and pain. *Deep sensibility* includes painless and painful pressure, postural sensibility, and vibration sense.

Each sensory mode has its own special end-organs and conducting fibres. The end-organs lie in small groups of two or more, each group being innervated by at least two branches of a dorsal root fibre. Each mode of cutaneous, and to a lesser degree of deep (painless and painful pressure) sensibility carries local sign: that is, the appropriate sensation is not only evoked but is localized, and when sufficiently separated in space two sensory stimuli can be felt as distinct. It was formerly taught that both localization and this "two-point" discrimination were faculties inherent in tactile sensibility only, and travelled in special anatomical pathways in the cord and brain-stem, but this, of course, cannot be the case. Both these aspects of sensation inhere in all modes of cutaneous sensibility and also in pressure sensibility, and are due in part to the complex nature of the grouping and innervation of the end-organs, and in part to integrative processes in the highest sensory centres in the cerebral cortex. The classification of cutaneous sensibility into "protopathic" and "epicritic" modes has been abandoned as not in accord with the anatomical basis of cutaneous sensibility, nor with the results of clinical observation (Fig. 5).

The end-organs subserving touch and pressure are stimulated by deformation of the skin, those subserving pain by a variety of potentially harmful stimuli, such as penetrating pinprick, chemical stimuli, severe degrees of pressure or of thermal stimulus. Those subserving cold are stimulated by stimuli which subtract heat from the skin, and those

c

subserving warmth by stimuli that add heat to the skin. Supramaximal degrees of both heat and cold evoke pain, as already mentioned.

Postural sensibility depends upon sensory end-organs in muscles, tendons and joints, and by means of stimuli excited in these the in-

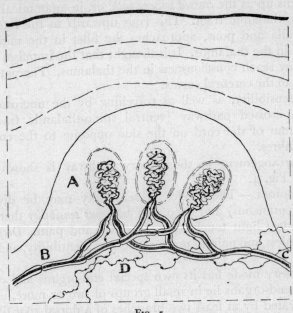

FIG. 5.

DIAGRAM OF A "TOUCH SPOT."

Diagram giving a simplified representation of a "touch spot" in the skin of the finger tip. This consists of a group of three Meissner's corpuscles (A). Each receives a dual innervation from two medullated fibres (B and C), each of these in turn arising from a distinct parent fibre. There is also an "accessory" innervation to each corpuscle by a beaded non-medullated fibre (D) which arises in a plexus of non-medullated fibres subserving cutaneous painful sensation. The function of the last-named fibre is to elicit pain when the touch spot is subjected to excessive stimulation. There are numerous such small groups of corpuscles in close proximity. Probably the capacity to localize a tactile stimulus depends largely upon this multiple grouping of end-organs and upon their multiple innervation. While the single corpuscle may be considered the anatomical unit of the sensory mechanism for touch, it is probable that the physiological unit of tactile sensibility comprises all the corpuscles innervated by a single dorsal root fibre. A comparable grouping and multiple innervation of end-organs obtains in the case of pressure and thermal (warmth and cold) end-organs, cutaneous pain being subserved by the non-medullated plexus.

dividual is able to ascertain the position of the body and its several parts (limbs, head) in space, and to appreciate the degree and direction of their movements. An important sensory end-organ in this connection is the labyrinth (otolith organ).

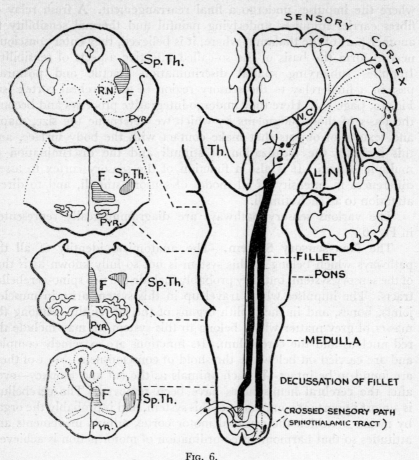

FIG. 6.

THE CENTRAL SENSORY PATHS.

On the right the sensory pathway is represented in its longitudinal course. On the left a series of transverse sections indicate the positions occupied by the components of the sensory path at the different levels of the brain-stem.

The uncrossed sensory path runs up in the dorsal white column, its fibres terminating in the dorsal column nuclei of the medulla (nuclei of Goll and Burdach). The path then decussates (decussation of the fillet) and runs up as the mesial fillet to the thalamus. The crossed sensory path travels upwards in the lateral column (lateral spino-thalamic tract) and in the ventral column (ventral spino-thalamic tract). These two meet in the medulla and run up together in the lateral region of the medulla and pons, gradually nearing the fillet and finally becoming continuous with it in the midbrain. The entire sensory pathway reaches the thalamus. Thence it divides, one component passing to the main thalamic nucleus, another passing to the sensory cerebral cortex. In dotted lines is represented a cortico-thalamic tract which, so it has been supposed, transmits cortical control of the thalamic component of the sensory mechanism. (Modified after Head and Holmes.)

Th., thalamus. N.C., caudate nucleus. L.N., lenticular nucleus. Sp. Th., spinothalamic tract. Pyr., pyramidal tract. F., Fillet.

All the sensory pathways enter the lateral part of the thalamus, where the impulses undergo a final rearrangement. A fresh relay of fibres carries impulses underlying painful and thermal sensibility to another part of the thalamus where, it is believed, they enter consciousness to form the basis of the so-called affective aspects of sensibility. Impulses subserving spatial discrimination (tactile and postural) pass in a final relay to the sensory region of the cerebral cortex (see Fig. 10, page 49). Here they undergo integrative processes and become the basis of those judgments by which we determine the size, shape, and texture of objects that make contact with the body surface, and this includes the localization of stimuli and the discrimination of multiple stimuli. It is also a function of the sensory cortex to assess differences in intensity of all modes of sensory stimuli, and to direct attention to all such stimuli.

The various sensory pathways are diagrammatically represented in Fig. 6.

The Non-sensory System.—The anatomical identity of all the pathways which belong to this system is not so fully known as is that of the sensory system, but they probably include the two spino-cerebellar tracts. The impulses which travel up in this system arise in muscles, joints, bones, and in the otolith organs of the labyrinths. Among the masses of grey matter which belong to this system we may include the red nucleus and the cerebellum. Its functions are extremely complex and are carried on below the threshold of consciousness. Most of them are found to be intact—in such animals as the cat and monkey—even after the cerebral hemispheres have been removed. The cerebellum is a most important component of this system, and is probably the organ by means of which the cerebral motor cortex adjusts movements and attitudes so that harmonious co-ordination of motor action is achieved.

THE SYMPTOMATOLOGY OF LESIONS OF THE SENSORY SYSTEM

The situation of a lesion on the sensory pathway chiefly determines both the topography and the quality of the sensory changes resulting, though—and particularly in the case of the peripheral part of the pathway—the nature of the lesion may markedly modify the quality of these changes. It follows from what has already been said of the sensory mechanism, that lesions of the peripheral pathway commonly affect all modes of sensibility, that systemic or localized lesions of the spinal cord may impair some modes while leaving others intact, that thalamic lesions may involve all forms though not always equally, and that cortical lesions tend to involve only what have been called the spatial and discriminatory substrata of sensibility.

In respect of *quality* of sensory change, lesions of the sensory pathway may lead to pain, to abnormal sensations (paræsthesiæ), to impairment or to loss of sensation. Disturbances of all three orders may be present simultaneously, especially in peripheral nerve injuries. Spontaneous pain as a result of central lesions is comparatively rare, and when it is found occurs usually in connection with thalamic lesions, of which it forms a characteristic symptom. Severe and persisting pain may arise from relatively slight injuries of certain peripheral nerves (median and internal popliteal) when irritation is set up at the site of injury. This pain, which is of an intense burning quality, goes by the name of *causalgia* and is associated with dryness and redness of the skin in the territory of the affected nerve and with extreme hyperæsthesia of this skin. Causalgia is commonly the sequel to a glancing injury which damages few fibres and may not lead to any considerable muscular weakness or objective loss of cutaneous sensation. This pain is further discussed in the chapter dealing with affections of the spinal nerves (page 280).

Paræsthesiæ.—The sensations of tingling and numbness so named may result from lesions of any part of the sensory pathway, though they are most obtrusive and uncomfortable in peripheral nerve affections. Their distribution will afford evidence as to the situation of the under-lying disturbance.

The measure of disability resulting from sensory loss varies not only in proportion to the depth and extent of the loss, but also according to the modes of sensibility involved. Very striking are the disability and disorder of movement ensuing upon defects in postural sensibility, and known as *sensory ataxy*. In these circumstances the subject is imperfectly aware of the position of the limbs and of the range and direction of movements. Up to a point this defect may be compensated for by the direction which vision may supply, and a measure of control of movement is achieved by its aid. When the eyes are closed, ataxy develops. In the case of the lower limbs the gait becomes ataxic, if not when vision is available, then when this is lacking, as in the dark or when the eyes are shut. The patient then begins to sway and stagger, a phenomenon familiarly known as Rombergism, from the original description of the symptom by Romberg. In the case of the upper limbs, the subject has difficulty in distinguishing by manipulation the size and shape of objects held in the hand. These, therefore, he cannot identify: a phenomenon known as *astereognosis*. In the finger-nose test usually adopted to test for the presence of loss of postural sense in the upper limbs, the patient with eyes closed endeavours to place his index finger-tip upon his nose. The limb is seen to deviate from its normal path and fails to reach its objective, showing an error of projection. The horizontally extended arms, the eyes being closed, are seen to fall away, and in severe loss the fingers perform slow flexion-extension movements, singly and irregularly, in a manner rather like the movements of athetosis.

The ataxy of cerebellar lesions is in contrast to this, in that while there is no trace of error of projection, the movements of the limb through space show an irregular and jerky progress, the so-called intention or action tremor. In the case of the legs, closing the eyes does not increase the ataxy.

It follows from what has been said that postural sensory loss is more disabling than purely cutaneous loss, though the combination of both still more deeply disturbs the normal use of the limbs.

(1) *Lesions of the peripheral sensory neurones.*—The consequences of these are more fully discussed in the chapter on affections of the spinal nerves, but the following generalizations may here be made. All modes of sensation tend to be affected and the topography of the region of change corresponds to the distribution of the nerve affected. In partial lesions, less than the full cutaneous distribution of a given peripheral nerve shows sensory change. There is usually a focus of complete cutaneous anæsthesia surrounded by a zone of partial loss, or there may be partial loss only.

Even in a total lesion of such a nerve as the ulnar we find a central zone of anæsthesia to all forms surrounded by a zone of partial loss, in which the loss deepens from the periphery towards the central anæsthetic zone. Within the peripheral zone, pinprick may have a diffuse burning quality.

(2) *Lesions of the sensory pathways in the spinal cord.*—Here the re-arrangement of sensory impulses into separate tracts according to quality may lead to some modes of sensation being lost while others are retained. Thus a lesion of the dorsal columns will cause loss of the sense of position and of vibration sense, while a lesion interrupting the decussation of the pain and temperature fibres (as occurs in syringo-myelia) will lead to loss of these forms of sensation with integrity of the others. Again, a unilateral lesion of the spinal cord involving the entire half above the level of the 12th thoracic segment gives what is known as the Brown-Sequard syndrome: loss of pain and temperature sense on the side opposite to the lesion, loss of postural and vibration sensations on the side of the lesion. Touch having a double (uncrossed and crossed) path may escape (Fig. 7).

(3) *Lesions of the sensory pathway in the brain.*—As the two spinal components of the sensory path near the thalamus they approach each other, and thus local lesions produce a crossed hemianæsthesia in which all forms of sensation are affected. Yet in the brain-stem dissociated forms of sensory loss may result from local lesions (see page 106 and Fig. 26).

Lesions involving the lateral part of the thalamus, if not so severe as to destroy sensibility produce a hemianæsthesia of characteristic quality. Postural sensation is most severely affected, and there is often

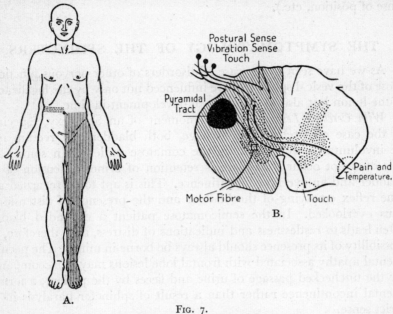

FIG. 7.

THE BROWN-SEQUARD SYNDROME.

Illustrating the Brown-Sequard syndrome from a lesion of the right half of the cord. In A the distribution of cutaneous sensory change is indicated. In B, the shaded (right) half of the cord is the seat of the lesion and the diagram indicates the pathways interrupted. The resulting disorders are given in the table below.

On the side of the lesion.	On the opposite side.
SENSORY.	
At level of lesion.—A band of cutaneous hyperæsthesia may be present. Alternatively, and only if three successive spinal segments are involved, there may be a band of impairment of cutaneous sensibility to touch, pain and temperature.	No abnormality.
Below level of lesion.—Tactile, painful and thermal sensibility normal. Postural and vibratory sensibility impaired or lost.	Impairment or loss of painful and thermal sensibility. Tactile, postural and vibratory sensibility normal.
MOTOR.	No abnormality.
Below level of lesion.—Spastic paresis of leg, increased tendon jerks, clonus, extensor plantar response.	

spontaneous pain at various sites on the affected half of the body, and to painful stimuli (pin-prick, heat or cold) there is an abnormal and very painful response (see page 105).

Lesions involving the sensory cerebral cortex are not characterized by loss of pain or temperature sensation, though different intensities of these may be imperfectly differentiated, but by loss of those aspects of sensation that underlie spatial discrimination (localization of touch, sense of position, etc.).

THE SYMPTOMATOLOGY OF THE SPHINCTERS

As we have seen in the case of disorders of other nervous functions, those of the vesical sphincters are influenced not only by the localization of the lesion but also by its mode of development in time.

With Cerebral Lesions.—At the moment of an apoplexy, especially in the case of cerebral hæmorrhage, both bladder and rectum may be involuntarily evacuated by the comatose patient. In some cases this does not occur, but there is retention of urine, distension of the bladder and an overflow incontinence. This is apt to be regarded as a true reflex emptying of the bladder and the presence of distension is thus overlooked. In the semicomatose patient a distended bladder often leads to restlessness and indications of distress, and, therefore, the possibility of its presence should always be borne in mind. The peculiar mental apathy associated with frontal lobe lesions may be accompanied by the unchecked passage of urine and fæces by the patient, a form of mental incontinence rather than a result of sphincter paralysis in the strict sense.

In general we may say that with cerebral disease incontinence is an accompaniment of disturbances of consciousness and is not due to any special localization of the lesion.

With Spinal Cord Lesions.—In acute transverse lesions causing total paraplegia there is retention of urine, followed by overflow, and finally by what is often called automatic micturition. But the true reflex incontinence of the baby in which the bladder is periodically emptied is never reproduced in spinal cord disease. What happens is that periodical sphincter relaxation allows the escape of some of the bladder contents but not of all. There is always some residual urine. In slowly progressive spinal cord compression the initial sphincter disorder may be precipitancy of micturition followed in due course by what we have spoken of as automatic micturition. Yet at some stage of such a condition retention of urine may suddenly develop and, as in the case of apoplexy already cited, may escape notice until with maximal distension there ensues an almost continual dribbling of urine. *Such a mode of leakage should always lead to an examination of the abdomen to detect whether or not the bladder is distended.*

In system degenerations of the cord, such as amyotrophic lateral sclerosis or Friedreich's ataxy, sphincter control remains intact.

The rectal sphincter shows disordered function by the appearance of constipation which gives place to fæcal incontinence after aperients. In total paraplegia from transverse lesions of the cord periodical fæcal incontinence occurs.

The paralysed bladder not infrequently becomes infected, and chronic infection leads to shrinkage of the organ and to almost continual dribbling of urine.

VISION : ORGANIZATION AND SYMPTOMATOLOGY

Anatomical.—The visual pathway extends from the head of the optic nerve to its termination in the cerebral cortex of the occipital lobe. The two optic nerves converge and meet at the optic chiasma. Here there is a partial decussation of the visual fibres, those from the two nasal half-fields crossing to enter the opposite optic tract, those from the two temporal half-fields entering the optic tract of the same side. Through their entire course from retina to occipital cortex, the visual fibres are grouped according to the retinal quadrants in which they arose. Thus, those from the two upper quadrants of each retina lie dorsal to those from the lower quadrants. In fact, the retinal origin and cortical destination of the visual fibres can be determined at every part of the visual pathway by the position of the fibres in it. The optic tract, containing fibres from the uncrossed temporal and the crossed nasal half-fields, enters and its fibres terminate in the lateral geniculate body of the thalamus. Here a fresh relay of fibres arises, and constituting the optic radiation (or geniculo-calcarine path) passes to the cortical region known as the area striata which surrounds the calcarine fissure at the occipital pole and on the mesial aspect of the occipital lobe. Some fibres of the radiation pass outwards and entering the temporo-sphenoidal lobe sweep round the descending horn of the lateral ventricle. These form the so-called temporal loop of the radiation, and the most anterior of these fibres represent the lower homonymous retinal quadrants (*i.e.* the upper homonymous quadrants of the visual fields). The course of the visual pathway is represented in Fig. 9. From this it will be seen that the macular region of the retina is represented at the posterior end of the area striata (*i.e.* at the occipital pole), the most peripheral parts of the retina at the anterior end. This relationship is indicated by the markings on visual fields and area striata in the figure.

In addition to the visual fibres, the optic nerve and tract contain the fibres that subserve the pupillary reflexes. These leave the tract to enter the superior quadrigeminal body, whence connections are established with supranuclear centres in the brain-stem and with the third nerve nucleus.

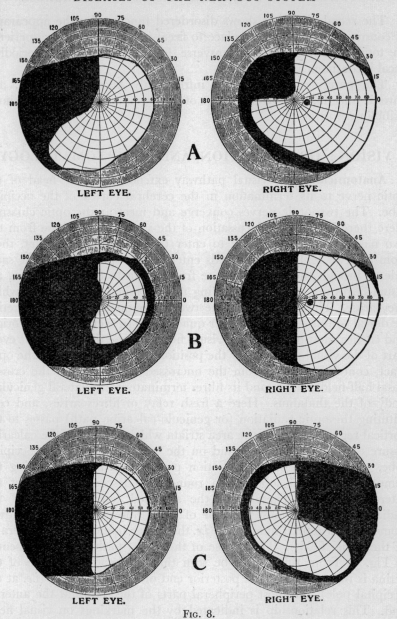

LEFT EYE.   RIGHT EYE.

A

LEFT EYE.   RIGHT EYE.

B

LEFT EYE.   RIGHT EYE.

C

FIG. 8.

A AND B. THE DEVELOPMENT OF A LEFT HOMONYMOUS HEMIANOPIA. C. A DEVELOPING
BITEMPORAL HEMIANOPIA.

A and B. Visual fields from a case of right-sided glioma of the temporo-sphenoidal lobe.
In A is seen the quadrantic mode of development of a left hononymous hemianopia, the
upper quadrants being those affected. InB, taken at a later stage, a complete homonymous
hemianopia splitting the macula is seen.

C. Visual fields from a case of pituitary adenoma with pressure on the chiasma, producing a bitemporal hemianopia. This appeared earlier and has progressed to an almost
complete loss of the temporal field of the left eye. In the right eye, the upper temporal
quadrant is lost and the lower quadrant just beginning to be invaded.

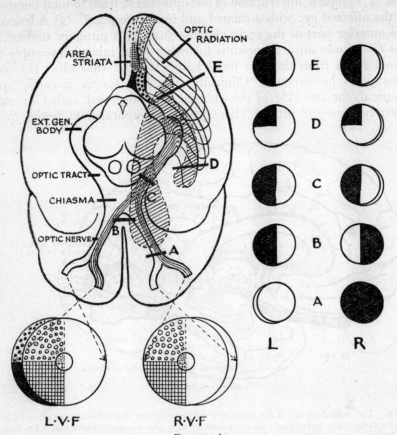

OCCIPITAL POLES

OPTIC RADIATION

AREA STRIATA

EXT. GEN. BODY

OPTIC TRACT

CHIASMA

OPTIC NERVE

E

D

C

B

A

L   R

L·V·F   R·V·F

Fig. 9.—A.

A. The Visual Pathways.

A. The course of the visual fibres from the right homonymous halves of the two retinæ to the right occipital pole is represented. The termination of the right optic tract in the external geniculate body can be seen and also the course of the optic radiation to the area striata surrounding the calcarine fissure. The relation of the radiation to the descending horn of the lateral ventricle in the temporo-sphenoidal lobe is indicated, the most anterior part of the radiation being the so-called temporal loop. The topographical representation of the different parts of the visual field in the area striata can be seen.

On the right of this anatomical diagram are represented the disturbances of the visual field resulting from lesions at different parts of the visual pathway.

(A)—A lesion of the right optic nerve, resulting in complete blindness of the right eye with immobility of the pupil.

(B)—A lesion of the anterior border of the chiasma, resulting in bitemporal hemianopia.

(C)—A lesion of the optic tract involving loss of vision in the left homonymous half-fields.

(D)—A lesion in the temporo-sphenoidal lobe, involving the temporal loop of the optic radiation and producing loss of vision in the left homonymous upper quadrants of the half-fields.

(E)—A lesion of the optic radiation leading to a left homonymous hemianopia.

(Modified from Bender and Kanzer.)

Symptomatology.—From these anatomical arrangements it follows that (1) complete interruption of one optic nerve leads to total blindness in the affected eye with a dilated and immobile pupil. (2) A lesion of the anterior part of the optic chiasma (usually a pituitary tumour, or less commonly an arachnoiditis following head injury) interrupts the visual fibres from the two nasal half-fields and thus gives rise to a bitemporal hemianopia. Clinically, this hemianopia is rarely symmetrical, for one side of the chiasma is compressed earlier or more severely than the other. Therefore one temporal field begins to be

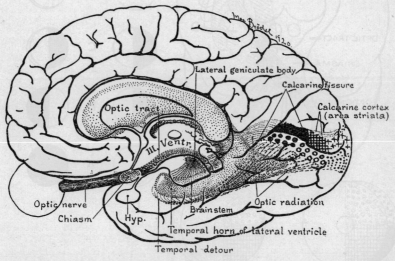

Fig. 9.—B.

B. The mesial aspect of the right cerebral hemisphere, the geniculo-calcarine pathway (optic radiation), particularly in its relations with the temporo-sphenoidal lobe and the descending horn of the lateral ventricle. The most anterior part of the radiation which surrounds the tip of the descending horn of the ventricle represents the lower homonymous quadrants of the left visual fields. Hence the earliest defect in the visual field is commonly an upper quadrantic hemianopia. (Modified from Cushing.)

(From *Transactions of the American Neurological Society, 1921.*)

invaded before its fellow, that is, vision is lost within it sooner and more extensively. Usually the loss of vision first appears at the periphery of the upper quadrant and advances towards the macular area. The lower quadrant is next invaded. Thus a full hemianopia may be established in one eye while in its fellow only the upper temporal quadrant shows a defect. Finally, as compression increases, the nasal field is invaded and vision in one eye is totally lost at a stage when the opposite field shows only a temporal defect.

(3) Lesions of the optic tract, commonly tumours, lead to a homonymous hemianopia of the crossed half-fields. This begins peripherally and extends centrally, finally "splitting the macula." It has been

taught that tract hemianopia differs from radiation hemianopia in that in the former the macula is "split," while in the latter macular acuity is spared. This is probably not the case, for the study of the progressive hemianopias of tumour indicate that ultimately in both instances the macula is finally involved.

(4) Lesions involving the optic radiation (tumour or vascular lesion) also lead to a crossed homonymous hemianopia. Temporal lobe tumour or abscess may interrupt the temporal loop and yield this result, and frequently the defect first appears as an upper quadrantic defect in the crossed homonymous half-fields.

In both tract and radiation hemianopia, the impairment of visual function occurs in the following order: colour vision, form vision, and appreciation of movement. The accurate determination of the various defects in the visual fields requires the use of a perimeter or a Bjerrum screen, but a simple method of determining the presence and form of defects by confrontation is described on page 338.

In respect of the pupils it is usually taught that in a tract hemianopia, illumination of the blind half of the retina yields no pupil reaction (hemianopic pupil reaction), while illumination of the seeing field yields a normal reaction of the pupil to light. The difficulties in restricting illumination to the half retina deprives this test of any great practical value. In rare cases of total blindness from a bilateral destruction of the visual cortex (occipital blindness) the pupil reactions remain intact.

Ocular Movements.—Brief reference may here be made to the organization of these movements and to their disorders, because the generalizations already made in respect of the motor system do not apply without qualification to them. Their cortical representation is topographically separate and distinct from that of other movements, and is situated in the frontal lobe cortex anterior to the so-called "motor cortex" (see Fig. 10). The division of ocular muscle innervation into upper and lower motor neurone types holds, as for other voluntary movements, but under normal conditions perhaps the majority of eye movements are reflex and not purely voluntary. Put in another way, we may say that attention plays relatively little part in their initiation, and they are largely reflexly induced; the exciting stimuli arising in the retinæ and vestibular and auditory nervous apparatus. There have arisen in consequence "centres" for the co-ordination of ocular movements in the brain-stem, closely connected with and adjacent to the nuclei of the 3rd, 4th, and 6th cranial nerves. The movements innervated from the cerebral cortex and from the brain-stem centres referred to are co-ordinated movements, involving the harmonious action of several external ocular muscles, and of internal ocular muscles (*e.g.* the contraction of the pupils in convergence), and they consist in conjugate movement of the eyes in a lateral or vertical direction in which the visual axes remain parallel, and in convergence. The nuclei and issuing nerves (3, 4, 6), on the other hand, constitute the lower motor neurone and innervate muscles as such and not movements in the sense of co-ordinated movement involving reciprocal innervation.

Symptomatology.—From all this it follows that we have two types of paralysis where ocular movements are concerned, an upper and a lower motor neurone type, the former a paralysis of movement, the latter a paralysis of muscles. In the former, since only co-ordinated movements are lost, there is neither diplopia nor squint, while in the latter both are characteristically present unless there is complete external ophthalmoplegia. It is usual to speak of the upper motor neurone type of paralysis as *a supranuclear paralysis*, and of this there are two varieties, one when the voluntary initiation of conjugate movements is lost, but such movements can still be evoked by reflex stimulation; the other when such movements are totally lost and cannot be elicited by any means. The former occurs, usually as a temporary phenomenon, in lesions producing sudden hemiplegia (apoplexy from vascular lesion), and consists in a weakness or loss of conjugate deviation of the eyes to the side away from the lesions. The latter is seen in lesions of the dorsal (tegmental) region of the midbrain and pons.

A characteristic sign of a lesion involving the quadrigeminal region of the midbrain (such as pressure from a superjacent pineal tumour) is a loss of upward deviation of the eyes, the pupils being often dilated and immobile. In pontine lesions near the sixth nerve nucleus there may be paralysis of conjugate deviation of the eyes to the side of the lesion, indeed the eyes may be permanently deviated away from this side. Gross lesions in the brain-stem may, of course, produce supranuclear and lower motor neurone types of paralysis, and in this case squint and diplopia may be added to the conjugate paralyses.

The symptoms that ensue upon paralyses of isolated ocular muscles are described on page 258 in the chapter dealing with cranial nerve affections.

THE SPEECH FUNCTION: ORGANIZATION AND SYMPTOMATOLOGY

1. **Organization.**—Physiologically considered speaking and writing are movements, but psychologically considered they are the production of symbols that in the expression of thought we use to refer to things. A word has no meaning until it is used by a thinker to refer to, that is, to stand as a sign for, something.

In addition to what we may call this referential function of speech it has also an emotive function in which words are used not to make a proposition but to express or to arouse feeling. The simplest example of this usage is an oath which is an interjection, an explosive sound.

In general our use of words combines both these functions more widely than we commonly suppose. Many propositions are verbally elaborated so as to create some desired impression, or are cast in verse to arouse emotion. In a purely scientific statement the referential use of words is paramount, but in politics, poetry, and philosophy their use is often largely emotive.

Clinically, as we shall see, the distinction is of some importance, for in disease affecting the speech function referential speech is much more severely impaired than emotive.

While speech is thus ultimately a psychological function it has an anatomical and physiological basis: anatomical in respect of the neurones concerned in the reception of speech sounds and in the performance of speech movements, and physiological in respect of the activity of these neurones; a fact illustrated by the speechlessness that may ensue upon a small local lesion in a certain part of the left cerebral hemisphere.

Acquisition of speech by the infant.—The physiology and psychology of the speech function are thus seen to be but different aspects of the same problem, and while neither aspect is yet fully understood, a few quite simple generalizations may be made concerning the acquisition of speech by the infant. The articulate sounds he hears become associated in his mind with the objects and events that come to occupy his attention at the time these sounds are uttered by those who care for him. These sounds leave their traces in his cerebral cortex, or to speak psychologically, are remembered by him. They become part of a context in his mind, so that the repetition of the sound calls up in his mind the associated object or event. Thus, the articulate sound becomes a sigh or symbol which the infant interprets and in so doing makes the first step in the acquisition of speech.

The word "mummy" calls up in his mind his image of his mother, while conversely, the sight of his mother evokes the symbolic sound "mummy."

Later, under the directing influence of these auditory memories and associations, the infant himself attempts and finally learns to utter these symbolic sounds, thus making his first essays in the verbal expression of thought, which is articulate speech.

As his learning progresses, ever more sounds acquire symbolic value for him, while the traces of an increasing number of patterns of motor innervations of such sounds are laid down in his cortex.

In the acquisition of reading and writing, visual symbols and those patterns of motor innervation that underlie writing occupy the place taken by auditory symbols and articulate speech in the brief statement made above.

Both physiological and psychological terms have been used in this introduction. This mixture of categories has been deliberate and will serve to emphasize that in them we speak but of two modes of approach to a single problem.

So far nothing has been said of gesture, which may play a great part in the communication of thought and feeling. Within its somewhat narrow limits it remains the most unequivocal form of "speech" there is, but its further development as a chief means of communication, during the evolution of speech in the infancy of the human race, was probably halted by the fact that if one is using one's hands and arms for gesture one can do nothing else at the same time. Vocal speech does not hold up action.

In short, the study of speech is a science of symbols and of symbolic thought, and much of the difficulty and misunderstanding that arise in the communication of thought by speech are due to subtle and often unnoted differences in the meanings given to our symbols by different persons. How easily this may occur in the use of abstract names, such terms as "truth" and "beauty" with their numerous and often indefinite shades of meaning well illustrate.

Anatomically the neurones subserving speech lie within a fairly well-defined region of the left cerebral hemisphere, bounded anteriorly by the second and third frontal convolutions and by the angular and first temporal convolutions posteriorly, the whole having a roughly quadrilateral form as viewed on the convexity of the cerebral hemisphere.

Physiologically, the hearing and seeing of words are sensory impressions, while speaking and writing are co-ordinated movements. These sensory impressions and movements conform to the general laws characteristic of sensation and motion. Lesions interrupting the appropriate sensory or motor paths will interfere with the reception of speech sounds or with the performance of speech movements. The motor cortex and pyramidal tract innervate these movements and a lesion involving the latter will, as part of the ensuing paralysis, affect speech movements, producing a disorder of articulation (dysarthria, or anarthria) as well as of other movements in which the same muscles may take part.

A disorder of articulation is not, strictly speaking, a disorder of the speech function, nor is the cutting off of sensory impressions, auditory or visual, able of itself to produce a true speech disturbance. The speech function is not a property of the cortical projection areas, sensory or motor, that is, the areas to and from which the long projection tracts pass, but of association areas adjacent to them in the cerebral cortex. In these the traces of articulate sounds heard or written words seen, and the sensory impressions left by past speech movements are laid down and retained. Similarly, within association areas adjacent to the motor cortex are stored the impressions left by the performance

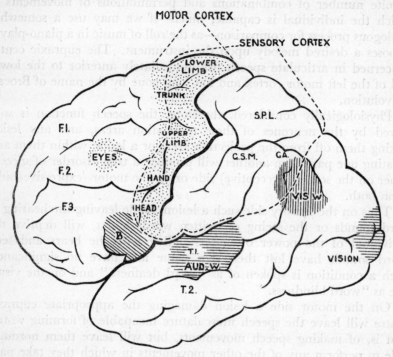

FIG. 10.

THE CORTICAL REPRESENTATION OF FUNCTION.

In this diagram the cortical functions described in this chapter are given their topographical representation.

The lateral aspect of the left hemisphere. *The motor area* extends over the ascending frontal convolution and the cortical region immediately anterior to it. At the posterior end of the second frontal convolution is a region in which eye movements are represented. Both this and the motor cortex proper are indicated by stippling. *The sensory cortex* is more extensive and includes the ascending frontal, superior parietal, and angular convolutions (After Henry Head).

At the foot of and anterior to the ascending frontal convolution is the so-called motor speech centre, Broca's convolution (B.).

In the first temporal convolution of this hemisphere is the auditory word centre (Aud.W.). and in the angular gyrus the visual word centre (Vis.W.).

The visual cortex just extends on to the lateral aspect of the hemisphere at the occipital pole. F.1, 2, and 3. First, second, and third frontal convolutions. T.1 and 2. First and second temporal convolutions. S.P.L. Superior parietal lobule. G.S.M. Supramarginal convolution, G.A. Angular convolution.

of previous speech movements; the patterns of speech movements. Such association areas (eupraxic centres) functionally connected with the motor cortex exist in respect of all learned purposive movements. In them are stored what we may call the motor habits of the individual,

D

and these they transmit to their executive mechanism—the motor cortex—under direction of the receptive association areas already mentioned. The movements represented in the motor cortex are at the disposal of the eupraxic centres which utilize them for the almost infinite number of combinations and permutations of movements of which the individual is capable, much—if we may use a somewhat analogous process for comparison—as the roll of music in a piano-player imposes a desired melody upon the instrument. The eupraxic centre concerned in articulate speech lies immediately anterior to the lower end of the left motor cortex and has long gone by the name of Broca's convolution.

Physiologically considered, therefore, the speech function is subserved by the neurones of these association areas, and any lesion cutting them off from the projection areas or a lesion within them and isolating one part from another will produce a true disorder of speech, either on the sensory (receptive) side or on the motor (expressive) side, or on both.

Thus on the sensory side such a lesion, while leaving the hearing of word sounds or the seeing of written words intact, will deprive the individual of the power of understanding what he hears and sees. Word sounds have lost their sign value and have no significance. Such a condition is spoken of as "word deafness," and on the visual side as "word blindness."

On the motor side a lesion damaging the appropriate eupraxic centre will leave the speech musculature incapable of forming words, that is, of making speech movements, but will leave them normally able to perform any of the other movements in which they take part. The traces of previous speech movements are lost and the affected individual cannot activate the motor cortex for their production though he can activate it for other movements employing the same muscles.

The condition in which the individual does not comprehend spoken or written words is known as *receptive or sensory aphasia*, that in which he cannot make speech movements is known as *expressive or motor aphasia*. In the case of writing movements we speak of *agraphia*.

Consideration will show that both sensory and motor aphasia are but special examples of more general defects. Thus we sometimes encounter a condition in which the subject no longer recognizes the nature or use of a familiar object which he sees perfectly. To this defect the name *agnosia* is given. Sensory aphasia (word deafness and word blindness) is but a special form of agnosia. We also see from time to time an individual who, knowing the nature of some familiar object and having neither paralysis, ataxy of movement, nor sensory loss, yet cannot perform the movements appropriate to the use of this object.

This condition is known as *motor apraxia*. Motor aphasia and agraphia are but special examples of motor apraxia.

Pathologically both motor and sensory aphasia are only symptoms and result from lesions of any kind—thrombosis, tumour, abscess, degeneration—within the appropriate cerebral region, that is, within what has been called the speech quadrilateral in the left cerebral hemisphere.

Lesions involving the anterior end of the quadrilateral affect expressive speech predominantly, those involving the posterior end the receptive aspect of speech. Thus cases of speech disturbance fall roughly into two groups, motor and sensory.

2. **Symptomatology.**—*Motor Aphasia* is associated with lesions involving Broca's convolution. In its mildest form it consists in a loss of names. The subject cannot find names in his spontaneous conversation, cannot give names to familiar objects presented to him, and seeks to remedy the defect by periphrasis. Thus he calls a pen "what you write with." Although thus unable to find names, he immediately recognizes the lost word when it is supplied to him. If some familiar object be presented to his view and he is asked to name it he is unable to do so; but when a series of names is said aloud to him he rejects the wrong ones and assents immediately he hears the correct one. That his memory for names is intact can be seen also by giving him simple orders. These, if he be not paralysed, he can carry out, thus revealing that the comprehension of spoken speech is intact.

In the mild degree of aphasia thus exemplified the capacity to construct a sentence, though one largely shorn of names, remains; but in more severe degrees even this is lost and the subject may be reduced to the recurring utterance of a single word such as "yes, yes," which he uses on all occasions, sometimes seeking to lend his utterance meaning by varying the inflexion of his voice or by accompanying gesture.

In addition to this loss of words, most aphasic subjects—though their comprehension of spoken speech is normal or relatively good—cannot read. This defect is most conspicuous in poorly educated persons not used to much reading. It is supposed that such persons when reading say over to themselves the words as they follow the lines of writing, and the motor aphasic not having the power even of this internal speech cannot read.

Sensory Aphasia.—The symptoms here also vary in severity. Essentially they consist in an impaired or lost comprehension of spoken speech. The subject hears the words said to him, but these are devoid of sign value; they mean nothing. He cannot read for he cannot understand the words he sees.

Since the motor side of the speech mechanism is directed by the receptive or sensory side, it follows that expression is also disordered in sensory aphasia. The subject may have plenty of words at his disposal, but they are the wrong words. The eupraxic centre is abnormally activated and in its turn transmits the wrong speech patterns to the motor cortex. Not only may wrong words be uttered, but words may be badly arranged and a jargon speech ensue. The patient being word deaf is unaware of his mistakes. Owing to his word deafness the subject cannot reply appropriately to questions and cannot carry out spoken orders. He may have names for familiar objects but they are the wrong names, though he fails to recognize his errors.

Pure forms of aphasia are not commonly met with: this is perhaps more especially the case with sensory aphasia, which is often accompanied by some loss of motor speech. A relatively pure motor aphasia, on the other hand, is not so rare. An inability to write, from loss of words in the motor aphasic and from errors in words in the sensory aphasic, accompanies the disorders of articulate speech.

In respect of other functions than speech the symptoms of motor apraxia and agnosia result from lesions involving association areas adjacent to but not identical with those for speech. Each purposive movement complex may be said to have its private eupraxic centre, and each group of sensory impressions that has acquired significance its private cerebral representation. Hence we may see a grade of motor apraxia in which some purposive movements are lost, others retained. The lesions underlying motor apraxia are situated in the frontal lobe immediately anterior to the motor cortex, those underlying agnosia in association areas adjacent to the sensory projection areas of the cortex. Agnosia and apraxia are investigated by giving the individual familiar objects and watching his capacity to recognize their nature and use, and his power of making the movements appropriate to this use. Also, in the case of motor apraxia, by asking him to perform certain familiar movements, such as clapping his hands, beckoning, turning a key, etc. These he cannot do to order, though he may be seen to perform them unthinkingly. The more fully deliberate and voluntary such a movement is the more seriously is it prone to be disturbed, the more automatic it is the less it is impaired.

This brings us back to the distinction already drawn between referential or intellectual speech on the one hand and emotive speech on the other. The former is most voluntary, the latter most automatic, the former most severely disturbed in aphasia, the latter least severely.

In all aphasic patients certain general features are to be noticed. The expression and exchange of thought are impaired and thought itself accordingly damaged, and this even though it may be possible to think without words. There is thus the appearance of some intellectual impairment in all but the mildest forms of aphasia. Further, there is a tendency in aphasic subjects to repeat words, and to repeat a movement already carried out to order when some other movement is asked for. Thus a man asked to close his eyes does so. He is then asked to put out his tongue. He may respond by again closing his eyes. This tendency which betrays some intellectual disintegration is known as perseveration.

Disorders of articulation fall, like those of other movements, into categories of upper and lower motor neurone types.

The terms dysarthria and anarthria are applied equally to both.

THE PITUITARY-HYPOTHALAMUS COMPLEX: ORGANIZATION AND SYMPTOMATOLOGY

Amongst the varieties of intracranial tumour that will engage our attention in a later chapter, are those that involve—either directly or by compression—the pituitary body and its stalk and the hypothalamus.

Not only are these structures related embryologically and topographically, but their functions are closely linked. Our knowledge of the last-named is recent and as yet incomplete, while, taking them as a whole, their apportionment between pituitary body and hypothalamus has not yet in all respects been conclusively decided. Further, the lesions of disease rarely affect one of these structures, leaving the other intact. This is particularly true of tumours which characteristically produce disorders of function over a wider region than that of their anatomical extent. Therefore a full discussion of pituitary and hypothalamic activities is not within the compass of this book. Nevertheless, the following brief summary of what is now generally believed may be given.

ANATOMY AND PHYSIOLOGY.—The pituitary body consists of a glandular *pars anterior* and a *pars intermedia*, both derived from the embryonic cranio-buccal (Rathke's) pouch, and a neural *pars posterior* derived from a downgrowth of the floor of the third ventricle which also provides the pituitary stalk. A collar of cells derived from the pars anterior surrounds the base of the pituitary stalk and is known as the *pars tuberalis*.

In the *pars anterior* are cells of three types, named according to their reaction to dyes as chromophobe, acidophile, and basophile cells. The chromophobe cells are ordinarily the most numerous, possess a non-granular cytoplasm and, as far as is known, have no secretion. It is believed that they are precursors of both acidophile and basophile cells, and that in a normal secretory activity they become either acidophile or basophile according to the physiological conditions prevailing at the time (*e.g.* puberty, pregnancy, climacteric), returning again to the chromophobe type when exhausted by secretory activity and the discharge of their granules.

The physiological activity of the *pars anterior* depends, therefore, upon that of the acidophile and basophile cells, which between them produce a number of hormones. These control bodily growth, the development and activity of the gonads and breasts and the activity of the thyroid gland. They also regulate carbohydrate metabolism. Each of these hormones has its appropriate name, and their allocation to the two types of cell present has not been finally decided, but it is probable that the acidophile cells are concerned in bodily growth and the basophile cells in that of the gonads. The hormone regulating carbohydrate metabolism is spoken of as "diabetogenic," and its role is to regulate the absorption of glucose from the gut and to control the utilization of carbohydrate reserves. Together with the secretion of the adrenal cortex it antagonizes the action of insulin.

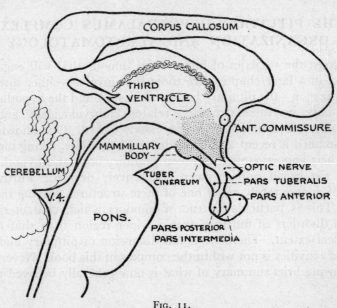

FIG. 11.

THE PITUITARY AND HYPOTHALAMUS.

A diagram representing a mesial sagittal section of the brain-stem and region of the third ventricle. The situation of the nuclei of the hypothalamus in the walls and floor of the third ventricle is represented by the dotted area. The stalk and three portions of the pituitary body are also diagrammatically represented.

Of the physiological activity of the *pars intermedia* and *pars tuberalis* nothing precise is known.

The neural *pars posterior* is closely associated with the hypothalamus and receives an innervation from the supraoptic nuclei which regulates its secretory activity, for the pars posterior is also a gland of internal secretion. Its two hormones are the oxytocic which influences uterine contraction, and the vasopressor or "antidiuretic" hormone. This controls water balance by regulating the retention of water by the kidney tubules. Carbohydrate metabolism is also influenced by the secretions of the *pars posterior*.

The *hypothalamus* is the small region of the brain beneath the thalamus and surrounding the third ventricle. Not only does it regulate pituitary activity, but it has important functions as a subcortical co-ordinating centre of the autonomic nervous system. This system probably has two distinct representations within the hypothalamus, one for the sympathetic and one for the parasympathetic component, and between the two there are reciprocal functional relationships. Temperature control and the regulation of sleep are functions of the hypothalamus.

Together, the pituitary body and the hypothalamus have been called the diencephalo-hypophyseal mechanism, and it is the functions of this as a physiological whole that are commonly disordered by tumours, rather than the functions of either component singly.

Symptomatology.—From the foregoing it is clear that a number of defect symptoms must arise from disease or injury of the pituitary and hypothalamus. The most important of these are as follows:—

Diabetes insipidus.—This ensues when the nerve fibres from supraoptic nuclei to *pars posterior* are interrupted, provided that the *pars anterior* remains intact. The polydipsia that accompanies polyuria is probably secondary to this. *Glycosuria* is a less common defect symptom.

Genital dystrophy.—This includes failure of the sexual glands and of the secondary sexual characteristics to develop, or, if these are already mature, their regression. Impotence and amenorrhœa are expressions of this failure.

Disorders of growth.—These are attributable to involvement of the pituitary, and include the effects of diminished function, *e.g.* infantilism and Fröhlich's syndrome (dystrophia adiposo-genitalis). The latter syndrome consists of absence of sexual development, obesity and sometimes diabetes insipidus and somnolence. Excess of acidophile secretion leads in infancy to gigantism and in later life to acromegaly.

Disorders of sleep and of temperature regulations are regarded as hypothalamic symptoms. Somnolence is the common sleep disturbance. Hyperthermia may be seen after operations involving the hypothalamic region.

The pathology of these various symptoms and symptom-complexes is discussed in Chapter III (page 79).

THE CEREBROSPINAL FLUID

This fluid is a secretion of the choroid plexuses. It escapes from the ventricular system via the foramina in the fourth ventricle and enters the basal cisterns of the subarachnoid space. It passes thence through the opening in the tentorium and over the surface of the cerebral hemispheres. It leaves the subarachnoid space through the arachnoid villi which penetrate the walls of the dural sinuses and deliver the fluid into the venous blood. The main function of this fluid is probably to provide a water bed for the brain and cord, but it is also a medium into which cells and substances in solution may pass from the perivascular spaces of the brain.

It is a clear, colourless saline fluid at a normal pressure of from 60 to 150 mm. of water. As obtained by lumbar puncture it contains up to 5 lymphocytes per c.mm. and its chemical composition is as follows:—

Protein　.　0·02–0·04 per cent. (20 to 40 mgm. per 100 c.c.)
Glucose　.　0·05–0·08 per cent. (50 to 80 mgm. per 100 c.c.)
Chlorides .　0·72–0·75 per cent. (725 to 750 mgm. per 100 c.c.)

Of the protein content albumin is the main constituent, being always above the globulin content even when both are in excess. Changes may occur in the fluid either as a result of altered secretion, or because of the additions to it as it fills the subarachnoid space. Apart from such changes in composition, its pressure, as determined by the manometer on lumbar puncture, may also vary, rising with raised intracranial tension.

To say that lumbar puncture and the examination of the cerebro-spinal fluid should be a routine part of a neurological examination would be to overstate the case. In many circumstances diagnosis is possible without this procedure, in others it is not capable of throwing additional light upon the clinical problem under consideration. To take but two common affections of the nervous system, epilepsy and disseminated sclerosis, lumbar puncture can but rarely be essential to diagnosis, and when the clinical evidence is conclusive there can be no justification for performing it. It is often a painful procedure for the patient, and occasionally a dangerous one. On the other hand, it may be essential for complete diagnosis to determine the composition or the pressure of the fluid, or to drain the theca as a measure of treatment. The object of this comment is to stress that discrimination should govern the employment of lumbar puncture. It is an accessory method of diagnosis, designed to complete the evidence afforded by clinical examination when this evidence is insufficient. It is not a short cut to diagnosis, nor a substitute for clinical investigation.

The various significant changes in the fluid will be discussed under the appropriate headings.

The Performance of Lumbar Puncture.—The patient should remain in bed for from 12 to 24 hours after puncture. The needle used should be about 8 cm. long and from 1·2 to 1·5 mm. in diameter. It should have a short bevel, and the handle should be flattened in the same plane as the bevel so that this can be passed into the theca facing downwards. The stylet should fit and should not be withdrawn until the needle has reached and penetrated the theca. The patient is placed lying on his side with the hips near the edge of the bed and his legs fully drawn up. The head should be on the same horizontal level as the sacrum and the chin as near the knees as possible.

The plane of the back should be vertical. The needle is then passed in between the 3rd and 4th lumbar vertebræ and this interspace usually lies on a line drawn between the highest points of the iliac crests. The needle is thrust forwards and slightly upwards and should reach the spinal canal at a depth of from 4 to 6 cm. When it is thought that the theca has been pierced, the stylet should be withdrawn. If no fluid is obtained, the bevel should be turned through a quarter circle. The needle should not be partly withdrawn and pushed in again if fluid does not escape at once, as this often leads to damage to veins, a blood-stained fluid, and severe headache for the patient. If the needle encounters bone, it should be almost wholly withdrawn and thrust in again.

It is advisable to anæsthetize the skin and the track of the needle by the injection of 2 or 3 c.c. of a 1 per cent. solution of novocain before inserting the lumbar puncture needle.

Intrathecal Pressure.—The information yielded by lumbar puncture is increased by the routine use of a manometer. The manometer devised by Greenfield consists in a 30 cm. length of thermometer tubing of such a bore that it will hold from 1·5 to 2 c.c. It is graduated in half centimetres, and can be attached by a piece of fine bore rubber tubing to a two-way stopcock which fits into the handle of the puncture needle.

When a block in the spinal subarachnoid space is suspected, as in the case of spinal cord compression, it is advisable to test the presence or absence of normal communication between the ventricular system and the intracranial subarachnoid space on the one hand and the lumbar cistern on the other. This is effected by compressing both jugular veins in the neck when the manometer is connected with the lumbar cistern through the needle. Normally this compression is at once followed by a quick rise in the intrathecal pressure and an equally rapid fall when the compression is relieved (Queckenstedt's phenomenon). With spinal subarachnoid block the rise is slight and slow. This test should not be performed until the level of the fluid in the manometer has become stationary and the patient is quiet. The contra-indications to lumbar puncture are considered on pages 56 and 68, and should always be carefully borne in mind.

THE TISSUE REACTIONS OF THE NERVOUS SYSTEM

The nervous system consists of nerve cells and their processes set in a supporting framework of neuroglia and blood-vessels. A disease process may originate in any one of these elements, but the remaining elements become secondarily involved sooner or later, and in some chronic processes this secondary reaction, when it is of the neuroglia, may dominate the histological picture.

Amongst the various structural abnormalities to be found in the nervous tissues we have defects of development (agenesis), defective vitality and premature decay, changes due to chemical action (anoxæmia, toxins, chemical poisons), inflammatory changes, new growth formation and meningeal lesions.

These various abnormalities are revealed by changes in the appearance of nerve cells, nerve fibres, and neuroglial elements.

ANATOMICAL.—The nerve cell varies in appearance according to the staining reagents used to demonstrate its features. Thus, when stained with toluidin blue (Nissl method) the cell shows a nucleus with contained nucleolus, and the cytoplasm may contain large granules—the Nissl granules. These granules are largest and best developed in the giant pyramidal cells of the Rolandic cortex, and are also seen in some of the ventral horn cells of the cord. The majority of nerve cells, however, show only a finely granular cytoplasm by this method. In fact the normal appearance of Nissl-stained nerve cells varies widely throughout the nervous system, and the detection of pathological appearances calls for considerable experience in the case of most of them. Stained by another method, the cell body is seem to be traversed by fine neurofibrils which are continuous with those in the axones and dendrites. Other structures in and immediately around the cell are revealed by other methods, but of these it is not here necessary to speak. The nerve fibre consists of fine neurofibrils embedded in a fluid axoplasm. At each node of Ranvier the fibre undergoes a narrowing which gives it as a whole a segmented appearance. In the central nervous system, as in the peripheral, all but the very finest fibres have a myelin sheath, while the peripheral fibres have also the neurilemmal sheath with its nuclei.

The neuroglia contains cells of three main types: *astrocytes, oligodendrocytes,* and *microglia.* The first-named cell possesses fibrillar processes at the distal ends of which are "sucker feet." These feet are attached to adjacent nerve cells or to capillary walls, and by means of these attachments the astrocytes and the blood-vessels form a sort of skeletal framework for the nervous system. The *oligodendrocytes* are the most numerous cells in the nervous system and they are most abundant in white matter, where they lie in rows between the nerve fibres. In the grey matter they lie around nerve cells. To them has been attributed a nutritive function in connection with the myelin. Both these types of cell are ectodermal in origin. The *microglia,* on the other hand, is a cell of mesodermal origin which first migrates into the central nervous system of the embryo at full term. From the microglia are derived the phagocytic cells of the brain and cord (compound granular corpuscles, or scavenger cells).

PATHOLOGICAL.—The study of the nerve cell by the Nissl method reveals a small number of types of abnormal change in disease and injury of the nervous system. The most familiar of these goes by the name of *chromatolysis* and corresponds to the cloudy swelling of cells elsewhere in the body. The cell becomes spherical, the nucleus also swells and may become eccentrically placed. The Nissl granules become indistinct and undergo some degree of dissolution. This change is produced by a great variety of disease processes, by high fever and by exhaustion. In its milder grades it is a reversible change, but it may also be the initial stage of a destructive process. Under the influence of various intoxications and infections the cell shows what is known as *the chronic cell change*. In this the cell body and nucleus are shrunken and the Nissl granules may disappear. The process may go on to the destruction of the cell. Since it is also seen as a result of ischæmia it is sometimes spoken of as the ischæmic cell change. In *acute necrosis* of the cell, as in cerebral thrombosis with infarction, the cell swells, its Nissl granules and neurofibrils disappear, and the nucleus and cytoplasm take on a homogeneous appearance. Dead nerve cells undergo liquefaction and the products of destruction are removed by phagocytes. In elderly persons the cell body contains brown pigment granules.

A characteristic reaction of the white matter of the central nervous system to diverse noxious agencies insufficient to cause complete tissue necrosis is *demyelination*: *i.e.* destruction of the myelin sheaths, the axis cylinders remaining intact. There are several maladies of the nervous system in which this process is the essential one, and of these disseminated sclerosis is the most familiar. Others are briefly discussed on page 187. Ætiologically, the demyelinating diseases do not form a homogeneous group.

The other typical reaction of white matter is Wallerian degeneration, in which the breaking down of the myelin sheath is followed by fragmentation and disappearance of the axis cylinders and, in the peripheral nerves, proliferation of the cells of the sheath of Schwann.

The neuroglia always reacts to nerve cell damage, and all three elements are involved in the response. Whereas the reaction of the nerve cell to noxious agencies is either to perish or to survive in a more or less damaged condition, showing no capacity for regeneration or multiplication, the neuroglia responds in more varied fashion. The cells may either perish rapidly or may be stimulated to hypertrophy and hyperplasia. In inflammatory, degenerative, and vascular lesions the astrocytes swell, lose their processes and multiply amitotically. The new cells then form fibrils and become what are known as "spider cells." Their function is to replace destroyed parenchymatous tissue and to surround and wall off infective and degenerative foci. In an infarct the spider cells form a glial scar in which, when it is of some duration, the fibrils predominate.

The oligodendrocytes are very sensitive to any pathological process in the brain, and swell and proliferate in response to it. They may collect round damaged nerve cells. The microglia cells also react to damage to nerve cells and fibres. They swell, proliferate and become amœboid. They ingest particles of broken-down cells and myelin and carry these to the perivascular sheaths of the blood-vessels, forming an important element in the perivascular infiltration seen in inflammatory and other destructive lesions. In severe pathological changes, cells of vascular origin also appear in the nervous system, namely, lymphocytes and plasma cells, and these are also to be found in the cuffs of cells which fill the perivascular sheaths and surround the small blood-vessels.

After infarction, the glial reaction forms a network of fibrils which fill the place left vacant by destroyed nerve cells, or form a filamentous network in cystic cavities.

The changes thus briefly summarized are seen in varying form throughout the entire range of diseases of the nervous system, and thus the microscopic appearances encountered are relatively limited in character. We cannot always correlate any particular mode of reaction with a single ætiological factor, and the abnormal appearances in nervous tissue may change considerably during the course of a single pathological process if this lasts long enough. Thus in an early focus of disseminated sclerosis we see a region of demyelination of nerve fibres, the myelin globules being ingested by amœboid microglia cells which tend to collect in local perivascular spaces. The astrocytes in the focus are swollen and multiplied, and lymphocytes and plasma cells may be seen. The blood-vessels are normal and the denuded axis cylinders for the most part intact. In an old focus, after the secondary glial reaction has developed, we see the typically sharply-outlined patch of sclerosis of irregular shape. The degenerated myelin has gone. The proliferated astrocytes with their fibrillary processes form a dense feltwork, a scar, and the blood-vessels may have undergone some hyaline change. A certain proportion of the denuded axis cylinders has disappeared.

In such an essentially degenerative process as motor neurone disease the primary loss of pyramidal nerve fibres and of motor nerve cells is not followed by so active a response on the part of the glial elements as in the disease just described, but even here there is some gliosis.

Another factor in the variations seen in the morbid histology of nervous diseases is the wide variation of normal structure. Thus, the cerebral cortex itself varies widely from region to region in its cell forms, cell arrangements, nerve fibre and glial content and arrangement. Still greater are the differences between this region and the cerebellar cortex, or the basal ganglia. Therefore, in assessing the changes seen under the microscope, due emphasis has to be laid upon the regions of the brain in which the changes are found.

PART II

DESCRIPTIVE ACCOUNT OF THE MORE COMMON DISEASES OF THE NERVOUS SYSTEM

CHAPTER III

Space-occupying Lesions within the Skull: Tumour, Hæmatoma, Abscess

GENERAL CONSIDERATIONS.—New growths of the brain and its coverings provide the majority of such lesions, but abscess and hæmatoma have also to be included in the category of space-occupying or expanding lesions. With a reservation in the case of certain gliomas, all these lesions form an addition to the normal bulk of intracranial contents, and since the skull is a rigid container of fixed volume, certain mechanical consequences follow from their presence and expansion. Hence all three have much in common in their symptomatology and may at times be difficult of clinical differentiation.

THE MECHANISMS OF SYMPTOM PRODUCTION

It is impossible to give a simple generalization as to the sequence of events by which, in the presence of a space-occupying lesion within the skull, a rise of intracranial pressure is produced. Although the sum of the factors involved may be the same in every case when its entire course is considered, the relative importance of each factor and the sequence in which each comes into play must vary from case to case according to the situation and nature of the lesion. Thus, a tumour that from the outset blocks the cerebrospinal fluid outflow from the ventricular system must act somewhat differently from a tumour in one cerebral hemisphere that can produce such a block only late in its development. Therefore all simple mechanical explanations, whatever their inherent charm, should be distrusted.

Room for an expanding lesion is first found by the expulsion of cerebrospinal fluid from the cranial cavity, and then by that of the fluid at the next lowest pressure, namely, the venous blood. As the total volume of the veins is much greater than that of the arteries, they can be compressed to about the volume of the arteries before any venous congestion occurs.

Sooner or later this point is reached, the circulation of both blood and cerebrospinal fluid is interfered with and pressure within the skull begins to rise.

Venous congestion leads to an increased secretion of cerebrospinal fluid from the choroid plexuses, and necessarily also to a diminished re-absorption of this fluid into the dural venous sinuses. The volume of cerebrospinal fluid therefore begins to rise, and as the cranial and spinal dural sac is relatively fixed in volume, pressure within it rises. This leads to still further venous compression, and a vicious circle is established.

Further complication is added to the situation when, owing to obstruction produced by the lesion, the outflow of cerebrospinal fluid from the ventricular system, or from some part of it, is reduced or blocked. The ventricles then distend, compressing the surrounding brain, and a condition of internal hydrocephalus is produced. Again, the great vein of Galen may be compressed and venous congestion thereby still further increased. As has been stated, the sequence in which these different factors come into operation varies from case to case.

Again, an asymmetrically placed tumour above the tentorium will tend to force one cerebral hemisphere against the dural partitions within the skull and thus to produce an obstruction to the flow of the cerebrospinal fluid to the arachnoid villi round the dural sinuses, through which it is absorbed into the blood.

The heightened intracranial pressure thus produced gives rise to what are known as the general symptoms of a space-occupying lesion. The so-called localizing signs which indicate the seat of the lesion owe their production to two factors: namely, to local interference with blood supply and to the destructive activity of the lesion itself upon nervous tissue. Of these two, the first-named is usually the more important, and it is probable that an impaired blood supply with its resulting anoxia is mainly responsible for the disorders in brain function that ensue. If localized compression predominates at the outset the clinical picture may open with the signs of a progressive local lesion of the brain, signs of a general rise of intracranial tension being sooner or later superadded; but if this raised pressure is fairly generalized from the outset the symptomatology is mainly or wholly such as to indicate raised intracranial tension perhaps giving no clue to the localization of the original expanding lesion. The remarkable absence of localizing signs in the early clinical stages of many cases of intracranial tumour may thus be accounted for. The normal range of intracranial pressure, as measured by lumbar puncture, is from 60 to 170 mm. of water. In the presence of an intracranial tumour it may range from 200 to 600 mm.

Of the symptoms of raised intracranial pressure not directly due to interference with the functions of the brain, headache is the most important. The mode of its production is still matter of controversy, some regarding it as due to stretching of the dural partitions, others as due to abnormal tension in the walls of the cerebral blood-vessels. It cannot be *directly* correlated with a general rise of intracranial tension since it may develop in a case of tumour when such general rise is not present, and it may be produced or increased by a lumbar puncture which lowers this pressure. It remains true to say, however, that headache is prominent amongst the general symptoms of a space-occupying lesion within the skull.

THE SIGNS AND SYMPTOMS ASSOCIATED WITH RAISED INTRACRANIAL PRESSURE

These consist of headache, papilloedema with failure of vision, sickness, progressive blunting of mental alertness and, less constantly, a slowing of the pulse rate.

Headache.—Since we must regard headache as a common early symptom of a space-occupying lesion within the skull, sometimes as the initial symptom, it is clear that in the first place the diagnosis of such a lesion may involve *the assessment of a complaint of headache in a subject who may present no abnormal physical signs on examination.* The possible complexity of the task needs no emphasis when we recall that a complaint of headache is amongst the commonest of all subjective symptoms, alike in the subjects of physical disorder as in the psycho-neurotic. In the latter it is a symptom of the greatest frequency, and a brief account of the features of psychologically determined "headache," as encountered in the hysteric or in the subject of an anxiety neurosis, is an important first step in our present connection.

Certain general statements can be made of psychogenic headaches. They are commonly spoken of as continuous and unremitting over long periods of weeks, months, or even years: they respond to none of the usual analgesic drugs: they are described in a wealth of metaphor, and by a lavish use of superlatives. Thus, they are "terrible," "agonising," "frightful," they are like corkscrews, knives, needles, etc., piercing the head. When questions as to their locality and quality are pressed, the patient's answers become ever more florid and vague, and "pains" are suddenly found to have become sensations of weight, pressure, or constriction and not real pain at all. In the hysteric these accounts are commonly given with animation and evident satisfaction, while the anxiety neurotic is plunged in gloom and self-pity. In both circumstances, the eager desire to impress at all costs and the almost wholly emotive character of the language used are evident. It is not information that these patients wish to convey, but an impression that they wish to create. In short, the story is not one to be accepted at its face value, but one to be regarded as a dramatization designed to express the patient's notion of how pain ought to be described and of

E

how its victim might be expected to react. The patient has to carry conviction to herself on the one hand, to her friends and to her doctor on the other. She achieves the first by repetition, the latter by over-statement and gesture. What we are dealing with is not true pain, but an image of pain conjured up by the patient and subjected to those processes of progressive elaboration to which mental images are prone. This is a state of affairs that analgesic drugs cannot be expected to mitigate, and with the exceptions mentioned they do not mitigate it.

A strikingly different picture is presented by the victim of severe headache of physical origin. The sufferer is clearly intensely pre-occupied with his pain, and the questions and physical examination of the doctor are as clearly an addition to his burden. He observes a marked economy of movement and of speech, since the effort of both aggravates his pain. This is never spoken of as continuous over long periods, since organically determined headache is never so continuous, but always subject to intermission over varying periods of time if it be of long total duration. Freedom from pain is admitted without emotional difficulty by the patient, and in his free periods he may wish, or attempt, to make some return to physical activity.

These two widely contrasting clinical pictures must be within the experience of every practitioner of medicine. The primary differentiation of psychogenic "headache" from true headache once achieved, it remains to consider the features usually presented by the headache of raised intracranial tension.

Its situation of maximal incidence varies from case to case and has no reliably localizing value in respect of the underlying lesion. It is throbbing in character, is apt to be increased by physical exertion of any kind or by stooping, it frequently develops during the night, awaking the subject in the early morning. He may obtain relief by propping himself up in bed. Although at first intermittent, the paroxysms become more frequent and more severe, and are at times accompanied by vomiting, the effort of which aggravates the headache still further. With great rise of tension within the skull the paroxysms may be of frightful intensity, the patient clasping his head in his hands and crying out. Such accesses are of grave import and herald an early fatal issue unless effective and radical measures to relieve pressure can be adopted. From such an attack the patient may pass into coma.

This progressively downward course may be compressed within the period of very few weeks, or may spread over many months. Gradually there are added to it other indications of the presence of an expanding lesion: sickness, apathy, drowsiness, blurring of vision, defects in memory and attention, and finally the signs of some progressive local lesion of the brain.

The other common variety of headache of physical—or at least of physiological—origin that may be found in the absence of abnormal physical signs is *migraine*. Here diagnosis should not be difficult. There is the long history dating probably from puberty, sometimes a familial history. The headache is preceded by a number of sensory symptoms, visual and cutaneous, for some ten to twenty minutes. The pain dawns in one temple and gradually extends over the forehead or vertex to the opposite side and is rapidly followed by the development of nausea and perhaps of sickness. After some hours the attack passes, leaving the patient in his usual health until the next attack.

In the case of both tumour and of migraine the headache itself is throbbing in character, and at its point of maximal severity the scalp may be tender to pressure, movement of the eyes may be painful, the eyeballs themselves tender, and strong light unpleasant to bear.

Paroxysmal headache without sensory preliminaries is not uncommon in healthy persons in association with gastro-intestinal disturbances, fatigue and eyestrain, but it lacks the dramatic background of psychogenic pain, and has not the progressive quality of the headache of raised intracranial tension.

Vomiting.—The vomiting associated with raised intracranial tension is usually referred to as "projectile." Frequently, however, it is not so, but is preceded by nausea and retching. Like the headache it is prone to occur in the early morning, and to be precipitated by exertion or by stooping. In these circumstances, too, transient amaurosis may be added to the headache and sickness. Vomiting is not found in every case of intracranial hypertension, but it is probably true to say that the more rapidly tension rises within the skull the more severe are both headache and sickness.

Papilloedema.—The raised cerebrospinal fluid pressure within the subarachnoid space is communicated to the fluid within the sheath of the optic nerve, where sooner or later it interferes with the venous return from the eye. The optic disc then begins to swell and the retinal veins become engorged and distended. The disc edges become hazy, usually in the upper and inner quadrant first. The disc swells, becomes highly coloured and less readily marked off from the surrounding red fundus. Finally the physiological pit is obliterated and the disc is replaced by a reddish protrusion on the fundus. The emerging vessels may for a short stretch be buried in the swelling and become invisible there. Flame-shaped hæmorrhages appear outside the disc edges, and the retina between disc and macula may become œdematous, rising into folds which spread fanlike from macula to disc. On the summits of these folds appear tiny spots of white exudate, the whole producing the macular fan, which is a common part of an intense and rapidly developing papilloedema.

It is difficult to correlate disturbances of visual acuity with ophthalmoscopic appearances. Vision may fade gradually, transient blurring occurring during physical exertion, or it may go suddenly and finally. It cannot be assumed that because the patient makes no spontaneous complaint of visual defect that no papillœdema is present. Examination of the fundus is necessary in all suspected cases, and with an electrically-illuminated ophthalmoscope is so easy that it should be regarded as much a matter of routine in the examination of patients complaining of headache or of failing vision, as the use of the stethoscope in the examination of the chest. Papillœdema is not an invariable concomitant of a space-occupying lesion. It may be absent throughout the whole course of the case, or be of late development. On the other hand, it may develop early and rapidly. If the raised intracranial pressure be not relieved, papillœdema proceeds to post-papillitic or, "consecutive" atrophy of the optic nerve. The disc becomes white, the physiological cup is filled with white exudate and thus concealed, while the disc edges are blurred. When this ensues vision is permanently lost.

Mental Change.—This, even more than headache and vomiting is a factor of variable diagnostic value. In some instances, particularly perhaps when a frontal lobe tumour is in question, changes in mental alertness and in disposition may usher in the clinical picture. In this case such symptoms are local rather than indicative of a general rise of intracranial tension, but sooner or later in all cases of increased tension within the skull a gradual blunting of alertness, of memory, and of power of attention develops.

Slowing of the Pulse Rate is perhaps the most inconstant of all indications of raised intracranial tension, and it seems probable that *the rate of rise* is a factor of importance in determining this symptom. Thus, it is common in head injuries associated with raised intracranial tension, in some cases of subarachnoid hæmorrhage, in abscess and subdural hæmatoma, and in tumours which develop general signs of raised intracranial tension quickly. In many cases of more gradual development, intracranial tension may reach a high level without any slowing of the pulse. In extreme high levels of pressure it may fall to 50 or even below, such a fall being of grave import. The systemic blood pressure does not rise above normal, but with a sudden exacerbation of tension within the skull, it may rise to 170 or thereabouts.

DANGERS ATTENDANT UPON LUMBAR PUNCTURE WHEN INTRACRANIAL PRESSURE IS RAISED

It does not need much thought to realize that in a suspected case of intracranial tumour, when there are signs and symptoms of raised intracranial pressure, there can but rarely be any necessity for lumbar puncture or the withdrawal of cerebrospinal fluid. Diagnosis is usually possible without this procedure, and since in these circumstances it is generally known to be dangerous, *it should never be performed except for some precise and compelling reason when there are clinical indications of raised intracranial pressure.* Even the insertion of a needle into the theca for the purpose of taking a manometric measurement of the fluid pressure is fraught with danger because there is so commonly a leakage from the hole in the theca that fluid escapes into the extradural space, just as surely as when it is drawn off by the operator into a test tube.

The alarming or even fatal issue of lumbar puncture in these circumstances is due to the displacement of the brain that follows the escape of fluid from the subarachnoid space. This displacement may take place at the tentorium when the uncus herniates through the opening, or less commonly at the foramen magnum when, in the case of subtentorial tumours, the escape of fluid from the theca allows the medulla to be forced down into the foramen. Thus, whether a tumour be above or below the tentorium, lumbar puncture is strongly contra-indicated.

Therefore, it cannot be too strongly emphasized that lumbar puncture is a procedure to be adopted with discretion at all times, and not blindly out of any notion that it is an essential part of investigation of every case of nervous disease.

EPILEPTIFORM FITS AS A SYMPTOM OF SPACE-OCCUPYING LESIONS

It is widely believed that when epileptiform fits usher in, or occur during the course of, an intracranial tumour, they are usually of Jacksonian type. It should be remembered, therefore, that even more common are generalized fits indistinguishable from those of idiopathic epilepsy. These may be the initial manifestation, occurring when physical examination of the patient reveals no abnormal physical signs. Therefore, when this happens at a period of life later than that at which idiopathic epilepsy commonly begins, namely, after the early twenties, the possible presence of tumour should be borne in mind and the course of the case carefully observed. Such generalized fits can hardly be said to have localizing value, or to indicate raised intracranial tension. On the whole they are most common in diffuse astrocytomas of the cerebral hemispheres.

Of the pathological range of intracranial tumours, it is perhaps the meningioma that is most frequently associated with the Jacksonian type of fit. In this connection the reader is referred to the section on symptomatic epilepsy (page 127) where the role of cortical atrophy in producing epileptiform fits is briefly discussed.

Some separate consideration may now be given to each of the three types of lesion capable of expansion within the skull, and thus of giving rise to increased intracranial tension.

INTRACRANIAL TUMOUR

That the brain is one of the commonest seats of new growth in the body is not as widely appreciated as it should be, with the result that the diagnosis of intracranial tumour is often unduly delayed, since what is thought to be rare is not readily recognized. Nothing certain is known of the factors that lead to the development of neoplasms within the cranial cavity. It has been suggested that there is some congenital factor that may be set in motion at critical periods of life, or perhaps by trauma. Trauma is too often and too lightly invoked as a factor in the causation of organic nervous affections of all kinds, yet there seems to be sufficient evidence to justify the conclusion that a head injury may occasionally act as a precipitating factor in the growth of both the glioma and the meningioma. It is not suggested that trauma by itself is an adequate cause of tumour development.

In addition to true neoplasms, infective masses (*granulomas*) are sometimes encountered. Of these the tuberculoma is perhaps the most familiar, though it is far less frequently encountered now than in former years. Gumma (syphiloma) is an extremely rare variety of intracranial granuloma. *Parasitic cysts* in the brain are extremely rare in this country, but hydatid, cysticercus, and schistosoma (Bilharzia) cysts in the brain are known.

Approximately 40 per cent. of all intracranial new growths are gliomas: that is, tumours arising within the brain in the neuroglia. Some 15 per cent. are meningiomas; that is, benign tumours arising in the arachnoid villi. Estimates vary widely as to the incidence of secondary carcinoma of the brain, some placing it as high as 20 per cent. of all tumours. Tumours of the pituitary body and stalk make up some 3 to 4 per cent., while the residue is composed of various rare varieties of new growth.

Hitherto it has been customary to discuss the pathology of these different varieties of tumour together and to describe the symptomatology of intracranial tumours as a whole and according to the localizing indications they give rise to: that is, upon a topographical basis. Yet it has become increasingly clear that the symptoms of a tumour are almost as much a product of its nature as of its site. Each variety of growth has its characteristic behaviour, even though all may have clinical elements in common. It is, therefore, proposed to describe each of the common varieties of tumour separately, both in respect of pathology and of clinical course.

GLIOMA

Pathology.—Elaborate subdivisions of the gliomas are current, based upon the various cell types they may be found to contain. They are largely academic, since a given glioma may contain cells of more than one type and may during its life-history change its prevailing cell type to assume characters of greater malignancy. Even the attempt to extirpate a slowly growing glioma may provide the stimulus to this change. Here we shall confine description to the three common varieties of glioma: the astrocytoma, the glioblastoma, and the medulloblastoma.

The *astrocytoma* is a slowly growing tumour composed of cells approximating in character to the adult normal astrocyte. It is commonly a truly infiltrating growth, and, at least in its early stages, may be thought of as an infiltration rather than as a space-occupying lesion. It tends to degenerate at its centre with the formation of a cystic cavity containing an albuminous fluid. In the cerebellum and less commonly in the cerebral hemisphere the actively growing part of the tumour may appear as a nodule on a cyst wall. This is especially likely to be the case in children, and is a fortunate mode of growth since the extirpation of the nodule may result in permanent relief of symptoms and cure. Again, a circumscribed and apparently encapsuled variety of astrocytoma, also removable, may be seen, but the truly infiltrating variety is always larger than it appears to the naked eye. The life history of an astrocytoma may extend over months or even years before its presence is clinically manifest (Figs. 12 and 13).

The *glioblastoma* is a rapidly growing, highly vascular and fairly circumscribed growth, reddish purple in colour and usually surrounded by an area of cerebral œdema. It consists of cells of relatively undifferentiated and embryonic type, and usually proves fatal within a few months of its clinical appearance. It may be the seat of hæmorrhage.

There are also gliomas composed of cell forms intermediate between those just described, and sometimes cells of different types are found in the various parts of a single tumour (Fig. 14). These gliomas have their different names, but it is beyond the scope of this book to enumerate them. Gliomas are usually single, but may be multiple, and a single growth may have several foci of active development. The convention that divides gliomas in benign and malignant has no precise pathological sanction, and may perhaps be called a surgical euphemism. It does, however, represent the fact of clinical experience that it is now possible to extirpate successfully certain varieties of astrocytoma, sometimes with permanent success and others for periods of several years.

The *medulloblastoma* calls for separate mention. It is a rapidly growing and metastatizing tumour, arising in the roof of the fourth ventricle, *i.e.* in the vermis, and often spreading outside the ventricle over the cerebellum, brain-stem, and cervical cord.

Age Incidence of Gliomas.—While the medulloblastoma is characteristically incident in the first decade of life, the cystic astrocytoma, particularly of the cerebellum, while not uncommon in later childhood and in adolescence may be found also in early or in middle adult life. The infiltrating astrocytoma occurs in early and middle

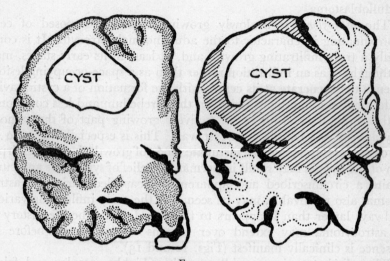

Fig. 12.

Macroscopic and Microscopic Aspects of a Glioma.

Diagrams of the two sections shown in Fig. 13. In the naked-eye slice there is no "tumour" but only a large cyst. The Nissl-stained section (cross-hatched portion) shows the neoplasm growing throughout the hemisphere. (After ▓ ▓ Scherer, Brain, 1940.)

adult life, while the glioblastoma falls mainly in the middle and later age periods.

Symptomatology.—An intracranial tumour may reveal its presence initially by (1) symptoms of rising intracranial pressure, (2) symptoms of a deepening and expanding local lesion, or by (3) recurrent epileptiform fits which may precede in point of time the two other orders of symptom. While these generalizations apply to all pathological varieties of intracranial tumour, what immediately follows applies especially to the gliomas. In the case of the astrocytoma the onset of symptoms is usually insidious and many weeks or months may pass before the nature of the patient's illness commands recognition. At first the patient begins to lose his normal degree of mental alertness.

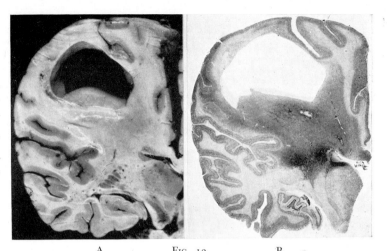

A   Fig. 13.   B

MACROSCOPIC AND MICROSCOPIC ASPECTS OF AN ASTROCYTOMA.

Photographs of (A) a coronal slice of a cerebral hemisphere, showing a cystic astrocytoma; and (B) a Nissl-stained section of the same specimen. The darker stained central tissue represents gliomatous infiltration.

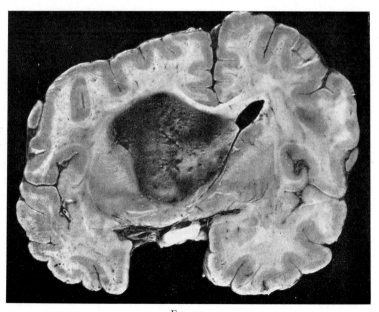

Fig. 14.

A CORONAL SECTION OF THE CEREBRAL HEMISPHERES.

Deep in the left hemisphere is a glioma which originated in the septum lucidum and was of a mixed character (oligodendroglioma and astrocytoma). (From Scherer, *Brain*, 1940, Vol. 63.)

To face page 72.

His energy and range of interests diminish and the fine edge of his judgment may become blunted. He tends to be apathetic and sometimes irritable. It is common for these symptoms to be attributed to overwork or to worry, but as they develop, and as headache and perhaps sickness are added to them a more serious view becomes inevitable. The headache tends to be most frequently complained of and most severe on waking in the morning, or upon stooping or muscular effort. Slowly, indications of a progressive local lesion of the brain develop, and the significant feature of these is that they indicate not only a deepening disturbance of function, but one extending to more functions, i.e. the lesion appears to be both deepening and expanding.

Gradually the headache becomes more obtrusive, and with the development of papilloedema some impairment of vision may be complained of. At first this commonly consists in transient blurring of vision during muscular effort or upon wide changes of posture: as when rising to the erect position from a chair or from bed, or when straining at stool. This sequence of events may be punctuated by generalized epileptiform fits showing no localizing characters. The localizing symptoms will, of course, vary in character according to the seat of the tumour.

The fact that an astrocytoma in its spread may leave within its borders nerve cells and fibres which are still active, tends to minimize the disturbance of function produced by its presence, at least in the early stages of the illness. During all this time the patient's general physical condition may remain so good that it is difficult to realize how grave his situation is, but as with rising intracranial tension and increasing disability the patient becomes prone to drowsiness, the presence of tumour is at last clear, sometimes only after several months. In the case of glioblastoma this sequence of events develops far more rapidly, and the sudden development of cerebral oedema around even a small glioblastoma may lead to a quick descent into stupor and semicoma.

The stage at which papilloedema develops varies according to the site and the rate of growth of the tumour. In frontal astrocytoma it may be long delayed, while in glioblastoma it may be early and rapidly productive of failing vision. Localizing signs also vary from case to case in the moment at which they make their appearance during the clinical course. The final stage of an unrelieved case is a lapse into coma and, especially in subtentorially situated tumours, to death from respiratory failure.

In the case of the astrocytoma, the clinically discoverable disorders of function may give a minimal picture and fail to reveal that the growth is already extensive. In such circumstances the evolution of the illness is apt to be long drawn-out. With the glioblastoma, on the other hand, events move much faster, the seriousness of the illness soon becomes manifest, and death commonly ensues within a year of onset of symptoms. In both types of growth, the rapid development of œdema of the brain surrounding the growth may bring matters to a head and cause the almost acute development of signs of raised intracranial tension. It has to be confessed, however, that length of clinical history is apt to be a fallacious guide when attempting to ascertain the nature of the intracranial new growth present in any case, for the most slowly developing tumour—an astrocytoma or even a meningioma—may remain clinically latent until it has reached a considerable size, when it suddenly manifests its presence by acute and grave symptoms.

It is not proposed to deal in any detail with localizing symptoms, but a few salient clinical features may be mentioned. Perhaps the commonest sites of a cerebral glioma are the frontal and the temporosphenoidal lobes. In the case of the frontal lobe, personality changes commonly usher in the clinical course of the illness and may for weeks or months dominate it before headache attracts attention. Here the change in temperament may be so striking as to lead to an initial diagnosis of "depression" or of "neurasthenia." Yet careful observation will show that the patient is not depressed, but profoundly apathetic and devoid of initiative. He may allow his bladder to empty in the most inappropriate circumstances, and this with no insight into his gross breach of the conventions. In such a case, papillœdema may be only a terminal event. In the case of temporo-sphenoidal tumour a comparable mental alteration may be present, though not usually as an initial manifestation. Pressure symptoms tend to develop earlier and more rapidly, and examination may reveal an upper motor neurone paresis of the face, sometimes with minimal signs of hemiparesis, a crossed homonymous hemianopia, usually beginning in the upper quadrants of the fields involved, and due to encroachment of the tumour upon the temporal loop of the optic radiations (see page 45). If the tumour be left-sided, aphasic symptoms may develop, while there may also be the focal fit characteristic of the region, namely the "dreamy state," which consists of a transient blunting of consciousness accompanied by an olfactory or gustatory sensation and sometimes by a smacking of the lips.

The medulloblastoma calls for separate description, since it is the common intracranial tumour of early life and also because its clinical picture is peculiar to it.

A previously healthy child begins to suffer from headaches of increasing frequency and severity. They may be referred either to forehead or to occiput. Their appearance is within a very few weeks followed by vomiting, which is apt to be associated with periods of severe headache and may or may not be "projectile." The child soon becomes listless, easily fatigued, and disinclined for exercise since this provokes or aggravates headache. He complains of recurrent and transient diplopia, which may become persistent and be accompanied by visible squint. He becomes a little unsteady on his feet and perhaps somewhat uncertain in the co-ordination of his hands. Within a few weeks in many instances, though somewhat later in others, it is clear that the child is seriously ill, though pulse and temperature remain normal. There may, in addition to the complaint of diplopia, be that of failing visual acuity. Examination reveals bilateral papilloedema, and commonly weakness or paralysis of one or both external rectus muscles of the eye with converging squint. The face is occasionally weak on one side. As a rule there is no nystagmus. All movements are somewhat unsteady, though a full-fledged cerebellar ataxy is uncommon. There is no paralysis, and the tendon jerks are often uniformly diminished, and may even be abolished. Percussion of the skull yields a "cracked pot" sound, and in young children there may be some enlargement of the head owing to progressive hydrocephalus.

As the condition develops, the child may have fits in which with loss of consciousness there is intense muscular rigidity with head retraction and opisthotonos. The appearance of these attacks heralds the final stage of the illness. Gradually the child loses weight, develops acidosis from recurrent vomiting, and lapses into a torpor which ends in the final coma. The entire illness from start to fatal issue is usually comprised within a period of from three to six months. Clearly, problems of differential diagnosis arise, and perhaps the most important of these is the differentiation from *tuberculous meningitis*. At first this may be difficult on purely clinical grounds. The general symptomatology is much the same: headache, sickness, and diminution of tendon jerks being common to both. There may also be some neck rigidity in both. In tuberculous meningitis, however, papilloedema is late and rarely more than slight in degree, whereas in medulloblastoma it is commonly early, develops rapidly, and presents the picture of choked disc with free hæmorrhages and much exudate. The examination of the cerebrospinal fluid on lumbar puncture also serves as a reliable differential procedure. In the case of tumour the fluid is normal in composition save sometimes for an increase in its protein content (up to 30 or 40 mgm. per 100 c.c.), whereas in tuberculous meningitis the characteristic changes are found: a lymphocytosis, a diminution of chlorides and glucose and a protein increase. Sometimes also the tubercle bacillus is found. The rise of pressure is greater in the case of tumour than that of meningitis. The dangers of lumbar puncture when there are clear indications of raised intracranial pressure are referred to on page 68.

SECONDARY CARCINOMA

Pathology.—Of growths within the substance of the brain, the secondary carcinoma may perhaps be considered as next in frequency to the gliomas, though estimates of its incidence, as has been mentioned on page 70, vary widely. Such metastatic growths are usually multiple and there may be as many as fifty or more nodules of sizes varying from the microscopic to those of one or more centimetres in diameter. The nodules are clearly defined, vascular and soft, and they may be accompanied by a microscopic infiltration of the pia arachnoid ("meningitis carcinomatosa"). Pulmonary growths of lung or bronchus are the commonest source of secondary carcinoma within the brain, but primary visceral carcinoma elsewhere sometimes gives rise to it.

Symptomatology.—Its clinical picture approximates to that of the gliomas, and it may be impossible to differentiate such deposits from this variety of primary growth. Yet there are often indications that serve to differentiate the two clinically. In general it may be said that the subject of a glioma may be in otherwise good general physical condition and does not look ill, at least in the early stage of his malady. The subject of carcinoma, on the other hand—even when the growth is pulmonary and as yet undiagnosed—tends to lose weight progressively and to become pale and cachectic, and such a state of affairs in any case of suspected intracranial growth should always lead to a search for a primary growth outside the skull. Further, mental symptoms such as confusion, sometimes even a muttering delirium, tend to occupy a more prominent place in the picture than in the case of primary brain tumour, while occasionally symptoms of meningeal irritation (severe accesses of headache, stiff neck, Kernig's sign, etc.) may be present. The localizing symptoms are apt to be complicated by the presence of multiple deposits. It is said that the cerebrospinal fluid may contain tumour cells, but this is rarely the case. Papilloedema may be late in appearance, or even absent throughout.

MENINGIOMA

Pathology.—This tumour arises as a proliferation of the cells of the arachnoid villi as these penetrate the dural walls of the venous sinuses. It is usually of firm consistence and poorly supplied with blood-vessels. It grows slowly and does not invade the brain, but pushes this before it. On the other hand, the bone overlying the tumour may be invaded by it, becoming thickened and appearing as a boss beneath the scalp, or it may react by a hyperplasia to the presence of the subjacent meningioma, in which case also it appears as a hard

and painless swelling beneath the scalp. These changes give characteristic radiographical appearances (Figs. 18 and 19).

Symptomatology.—From what has been said of its modes and
points of origin, it will be realized that the meningioma may be found
over the convexity of the cerebral hemispheres, or on the floor of the
anterior or middle fossæ of the skull. In the former case, signs of raised
intracranial pressure open the clinical picture and may for a long
period be the sole indications of the presence of a tumour. Relatively
late, minimal signs of local disturbance may make their appearance,
varying in form according to the region of the hemisphere compressed.
On the other hand a meningioma developing on the floor of the anterior

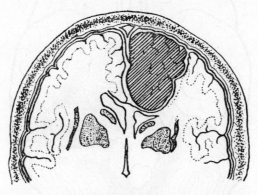

FIG. 15.
MENINGIOMA.

A coronal section of the skull and brain, showing
the mode of attachment of a meningioma to the
falx, and the manner in which this tumour pushes
the brain before it and, as it were, makes a nest for
itself. The resulting distortion of the lateral ventricles and basal ganglia can be seen. In this case
the bone overlying the tumour was not invaded.
(The tumour is cross-hatched).

or middle fossa may first reveal its presence by the appearance of cranial
nerve palsies. A meningioma growing from the ethmoidal plate of
the frontal bone will compress one optic nerve, giving rise to progressive
failure of vision in one eye with primary optic atrophy and with unilateral
loss of the sense of smell on the same side. As it increases in size, the
signs of raised intracranial tension develop: headache, papillœdema
in the other eye, and perhaps the symptoms of a frontal tumour already
mentioned. A tumour on the floor of the middle fossa will produce
diplopia, squint, and ptosis from progressive paralysis of the third,
fourth, and sixth cranial nerves. Here also the optic nerve may be
compressed, with failure of vision and primary optic atrophy. The eye
on the affected side is often proptosed. Occasionally, a slowly developing
unilateral exophthalmos, with some local pain and a later developing

defect of vision in the affected eye may be the first indications of a meningioma growing on the outer portion of the sphenoidal ridge. Ultimately, the signs of a general rise of intracranial pressure ensue.

It is in connection with these tumours in the middle fossa lying near the cavernous sinus that problems of differential diagnosis arise.

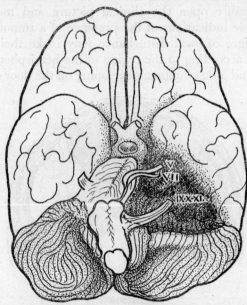

FIG. 16.

BASE OF THE BRAIN, SHOWING THE SITUATION OF AN AUDITORY NERVE TUMOUR.

An auditory fibroma has been removed from its bed beneath the temporo-sphenoidal lobe and cerebellum, its site being indicated by an interrupted line. The anterior part of the cerebellum is compressed and hollowed out, and the brain-stem is displaced to the opposite side and deformed. The pressure cone of cerebellum can be seen on each side of the medulla. The fifth and seventh nerves are greatly stretched and flattened as they passed round the anterior pole of the tumour, while the ninth, tenth, and eleventh nerves are comparably, though less, stretched round its posterior pole. The eighth nerve, embedded in the tumour, has been removed with it.

An unruptured aneurysm of the internal carotid artery may produce a comparable syndrome, though usually without the indications of raised intracranial pressure, but with severe pain in the territory of the ophthalmic division of the fifth nerve. Often, too, the onset of symptoms in aneurysm is sudden and accompanied by this pain around the eye. Finally, an epithelioma of the nasopharynx may invade the floor of the skull and produce this syndrome of cranial nerve paralysis of gradual onset. Careful examination of the nasopharynx is, therefore, part of the necessary investigation, and will in this case reveal the presence of a mass.

A variety of tumour allied to the meningioma occurs in the posterior fossa, where it develops in the arachnoid sheath of the eighth nerve and is known as the *auditory fibroma*, or *auditory nerve tumour*. It may develop as a single growth, or as part of a generalized neurofibromatosis. Such a tumour will first compress and stretch the eighth nerve (tinnitus, deafness, vertigo), the fifth nerve (loss of corneal reflex, numbness of the face), and the seventh nerve (weakness of the face). Then unilateral cerebellar ataxy, also on the side of the lesion, will develop, and finally the signs of a general rise of intracranial pressure. The sequence of events is commonly long drawn out and for months growing deafness with tinnitus may be the only symptoms. An intra-cerebellar tumour commonly gives early rise to general pressure symptoms, upon which background an incomplete picture of cerebellar ataxy develops.

GRANULOMA

Of the *granulomas*, the tuberculoma is the least rare. It may be found in any part of the brain, but perhaps its usual sites of development are the pons and cerebellum. Formerly it was regarded as the commonest form of expanding lesion in childhood, but now medulloblastoma is more frequently found. However, a generalization on this point is hazardous, for in some densely populated industrial urban centres the tuberculoma is still not uncommon.

Gumma of the brain is only exceptionally seen, and *the presence of a positive blood Wassermann reaction in a subject presenting the clinical signs of intracranial tumour is more likely to indicate the presence of a glioma in a syphilitic subject than to prove that the tumour is a gumma.* Before the latter may safely be diagnosed it is necessary also to find the appropriate changes in the cerebrospinal fluid.

Parasitic cysts are extremely rare in this country.

TUMOUR AND OTHER LESIONS OF THE PITUITARY BODY AND STALK

On page 53 a brief sketch of the anatomy and functions of the pituitary body and of the hypothalamus has been given, together with a summary of the most important defect symptoms arising from disease of these structures. The present chapter is strictly concerned with space-occupying lesions within the skull, but it is clear that lesions of other types may give rise to similar disorders of pituitary function, and it is, therefore, convenient to refer to the pathology of pituitary lesions in general at this point.

Pathology.—Syndromes of pituitary and hypothalamus disorder may arise from injury, from inflammatory lesions, and from direct involvement by, or compression by, new growths.

New Growths.—New growths of the pituitary include adenoma of the chromophobe, acidophile and basophile cells. Of these the chromophobe is the common pituitary tumour, the basophile adenoma the rarest. The two first-named varieties may reach a considerable size and thus give rise to pressure symptoms, the basophile adenoma is invariably minute and produces glandular disorders alone. A fourth variety is the stalk tumour (hypophyseal duct tumour) which commonly arises in the pars tuberalis and thus unlike the adenomata is usually suprasellar in situation. Further, since it arises in a rest of embryonic cells derived from the craniobuccal pouch it is characteristically a tumour of childhood or adolescence, the adenomata being tumours of adult life. A final generalization is that while acidophile adenoma usually first indicates its presence by signs of excessive secretion of acidophile cells (gigantism, acromegaly), the chromophobe adenoma and the stalk tumour reveal their presence by symptoms of a general depression of pituitary and hypothalamic function, and by an earlier appearance of local pressure symptoms than is common in the case of the acidophile adenoma; that is to say, the chiasmal syndrome (see page 81) is often the first sign of chromophobe adenoma or of a stalk tumour, but virtually never that of acidophile adenoma.

CHROMOPHOBE ADENOMA.—This expands in size and in so doing compresses and impairs the activity of the entire pituitary body. It may overflow the confines of the pituitary fossa and invade the interpeduncular space, compressing adjacent structures (cranial nerves and hypothalamus). It early presses upon the optic chiasma and expands the pituitary fossa and leads to rarefaction and erosion of the posterior clinoid processes, changes that are revealed in the radiogram.

ACIDOPHILE ADENOMA.—This is less common, but like the chromophobe adenoma may expand in size with the consequences enumerated above. Ultimately it tends to compress the entire pituitary body, so that the early signs of acidophile cell hyperactivity (gigantism and acromegaly) tend to be submerged by the indications of general hypopituitarism.

BASOPHILE ADENOMA is rare, usually requiring the serial section of the pituitary to reveal its presence. It is often accompanied by an overgrowth of the adrenal cortex, and the resulting syndrome is perhaps a polyglandular one.

PITUITARY STALK TUMOUR, arising as already indicated, may

grow within or above the pituitary fossa. It is commonly cystic and contains calcareous material. Its cell plan may resemble that of the enamel organ of the tooth. It may develop during childhood or adolescence: tends to give rise to the picture of hypopituitarism, and, when it grows upwards, may encroach upon the third ventricle and lead to hydrocephalus and the general symptoms of raised intracranial tension.

Rarely, a meningioma grows upon the dural diaphragm of the pituitary fossa, exerting local and general pressure, but not producing glandular disorder.

OTHER LESIONS.—A local arachnoiditis of the chiasmal and pituitary regions may ensue upon head injuries and give rise to local pressure symptoms and, less commonly, to those of pituitary defect. Meningitis involving this region may also lead to pituitary defect symptoms, and diabetes insipidus is occasionally seen. Finally, infarction of the pituitary, or tuberculous or secondary malignant deposits within it may develop.

Symptomatology. — In the case of an expanding lesion the symptoms fall naturally into three groups: (1) symptoms of pressure upon the adjacent optic chiasma and nerves, (2) symptoms of general rise of intracranial pressure, and (3) symptoms of disorder of pituitary function. Of these the second category is most often lacking, while in pituitary lesions other than tumour, the third group alone is present.

(1) Since a pituitary tumour lies below and usually somewhat posterior to the optic chiasma and is median in position, it tends to exert pressure earliest upon the mesial decussating fibres of the chiasma and thus to lead to the development of loss of vision in the temporal half-fields (bitemporal hemianopia). This rarely develops symmetrically, and the patient first notices a narrowing of the temporal field of vision in one eye, the same field in the opposite eye being later involved. Usually the upper temporal quadrants are the earliest impaired, and Figure 8 C traces the development of the loss as seen in perimeter charts. Unless relief be given, complete blindness ensues. As the direct compression of the chiasma and nerves also blocks the meningeal sheaths of the latter, papilloedema cannot develop, since any general rise of intracranial pressure cannot be transmitted by the cerebrospinal fluid past the block. Hence the ophthalmoscopic appearances are those of primary optic atrophy (see page 257).

This statement needs two qualifications. Stalk tumours in children may, as has been stated, grow backwards and give rise to internal hydrocephalus. Hence we occasionally do see papilloedema in stalk tumours. Again, we may in pituitary adenoma find a mild and early papilloedema superimposed upon a developing primary optic atrophy:

F

a combination suggested by the association of slight papilloedema with gross impairment of visual acuity, or with bitemporal field defects.

If the tumour overflows the confines of the expanded sella it invades the interpeduncular space, compresses cranial nerves and thus gives rise to the symptoms of third, fourth, fifth, and sixth nerve palsies, and also compresses the frontal and temporo-sphenoidal lobes so that cerebral symptoms ensue (hemiparesis, mental changes, generalized epileptiform convulsions, headache, and sickness). There may also be some proptosis of one or both eyes.

(2) The symptoms of general rise of intracranial pressure may be long delayed, may indeed never appear. Save in the circumstances already discussed, papilloedema is not part of this syndrome.

(3) From what has been said of the constitution and functions of the pituitary complex and of the effects upon them of an expanding lesion, it follows that the symptoms of glandular dysfunction we may encounter are a composite of several factors. *In chromophobe adenoma* there is a progressive loss of all pituitary functions and sometimes of diencephalic functions as well. Arising before the age of puberty this picture of hypopituitarism is commonly that known as *Fröhlich's syndrome* (dystrophia adiposogenitalis). The child is mentally alert. In the male the testicles do not develop and the penis remains small. The secondary sexual characteristics fail to appear and as the age of puberty is reached and passed, pubic, axillary, and facial hair do not grow. The child is plump, may even be obese, and has a feminine distribution of fat. Less constant symptoms are polyuria (diabetes insipidus) and somnolence. In the girl the menstrual function is not established. Developing after the completion of the changes of puberty, a chromophobe adenoma leads to a regression of the sexual organs and functions. The testicles atrophy, hair leaves the face, axillae and pubes, and in females the menses cease. With the appearance of obesity we see numerous striae on the skin of the buttocks and thighs.

In acidophil adenoma developing before the union of the epiphyses we see gigantism, but in older subjects acromegaly. This includes progressive enlargement of the hands, feet, facial parts of the skull, thoracic framework, and of the limbs generally. Kyphosis is common. The enlargement of the supraorbital ridges, malar bones and lower jaw, together with the characteristically coarse and thick skin, gives the patient a typical appearance (Fig. 17). From compression of basophil elements there ensues secondary atrophy of the genital organs and impotence or amenorrhœa, according to the sex of the patient. A slowly progressive hypopituitarism (shown mainly as obesity) may be superimposed upon this picture, sooner in some subjects than in others.

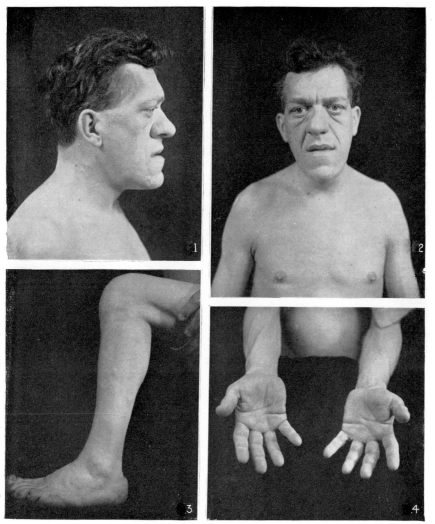

FIG. 17.
ACROMEGALY.
Showing the characteristic changes in facial skeleton and in the extremities.

To face page 82.

All the foregoing observations may be briefly summarized in the following table:—

	ADENOMA.		DUCT TUMOUR.	MENINGIOMA.
	Chromo- phobe.	Acido- phile.		
Age Incidence.	From adolescence onwards.		From 10 years to early adult life.	From 30 years on-wards.
Fundus Oculi.	Primary optic atrophy.		Papillœdema in children, usually primary optic atrophy in adults.	Primary optic atrophy.
Visual Fields.	Bitemporal hemianopia.		Bitemporal hemianopia.	Bitemporal hemianopia.
Pressure Symptoms.	Absent, or late.		Early and severe ex-cept in adults.	Absent, or late.
Glandular Symptoms.	Fröhlich's syn-drome.	Acro-megaly.	Hypopituitarism.	Nil.
Situation.	Intrasellar.		Suprasellar.	Suprasellar.
Radiological.	General enlargement and deepening of sella.		Shadows above and in sella. Sella shal-low and with un-even floor.	Commonly no change.

The general picture of pituitary stalk tumour is that of hypo-pituitarism, with the reservation that in children the symptoms of internal hydrocephalus (papillœdema, failure of vision, headache) may predominate.

The growth of all these tumours may be extremely slow and the evolution of their clinical pictures long drawn out.

After infarction of the pituitary, an extremely rare event, we see what is known as *pituitary cachexia*. The patient grows progressively thinner, loses hair and teeth, shows regression of the sexual organs and functions, a dry and wrinkled skin, and an increasing debility. There is also progressive mental deterioration and an abnormally low metabolic rate.

A form of hypopituitarism rarely found in children and adolescents, sometimes from tumour, is known as the *Lorain type* of pituitary dystrophy. There is general arrest of physical development, somatic and genital. The child is of delicate physique and slightly built, but mentally bright.

The syndrome of *pituitary basophilism*, already mentioned, consists of the following components. The face is of a bloated and dusky appearance and in women is abnormally hairy. The patient is obese as to the upper part of the body and the trunk, and there are many striæ on the skin of abdomen, buttocks, and thighs. The skin of the latter is brownish. The systemic blood pressure is abnormally high and there is polycythæmia. The condition progresses slowly to a fatal issue. Sexual activity wanes and disappears early.

The Place of Radiography in Diagnosis.—In general it may be said that the layman has exaggerated views of what may be expected from the radiography of the skull in intracranial tumour as in other diseases of the brain, and the doctor also tends to look for information from this source more often than it is available. There are four ways in which a simple radiogram of the skull may provide positive information. (1) In the case of long-standing increase of intracranial pressure, especially in a child, there may be an irregular thinning of the cranial vault which gives it what is called a "beaten silver" appearance, but this is not rarely present even in normal infants and young children, and in the absence of clinical signs of raised intracranial pressure is of no significance. On the other hand, separation of the sutures is indicative of increasing internal hydro-cephalus, but it must be rare indeed for this to occur without there being ample clinical evidence of this rise of pressure within the skull. Some erosion of the posterior clinoid processes may also be seen when intracranial pressure has been raised for some length of time. (2) A meningioma may invade the skull and produce a characteristic thickening and alteration in texture of the bone in the affected region (Fig. 15). The skull over a meningioma, even when not apparently invaded, may show a markedly increased vascularity—*e.g.* numerous and enlarged diploic channels (Figs. 18 and 19). (3) A tumour may contain calcareous material which casts a shadow and thus reveals both the presence and the site of the growth (Figs. 20 and 22). In and after middle age the normal pineal gland often contains such material, and if a tumour be present in one cerebral hemisphere, the shadow cast by the pineal may be displaced laterally. (4) A pituitary adenoma or a stalk tumour may produce enlargement and deformity of the sella turcica (Figs. 21 and 22).

It should be emphasized that the commonest of all intracranial tumours, the glioma, very rarely gives any radiographic indication of its presence, and this is also true of the secondary carcinoma. Thus, in the majority of cases, the simple radiogram gives a negative result. Finally, it should be remembered that there is a wide range of variation in the appearances of the normal skull in a radiogram, and the observer not experienced in interpreting these should be careful to avoid the error of ignoring clinical indications in favour of what may seem the more direct information revealed by a radiogram.

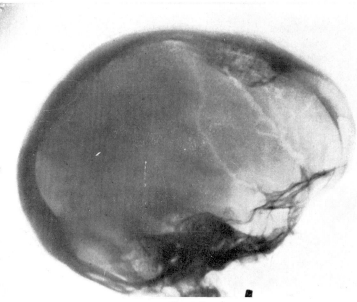

FIG. 18.

RADIOGRAM OF SKULL, SHOWING INVASION OF BONE BY MENINGIOMA.

A meningioma arising from the falx has invaded the frontal bone. Dilated diploic channels leading to the region of the tumour can be seen.

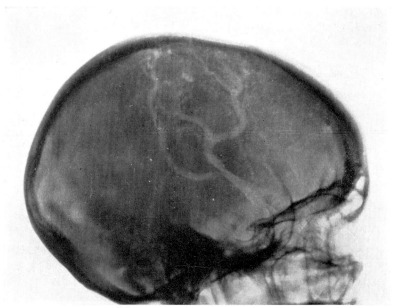

FIG. 19.

RADIOGRAM OF SKULL, SHOWING DILATED DIPLOIC CHANNELS.

A meningioma at the vertex. The skull has not been invaded, but greatly dilated diploic channels can be seen.

To face page 84.

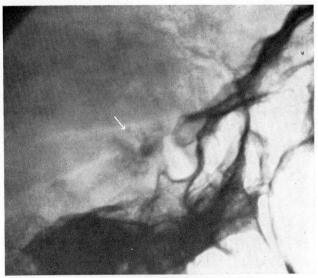

Fig. 20.

RADIOGRAM OF PITUITARY FOSSA, SHOWING CALCIFIED TUMOUR.

Above the pituitary fossa the irregular shadow (↑) of a calcified
pituitary stalk tumour can be seen. There is some erosion of the
posterior clinoid processes.

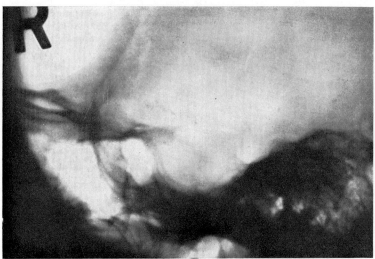

Fig. 21.

RADIOGRAM OF PITUITARY FOSSA IN CASE OF ADENOMA.

Enlargement of the pituitary fossa with disappearance of the posterior clinoid
processes. The case was one of pituitary adenoma.

To face page 85.

It should be mentioned, however, that if the ventricles are filled with air, either directly or by the lumbar intrathecal route, the resulting radiograms (ventriculogram, encephalogram) may reveal deformity or displacement of the ventricles and thus indicate the situation of a new growth that clinical examination may have failed to place. In many cases of intracranial new growth, one or other of these procedures may be an essential step in localizing diagnosis. It is then best carried out by the surgeon who will undertake any operation that may prove necessary, and under conditions that will allow of immediate operation should any sudden increase of symptoms follow the introduction of air into the skull.

Prognosis and Treatment.—An intracranial growth that cannot be removed must, sooner or later, end in death. Palliative decompression, once so common, may relieve symptoms of raised intracranial tension, and may in rare instances provide time for the planning and performance of more radical measures. As a rule, however, decompression merely prolongs for weeks or months a life of increasing disability and distress, and those old enough to remember the time when this procedure was almost a routine for cases of glioma will retain a horror of this mode of treatment of inoperable tumours. Surgical removal of the growth, therefore, provides the surest hope of permanent relief, though some varieties of glioma do respond, if only temporarily to X radiation.

The glioma and the secondary carcinoma together make up some fifty per cent. of all intracranial tumours. The latter, being almost always multiple, offer no solid hopes from surgery, but prognosis in the case of the gliomas is on the whole more favourable now than formerly, but in respect of certain varieties only. The glioblastoma is inoperable and death commonly ensues within six months of the appearance of symptoms. The cystic astrocytoma of cerebellum or of cerebral hemisphere may be completely and successfully extirpated. Occasionally, too, an encapsuled astrocytoma may be removed *in toto*. The infiltrating type, however, is irremovable, partly because it is not wholly visible to the naked eye. Further, the situation of a "benign" glioma is a factor in prognosis, for while a frontal or right temporal growth may be removed without producing disabling mutilation of the brain, a pathologically similar growth in other situations may be incapable of removal without the production of gross physical disabilities that make the life thus prolonged a torment. It has been necessary to state the position thus frankly in order that it may be realized that neither decompression nor the attempt at removal of a tumour should be regarded as routine measures in a case diagnosed as intracranial tumour. Each case must be considered on its localizing and pathological merits, and, not rarely, genuine humanity would allow the subject to pass to his inevitable end undisturbed by fruitless surgical intervention, and spare him a brief reprieve that is as painful to the patient as it is distressing to his relatives. On the other hand, until it be established by adequate investigation that a tumour is inoperable, steps should be taken to avert a lapse into coma and to relieve headache until a thorough assessment of the situation can be made. These steps consist in reducing the intracranial pressure by the intravenous administration of 100 c.cms. of 50 per cent. sucrose, or the rectal administration, up to twice or thrice a day, of 2 ounces of a 50 per cent. solution of magnesium sulphate. For the relief of headache, the latter method may be more effective than the use of an algesicdrugs, and, in addition, it is a valuable precaution to take before a patient with a considerable rise of intracranial tension is transported for any distance from home to hospital or nursing home.

The further clinical and radiological investigations that may have to be undertaken before operation is decided upon are not within the scope of this book. The treatment of pituitary adenoma is surgical and especially in early cases of chromophobe adenoma may be very successful. Eosinophil adenomas and stalk tumours are much less amenable to treatment, while the non-tumour syndromes do not respond to glandular therapy, save that polyuria may be controlled by the administration of pituitrin (either as a nasal spray or a snuff).

CHRONIC SUBDURAL HÆMATOMA

The variety of subdural hæmatoma that may follow immediately upon a severe head injury with concussion, contusion, or laceration of the brain is manifestly from the outset a surgical problem, but a subdural hæmatoma may follow an injury to the head of such an apparently trivial nature as not to come under medical observation. A simple fall on forehead or occiput without indications of concussion may lead to rupture of cortical veins as they cross the subdural space on their way to the dural venous sinus. From this rupture blood leaks into the subdural space and forms a collection in this space, usually over the convexity of the brain, and in about a third of all cases of the kind bilaterally.

It is with this variety of subdural hæmatoma that we are here concerned. In general its clinical picture is that of an expanding, space-occupying intracranial lesion, and its differentiation from intracranial new growth may be difficult.

Pathology.—The hæmatoma may form gradually if there be recurrent leakage from the veins. It may contain pure blood, but if there be a tear in the pia-arachnoid it may consist of a mixture of blood and cerebrospinal fluid. Shortly after its formation a fibrinous clot

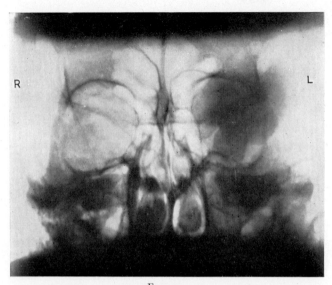

FIG. 22.
ANTERO-POSTERIOR RADIOGRAM OF SKULL.
On the left side can be seen the shadow of a meningioma on the
wing of the sphenoid bone.

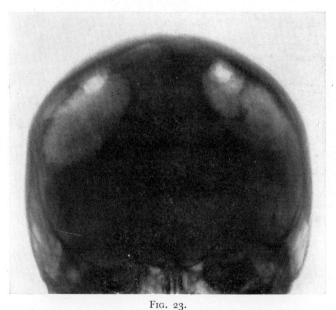

FIG. 23.
RADIOGRAM OF SKULL IN CASE OF SUBDURAL HÆMATOMA.
Antero-posterior radiogram of the skull. A bilateral chronic
subdural hæmatoma has been evacuated through two burr holes.
Air has entered through these and revealed the bilateral depression
on the convexity of the cerebral hemispheres produced by the two
hæmatomas.

To face page 87.

usually surrounds it, and from the overlying dura come fibroblasts which form a membrane round the clot and envelop it. The centre of the hæmatoma may contain stained fluid surrounded by clot and membrane. Usually the hæmatoma overlies the fronto-parietal cortex and, as has been said, there may be two hæmatomata, one on each side of the middle line. Rarely, such a hæmatoma may form subjacent to the temporal pole, when its presence is difficult to detect clinically.

Chronic subdural hæmatoma was formerly believed to be an inflammatory process known as chronic pachymeningitis hæmorrhagica, found in demented and alcoholic persons. It is now known to be

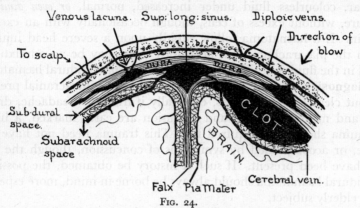

FIG. 24.

DIAGRAM OF SUBDURAL HÆMATOMA.

A coronal section showing a subdural hæmatoma on the right side. When the skull is struck the lateral movement of the contained brain may lead to the rupture of a communicating vein on its passage from the pia-arachnoid to the superior longitudinal sinus. The X-ray appearances of a bilateral hæmatoma are shown in Fig. 21.

(With permission from Rowbotham's *Acute Injuries of the Head*.)

traumatic, and its occurrence in the types of subject named above means no more than that such persons are the most liable to fall about and injure their heads, and the least likely afterwards to be able to give a history of trauma.

Symptomatology.—Clinically there is a latent period before symptoms appear that may range from a period of days to one of weeks or months; the more severe the causative injury the shorter the latent period. There then ensues a sequence of symptoms resembling in essence those described in connection with an intracranial tumour, but differing very commonly in the wide fluctuations in their severity from day to day, or even from hour to hour. Headache develops and increases in frequency and severity. The patient has accesses of drowsiness, is forgetful and at times confused. As the condition develops these accesses may develop into stupor, even to coma, from which he again emerges. The pulse rate tends to become slower, falling to 60, or even 50.

In the earlier stages physical examination may reveal no abnormality, but later some œdema of the optic discs, perhaps a unilateral increase of tendon jerks, perhaps the extensor plantar response—unilaterally or bilaterally—may be found. Even while under examination the patient may be overcome by uncontrollable drowsiness. The tongue is commonly coated. In the late stages, transient diplopia may develop, or inequality of the pupils, or even minimal signs of a hemiparesis. Unless surgically relieved, a final coma and death ultimately ensue, though it has to be said that occasionally in elderly persons a very old hæmatoma may be an unexpected post-mortem finding. Lumbar puncture yields a clear, colourless fluid under increased, normal, *or even diminished* pressure, without excess of cells, though occasionally with an excess of protein. If a hæmatoma follow rapidly upon a severe head injury in which the pia-arachnoid has been torn there may be an admixture of blood in the fluid, but this is not found in chronic subdural hæmatoma.

Diagnosis.—In all cases of rapidly developing intracranial pressure, without clear localizing signs, especially if frequent headache, drowsiness, and mental slowness and confusion are early marked, a history of trauma should be enquired for. This trauma need not have been severe, or accompanied by symptoms of concussion, though the latter may have been present. If such a history be obtained, the possibility of subdural hæmatoma should always be borne in mind, more especially in an elderly subject.

Treatment.—This is surgical and consists in the evacuation of the hæmatoma, through trephine holes if it be liquid, otherwise after bone flaps have been turned down. Thus treated, the prognosis as to recovery is good unless relief has been too long delayed. When the contents of the hæmatoma have been evacuated, they may be replaced by air, and a radiogram (antero-posterior) will then reveal the degree of depression of the hemisphere (Fig. 23).

ABSCESS OF THE BRAIN

As a space-occupying and expanding lesion within the skull an abscess may be expected to develop a clinical picture comparable with that of a tumour, yet in the ordinary way there are clinical features peculiar to abscess by which it may be recognized.

Pathology.—The majority of brain abscesses arise as a complication of chronic suppuration in the middle ear or mastoid antrum, usually in association with a cholesteatoma. When caries of the tegmen tympani ensues, infection reaches the under surface of the temporosphenoidal lobe, and when the petrous portion is carious, infection may spread posteriorly into the cerebellum. In both cases a brain abscess may develop. This may be closed, or may lead by a narrow track to the original septic focus in the bone. Frontal or ethmoidal sinusitis may, especially in young children, lead to frontal lobe abscess. Less common is the pyæmic brain abscess, which may be multiple and is usually a complication of suppuration in the chest; as in a chronic empyema, especially when this is subjected to surgical intervention, or in bronchiectasis.

Symptomatology.—Perhaps the most striking early indication that an abscess has formed within the brain is a change in the patient's mental alertness and emotional tone. Difficult as this is to describe, for it may involve no gross departure from the normal, it is yet quite distinctive to the careful observer. The patient tends to be an ineffective witness when questioned as to his illness, his memory is poor, and his capacity to sustained attention manifestly impaired. He is apathetic and may even be drowsy. The attempt to employ clinical tests involving his co-operation may prove unsuccessful, as, for example, the testing of the visual fields or of muscular co-ordination.

He may confess to headaches, but no very precise account of his symptoms can usually be obtained from him.

On examination nothing more definite than this may be found, and although quite a large abscess is subsequently revealed by operation there may be complete absence of localizing symptoms. Papillœdema is inconstant, save in the case of cerebellar abscess in which some œdema of the disc ultimately develops. The temperature may be raised and swinging, though with chronic thick-walled abscess it may be consistently subnormal. In the latter case the pulse is usually slower than normal. There is often a progressive loss of flesh and the patient looks ill. A coated tongue is usual. If localizing signs are present they tend to be minimal, and in the case of temporo-sphenoidal abscess include one or more of the following: slight paresis of the lower half of the face, diminution or loss of the abdominal reflexes, an extensor plantar response —all these signs being on the side opposite to the abscess. In a left-sided abscess of this lobe there may be aphasic speech defect, and if the patient's state allows of its examination it will be found that he tends to use wrong words, to muddle his words in a sentence, and to be at a loss for names. Such an abscess—if it involve the optic radiations as they traverse the temporo-sphenoidal lobe—may produce a crossed homonymous hemianopia, sometimes, complete but more often involving only the upper quadrants (see Fig. 8, page 45). In the case of a cerebellar abscess the patient's mental state may make complete demonstration of ataxy impossible, but certain signs are usually easy of elicitation: if the arms be horizontally extended the arm on the side of the abscess tends to droop, and if both extended arms be sharply tapped on the wrist, this arm is more widely displaced and swings pendulum-like before regaining its previous position.

Alternating movements of pronation-supination are more slowly and clumsily performed on the affected side. There may be a difficulty in turning the eyes to the side of the lesion, or alternatively a coarse nystagmus. Turning them to the opposite side is easier, but may show a finer, quicker nystagmus.

Diagnosis.—In the presence of signs of raised intracranial pressure enquiry must always be made as to whether or not there is otorrhœa or other indications of middle ear disease. If there be such, the possibility of intracranial abscess has to be considered. The history of cerebral symptoms is usually much shorter than in the case of tumour and the mental change described not quite of the same quality. Moreover, such as it is, it is not accompanied by the same marked grade either of general or of local signs as in the case of tumour. Also, accompanying an abscess there may be clinical indications of meningeal irritation: stiff neck, Kernig's sign, rigidity of the back. Once it is established that middle ear disease is present and that the intracranial symptoms are a complication of this, there still may remain the problem of differentiating local meningitis, with or without a subdural or extradural abscess, from brain abscess. With a *localized meningitis and extradural abscess* there may be signs of raised intracranial pressure, but the progress of the illness is apt to be more rapid than that of abscess within the brain. There is an irregular temperature and raised pulse rate and the signs of meningeal irritation are more marked.

Infective thrombosis of venous sinuses gives rise to greater constitutional disturbance than abscess: swinging temperature, rapid pulse, rigors, and indications of toxæmia. Apart from occlusive thrombosis of dural sinuses, there may arise infection of the lateral sinus in otitis media, and spread of infection with thrombo-phlebitis backwards to the torcular and thence into the superior longitudinal sinus.

In these circumstances the striking signs and symptoms described on page 114 under the heading of cortical thrombo-phlebitis may arise. On the other hand in children, what has been called *otitic hydrocephalus* may be the sole clinical expression of the spreading mural infection of the sinuses. The indications of this are headache, sickness, papillœdema and raised cerebrospinal fluid pressure. With repeated lumbar puncture otitic hydrocephalus usually clears up completely.

In making the differential diagnosis between these conditions the examination of the cerebrospinal fluid may be of crucial value. The relevant findings in the fluid are as follows. With an encapsulated abscess and no local meningitis, the fluid may be normal except that it is found to be under increased pressure, but in most cases of abscess the cerebrospinal fluid shows a slight increase in cell content above the normal range of 3 to 5 mononuclear cells per c.cm., the count rising to 20 or 30 cells per c.cm., almost all of the cells being mononuclears.

The glucose and chloride contents are normal, but the protein is commonly raised to as much as 40 to 80 mgms. per c.cm.

If there be localized meningitis, the chloride and glucose contents fall, the level of the chlorides being the most valuable index in prognosis. A progressive drop in the chlorides indicates a spread and generalization of meningitis, and if they fall as low as 650 mgms. per 100 c.cm., a fatal issue is likely. In these circumstances, too, the cellular content may rise considerably. It is only when the presence and extent of meningitis has to be determined that repeated lumbar puncture is indicated. With simple abscess it is not advisable to draw off more fluid than is essential for examination. A subdural abscess presents a cerebrospinal fluid like that of a local meningitis. In otitic hydro-cephalus the fluid is normal in composition, but is under increased pressure.

Course.—A chronic well encapsulated abscess may be clinically latent for weeks or even months. Indeed, in some cases of abscess following gunshot wounds of the skull and brain during the war of 1914–1918, years elapsed before clinical symptoms developed, and these were sometimes due to the bursting of an old abscess into the ventricles and the rapid development of an acute and fatal meningitis. In most cases of otitic and pyæmic abscess, the latent period is at most a matter of from two to six weeks, and the course thereafter is steadily progressive.

Treatment.—This is purely surgical, and in the skilled hands of the neurosurgeon the results are very much more favourable than was formerly the case.

DIFFERENTIAL DIAGNOSIS OF TUMOUR, HÆMATOMA AND ABSCESS

From this brief account it will be seen that while these three lesions present the same general features of symptomatology, yet there are differences in history, symptoms, and clinical course that give to each a certain individuality by which they may be differentiated. The routine of history-taking in a case presenting signs of raised intracranial pressure should include enquiries as to recent head injury, even though this be trivial, and as to old or recent ear discharge. The presence of suppuration within the chest, or indeed of recent suppuration elsewhere in the body, should bring the possibility of pyæmic abscess into consideration. It may usefully be remembered, also, that in young persons plumbism may present many of the signs of intracranial tumour. Lead encephalo-pathy may be accompanied by headache, convulsions, coma, hemiparesis, and papillœdema. Finally, the so-called acute hyper-tensive attack sometimes seen in the subjects of essential hypertension has to be borne in mind should an abnormally high blood pressure be found in association with signs of raised intracranial pressure. This clinical condition is discussed in more detail in connection with vascular disorders of the brain.

Lumbar puncture and the examination of the cerebrospinal fluid may upon occasion provide information of value, but it must be emphasized that this procedure has its dangers when there is a high intracranial pressure. Here, therefore, as elsewhere, lumbar puncture is not a routine method of investigation, but one to be used with discretion and for some clearly thought-out end.

CHAPTER IV

Vascular Disorders of the Brain

INTRODUCTION

DISEASE or disordered function of the cerebral arteries probably provides the bulk of cases of organic brain affection seen in the general practice of medicine. For the most part the illnesses so caused are of sudden onset and come under the clinical heading of apoplexy, yet the processes of arterial degeneration not infrequently lead to a state of slowly progressive impairment of cerebral activity. We have to remember that the blood supply to the brain is largely controlled extra-cerebrally and is a resultant of the combined functions of the heart and blood-vessels. Thus, even in the presence of diseased arteries an adequate cerebral circulation may be maintained until some transient or progressive impairment of cardiac efficiency just turns the balance and allows of cerebral softening from temporary diminution of blood supply, and thus of oxygen, to a greater or smaller region of the brain. Further, cardiac disease, by the mechanism of embolism, may lead to grave disorders of cerebral structure and function. Finally, certain transient disorders of cerebral function not associated with residual structural damage may result from general circulatory disorders: as, for example, the simple fainting attack that ensues upon a sudden and considerable fall in systemic blood pressure, and the hypertensive attack associated with essential hypertension.

In all these varied conditions the essential factor is an interference with the cerebral blood supply, either transient or persisting. The nerve cell is highly sensitive to variations in its blood supply, that is, in its oxygen supply. The cerebral circulation is so controlled as to maintain as constant a level of oxygen supply to the brain as possible, and even its anatomical arrangements seem specially designed to this end. In the circle of Willis and in the free anastomoses between the cortical branches of the cerebral arterioles we see an arterial system planned to secure an adequate collateral circulation in the event of local damage.

Complete ischæmia leads within a few minutes to irreversible changes in nerve cells. These changes are necrotic in character and may be of all grades of severity, from the slightest to the death of the cell. Hence, even transient interference with the cerebral circulation may lead to permanent residual symptoms.

93

To progressive oxygen deprivation the nerve cell reacts first by becoming hyperexcitable and then by diminution and loss of function. The convulsions of asphyxia, and those that may attend severe hæmorrhage elsewhere in the body, express this initial reaction of the nerve cell. In the last resort, then, vascular disorders of the brain produce their symptoms by reducing or abolishing the oxygen supply of nerve cells, though in the case of intracranial hæmorrhage there is also gross destruction of cerebral tissue by the issuing arterial blood.

A simple classification of vascular disorders of the brain from the clinical point of view may be made into:

(1) Those which are transient and recoverable and without structural damage to the brain. These include the simple fainting attack (vasovagal syncope) and the hypertensive attack of essential hypertension.

(2) Those which involve some degree of structural damage and thus lead to permanent sequels. These include cerebral hæmorrhage and softening.

THE FAINTING ATTACK—VASOVAGAL SYNCOPE.—When this is encountered clinically the associations which it arouses in the mind of the clinician are not those of vascular disorder of the brain so much as those of a "heart attack" or of epilepsy. In a text-book of neurology it is the latter that demands consideration, and, therefore, the description of the fainting attack is given in the chapter on epilepsy (page 125).

Ætiology and Pathology.—The causation and morbid anatomy of arterial disease, and the relation of this to the clinical states associated with it, nowhere present more obscure problems than in the case of the arteries of the brain. The difficulty that pathologists experience in finding those arterial occlusions by clot, and the arterial ruptures, that we have for so long supposed to underlie cerebral thrombosis and hæmorrhage respectively, imply that the accounts of these things given in text-books of neurology have become too conventional and oversimplified. It is probable that we have taken too little account of the possible roles of vasomotor disorders in these arteries in leading to cerebral softening and hæmorrhage. On no hypothesis of arterial occlusion by clot can we account for the fugitive hemiplegias and other transient paralyses of cerebral function that we encounter in hypertensive subjects, often preceding the later development of more severe and persisting paralyses. It may be that the familiar triad, hæmorrhage, embolism, and thrombosis, should be replaced by the two main categories of hæmorrhage and softening. Subdivisions of the latter would include softening from embolism and also from vasomotor disorders (vasospasm and vasoparalysis). The hypertensive crisis and the state known as hypertensive encephalopathy may also, in part at least, be expressions of vasomotor disorder, preceding or accompanying structural lesions in cerebral arteries and arterioles. In short, we may suppose that underlying cerebral disorders from vascular disease there are three essential factors, two cerebral, one extracerebral, namely, (1) abnormal vasomotor disorder in cerebral vessels, (2) structural disease of cerebral vessels, and (3) fluctuations in cardiac efficiency from heart disease. Some would now add a fourth—a psychological—factor, which they regard as capable of initiating vasomotor disorders, whence structural lesions may follow. How this may happen is neither known nor suggested, but there is some evidence that it may so happen.

With at least four factors in operation, varying in their relative importance from case to case, it is not surprising that the clinical pictures of cerebral vascular disease are very numerous, and diverse in form and behaviour.

This is not the place to discuss in any detail the morbid anatomy of arterial disease, but brief reference is necessary to the two main varieties found in the arteries of the brain.

Atherosclerosis (or atheroma) is the process found in the large cerebral arteries. It is a patchy and nodular process, leading to distortion of the vessel and even to narrowing or occlusion of its lumen. The intima is the seat of the essential lesion, which consists in fatty deposition, followed by sclerotic changes in the intima and some calcification. These lead to aneurysmal dilatation and even to rupture as well as to narrowing.

Arteriolosclerosis (or hyperplastic sclerosis) is a diffuse process characteristic of the intimate vasculature of organs, pre-eminently of the kidney, but found also in the brain. It is the change found in association with hypertension, and has been thought to be a response to this. A hyaline change and thickening of the subendothelial layer of the intima is the essential lesion, and it leads to narrowing and even to occlusion of the arteriolar lumen.

We see, therefore, that the larger arteries of the brain become the seat of the patchy change known as atherosclerosis, while the arterioles show a diffuse change of a different character. In some subjects of cerebral vascular disorder both varieties of arterial change may be present, while in others one or other variety may predominate.

Too little is known of the role of vasospasm in producing cerebral hæmorrhage and softening to allow of dogmatic statements, but it is possible that when softening ensues upon atherosclerosis of the larger arteries we are dealing with occlusion of an already narrowed artery by blood clot, a true thrombosis, while the softening that ensues upon the sclerosis of arterioles may result as frequently, or even more frequently, from spasm as from clot formation. Throughout this section, therefore, the word thrombosis is used "without prejudice" as it were, and it is to be understood that in many instances of so-called cerebral thrombosis, the essential factor may have been a transient arteriolar spasm, leading to an ischæmia of sufficient duration to produce softening of cerebral tissue.

A further point remains: it is clear that if cardiac weakness supervenes in a subject with cerebral arterial disease, the addition of this further factor may lead to disaster by still further impeding the cerebral circulation. In these circumstances a failing heart may precipitate a cerebral vascular disaster, and thus it is that some cases of terminal heart failure present a strikingly cerebral symptomatology.

TRANSIENT CEREBRAL DISORDERS IN ESSENTIAL AND MALIGNANT HYPERTENSION : THE HYPERTENSIVE CRISIS

Whether or not hypertension is primary to, or consequent upon, what we have called hyperplastic sclerosis of the arterioles (arteriolosclerosis), the two are ultimately found together, and in these circumstances the symptoms of cerebral vascular disturbance are prone to occur. These may take the form of *sudden and transient paralyses*, monoplegia, aphasic speech disorders, hemianopia or hemiparesis, which clear rapidly leaving little or no trace, or of what is known as the *hypertensive crisis*.

There can be little doubt that both these categories of event are preceded by—and precipitated by—a further rise in the already high level of systemic blood pressure obtaining, a rise that in all probability is due to arteriolar spasm. Little is known of the factors that lead to this abnormal vasomotor activity, and we have no systematic information as to the blood pressure levels in the hypertensive subject immediately prior to a cerebral vascular episode. It may be found, however, for a period of a week or more after a hemiparesis, transient or slowly improving, that the systolic and diastolic levels fluctuate widely, finally reaching a steadily maintained level under uniform conditions.

Symptoms.—On the whole, cardiovascular symptoms are more common in the subjects of hypertension than are cerebral, yet certain cases tend throughout their course to present the latter. Symptoms premonitory to a hypertensive crisis or to a transient paralysis are headache, irritability, and a sense of fatigue physical and mental. When a crisis is developing the headache increases in severity, sometimes occurring in paroxysms of great intensity. The blood pressure is found to be of the order of 250/140. Sickness may accompany the headache, and giddiness also. In severe cases the patient may become drowsy or even semi-conscious. In the patient with essential hypertension, the blood urea and urea concentration tests reveal no renal inefficiency, and the urine may be normal. Ophthalmoscopic examination will show narrowing of the retinal arteries and perhaps some indications of a hypertensive retinitis. In patients in whom essential hypertension is giving place to the so-called malignant form, indications of renal impairment will be found, while the fundus oculi will show more advanced retinitis, and often œdema of the discs and numerous small retinal hæmorrhages. In these circumstances, the cerebrospinal fluid pressure is also abnormally high. Symptoms of focal cerebral disorder may ensue, paralyses, hemianopia, Jacksonian or generalized fits.

Such a crisis may maintain its level of maximal severity for periods ranging from hours to several days. It may end in complete subsidence, or, upon occasion, in a cerebral hæmorrhage.

Diagnosis.—To those who are not familiar with the cerebral hypertensive attack, the possibilities of error are considerable. If the presence of high blood pressure is known, a diagnosis of uræmia may be made, but in the uncomplicated hypertensive attack the blood urea is within normal limits and the urine may contain as its only abnormal constituent a small amount of albumin. When papillœdema is present and severe the possibility of intracranial tumour has to be considered, but while it need not be maintained that the systolic blood pressure is never raised in the subject of tumour, it can be said that it does not reach the high levels seen in essential hypertension. The course of events usually clears up any uncertainty within a week or so, for cerebral tumour is a progressive condition. One remote possibility of error yet remains, namely, lead encephalopathy. Plumbism in young persons may take this form, when it is characterized by headache, vomiting, papillœdema, convulsions, signs of local cerebral lesion, and sometimes also by a high blood pressure and albuminuria. In this case, careful history-taking and the search for the other indications of lead poisoning will serve to differentiate the two conditions.

Prognosis.—The prognosis as to recovery from the individual attack is good if treatment is early and energetic, but the underlying arterial and cardiac condition persists, and the ultimate prognosis is that of essential hypertension with this proviso, that the victim of what has been called "hypertensive encephalopathy" is perhaps more likely to succumb ultimately to cerebral hæmorrhage than to cardiac failure.

Treatment.—The subject of essential hypertension who develops a transient hemiparesis or other focal symptom should be put to bed for at least a week or ten days, however transient his paralysis. This is the most effective way of bringing his systemic blood pressure to a lower and more uniformly maintained level. The administration of nicotinic acid (50 to 100 mgms. daily) and of alcohol (whisky) has been recommended to induce cerebral vasodilatation. The long term treatment of hypertensive subjects with cerebral symptoms is considered on page 110.

G

With the development of a hypertensive crisis, venesection—up to a pint—is a useful measure, and if there be signs of cerebral œdema (papillœdema, high cerebrospinal fluid pressure, convulsions) the administration of sucrose solution, as in the case of intracranial tumour, or of rectal magnesium sulphate may be considered. Headaches are most effectively relieved by these means. Convulsions may be controlled by rectal paraldehyde (4 to 6 drachms in water) or by the hypodermic injection of phenobarbitone (3 grains, repeated as necessary).

CEREBRAL HÆMORRHAGE AND SOFTENING : APOPLEXY

In past editions, the heading of this section has included the terms "thrombosis" and "embolism." It has been pointed out, however, that, though exact knowledge on the subject is far from complete, there are reasons for thinking that cerebral softening may follow transient spasm of arterioles and that this may be the mechanism in many of the cases that in the past we have been content to regard as cerebral thrombosis from clot formation within the vessel. Embolism is a special case, but there is good experimental evidence that the impaction of a solid embolus within a cerebral artery or arteriole may be accompanied by widespread vasospasm within the brain. Even here, then, vasomotor factors may be operative.

Some further reference must, however, be made to cerebral embolism, and to the morbid anatomy of cerebral hæmorrhage and softening.

Pathology.—The common site of hæmorrhage is the region of the internal capsule, corpus striatum and thalamus: that is, the region supplied by the small central (lenticular) branches of the middle cerebral artery (Fig. 25). When profuse, the hæmorrhage may break into the lateral ventricles. When a horizontal section is made through the brain of a fatal case of hæmorrhage a dark gelatinous blood clot is seen to occupy the central region of the affected hemisphere, and when this is washed away the torn cerebral tissue surrounding the site of hæmorrhage can be seen. In old cases that have long survived such a lesion we find a cyst-like cavity containing a yellow fluid.

Massive cerebral softening usually involves the region already described as the common seat of hæmorrhage, but regions of the brain within the distributions of cortical branches of the three cerebral arteries, and within those of branches of vertebral and basilar arteries may also be involved. The appearances of the infarcted region varies according to the degree of collateral circulation obtaining. When this is scanty we have a white softening, when free the softened area is red. Phagocytic microglial cells ("compound granular corpuscles") soon enter the softened area and carry away necrotic material, leaving in the case of large softenings a cystic cavity crossed by delicate strands of proliferated glial fibres.

Except for the extra-cerebral (subarachnoid) hæmorrhage resulting from the rupture of a basal aneurysm, which may be seen at any age, cerebral hæmorrhage is found in elderly persons with atheroma, but

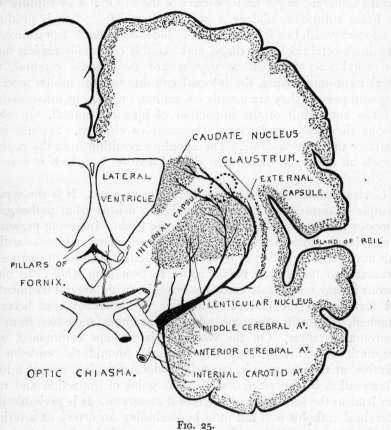

FIG. 25.

DISTRIBUTION OF THE MIDDLE CEREBRAL ARTERY.

Coronal Section of the Left Cerebral Hemisphere, showing the central branches of the middle cerebral artery. The region of the lenticulo-striate artery, which is commonly the seat of rupture and of cerebral hæmorrhage, is indicated by a circle of dots.

in young adults cerebral thrombosis may be found in association with syphilitic endarteritis, in septicæmia, and other infective conditions.

The cerebral aneurysms from which, upon rupture, subarachnoid hæmorrhage occurs are not the so-called miliary aneurysms found upon the perforating branches of the middle cerebral artery, but larger dilatations, usually saccular, which are found upon the arteries which enter into the circle of Willis. Such dilatations may never give rise to symptoms, they may be of such size and so situated to cause pressure symptoms within the skull, or they may rupture. When the last happens, the blood pours into the subarachnoid space at the base of the brain and may spread up over the convexity of the hemispheres and filter down into the spinal theca. Should such an aneurysm have become adherent to the under surface of the brain, it may rupture into the brain substance, and even into the ventricles, when it produces an apoplexy with hemiplegia clinically indistinguishable from the ordinary intra-cerebral hæmorrhage, and like this commonly rapidly fatal. The usual sites for such aneurysms are the middle cerebral, the anterior communicating, the internal carotid, and the basilar arteries. In young persons they are usually congenital, but may be inflammatory and the end result of the impaction of infective emboli. In older persons they may result from atheromatous changes. Syphilis is a relatively uncommon cause. The apoplexy resulting from the rupture of such an aneurysm has certain clinical features by which it may be recognized.

Cerebral embolism calls for a further brief mention. It is the typical example of disorder of cerebral circulation arising from pathological processes topographically remote from the brain. In young persons it is associated particularly with rheumatic or bacterial endocarditis, with auricular fibrillation at its onset, or when, as a result of treatment, it ceases and the auricle begins again to beat as a whole. In older persons it may complicate coronary thrombosis, as when a fragment of clot forming on the endocardium over the infarcted area becomes detached, or aortic atheroma when a thrombus separates from an atheromatous ulcer. On the whole, it is perhaps commonest with rheumatic endocarditis in young persons. Should the embolus be infective, as may happen in bacterial endocarditis, it produces a local inflammation in the arterial wall at its point of impaction and may thus lead to the formation of a cerebral aneurysm. It is probable that a cerebral embolus acts not only by occluding an artery or arteriole, but also in virtue of the widespread vaso-constriction it may cause in the brain upon impaction. There are thus reversible as well as irreversible changes set up in embolism.

APOPLEXY

Cerebral hæmorrhage and softening are commonly encountered in the elderly subjects of hypertension and associated with one or both the forms of arterial degeneration already described. It is often assumed that hæmorrhage is a concomitant of high and softening of a low systemic blood pressure. Yet the vascular conditions that underlie both are essentially the same, and it may be the precipitating factors that differ. Thus hæmorrhage may accompany effort, while thrombosis often follows upon fatigue or upon some debilitating illness when, for the time being, the blood pressure is below its customary high level. Indeed variations in blood pressure seem to occur more readily and frequently in hypertensives than in normal persons, and it is noteworthy that cerebral thrombosis often sets in during sleep or when the subject is unduly fatigued.

It is, therefore, not possible to determine the cause of an apoplexy, as between hæmorrhage and thrombosis by measuring the blood pressure of the comatose patient. Unless he be collapsed and moribund it will probably be found well above the normal in both instances. Of the two disasters, thrombosis is much the commoner and the less often immediately fatal. If two or more recurrences of apoplexy occur in the same subject, we may safely assume that all have been due to softening except the last and fatal one.

In both events we are dealing with a sudden interruption of the cerebral arterial supply involving a larger or smaller region of the brain. If only a small region be rendered ischæmic, the resulting disturbance of function may be confined to this region, but when a large region is involved the entire cerebral mechanism is thrown temporarily out of action and consciousness is suddenly lost. It is to this loss that the term apoplexy is applied.

The mode of onset of apoplexy and the depth and duration of the ensuing coma may provide clinical indications from which we may judge the character of the responsible lesion. The dislodgement of an embolus from heart or aortic wall is an instantaneous event, and therefore the apoplexy of cerebral embolism is the most sudden of all. Rapid in onset, though usually less instantaneous, is the apoplexy of cerebral hæmorrhage. With this, brief premonitory headache or paræsthesiæ of unilateral distribution may precede the rapidly developing loss of consciousness. In cerebral thrombosis, on the other hand, the mode of onset varies widely from case to case. It may be apoplectic, approximating in character to that of hæmorrhage, and a brief generalized convulsion may accompany the onset. Perhaps more often hemiplegia begins to appear and to deepen, and with this increase consciousness progressively wanes. This happens when a thrombosis beginning in a small artery spreads backward towards the parent trunk—probably the middle cerebral artery; such a process may take from one to more hours to evolve, the subject finally becoming comatose, though rarely so deeply as in the case of hæmorrhage. The profound coma, with relaxation of both sphincters and with vomiting, is more likely to be due to hæmorrhage than to thrombosis. A common mode of onset is that in which the subject retires to bed in his usual health, though possibly more fatigued than is customary, to awake next morning with a hemiplegia already present. Again, he may be found semi-conscious on the floor of his bedroom, having fallen when he attempted to get out of bed. It may usefully be remembered that in the subject of cardio-vascular degeneration, the onset of coronary thrombosis may, in virtue of its effect upon the cerebral circulation, be accompanied by cerebral symptoms due to local ischæmia and an ensuing softening. In such circumstances, one or other of these episodes, commonly the coronary thrombosis, may escape detection, and the patient be thought to have had a cerebral thrombosis alone.

In subarachnoid hæmorrhage the onset is almost invariably marked by the absolutely sudden development of intense headache, and whether consciousness is then lost depends upon the amount of hæmorrhage. In small leakages, a period of confusion or delirium, during which the headache persists, may occur, consciousness never being lost.

These varying modes of onset, taken in conjunction with the general background of the subject's cardiovascular state, will generally make a pathological diagnosis possible, but it has to be confessed that when the onset has not been observed and the subject is discovered already comatose it may be difficult to differentiate the possible under-lying pathological processes. In these circumstances the problem may resolve itself into the larger one of the differential diagnosis of coma.

The Differential Diagnosis of Coma.—In the differential diagnosis of any state of coma it should be borne in mind that, quite apart from structural lesions of the brain, changes in the reflexes may be found. Thus, in deep coma the tendon reflexes may be abolished, while in many forms of intoxication the plantar responses may be of the extensor type. This form of plantar response is found, for example, in barbiturate and aspirin poisoning, in the cholæmia of acute yellow atrophy of the liver and of delayed chloroform poisoning, and in hypoglycæmic coma. It is also present as a transient phenomenon in the flaccid coma that follows the convulsion of a generalized epileptiform fit. In all the above-mentioned states such abnormalities in the reflexes as may be found are bilateral.

(1) *Vascular Lesions of the Brain.*—In cerebral hæmorrhage, softening and embolism the signs of a unilateral lesion of the brain are present, *e.g.* hemiplegia. These signs have already been described in Chapter II, page 23. But in uncomplicated subarachnoid hæmorrhage hemiplegia is lacking. The features of this condition are fully described on page 112, and need not here be detailed.

In any progressive intracranial hæmorrhage the pupils tend to dilate progressively as coma deepens towards death, the paralytic dilatation appearing first on the side of the lesion when this is unilateral.

(2) *Non-vascular Lesions of the Brain.*—These rarely give rise to a sudden lapse into coma and thus commonly provide a medical history

from which information of great diagnostic value may be obtained. Such lesions are intracranial tumour, hæmatoma, and abscess, of which the signs have already been described. The polio-encephalitis of childhood may be ushered in by coma with convulsions, rapidly followed by the signs of hemiplegia in most instances. Here the fundus oculi is normal. Lead encephalopathy may also produce coma. The signs and symptoms of this intoxication have already been described on page 97.

(3) *Narcotic Poisoning.*—Opium and its derivatives no longer occupy pride of place in this category since the numerous barbiturate drugs have come into such general use. The signs of opium poisoning are familiar from countless descriptions in text-books and may be briefly summarized. The pupils are minutely contracted, the tendon reflexes may be absent, the skin is cold, the face livid and clammy, the pulse feeble and slow, respiration slow—later irregular and stertorous. The plantar responses are flexor.

In connection with barbiturate poisoning it is important to remember that a bilateral extensor type of plantar response may be present. If this be not known, such a finding is apt to lead to a diagnosis of some structural disease of the brain. For the rest, the clinical picture varies according to the depth of the coma and the severity of the poisoning. This skin is usually cold and clammy, the face pale, respiration is slow and finally irregular. The pupils are small, and in the lighter degrees of coma the eyes move irregularly, showing squint as they do so. The tendon reflexes are diminished and may be abolished. Severe aspirin poisoning may present a similar picture, including the presence of extensor plantar responses, but the patient has usually been very sick and he and his bed or his garments may reveal this by the presence of vomited material.

(4) *Diabetic and Hypoglycæmic Coma.*—Diabetic coma may most readily be identified by the examination of the urine and the detection of glucose and acetone bodies therein. The tendon jerks may be abolished from the presence of a peripheral neuritis, the plantar responses are of the normal, or flexor, variety. In hypoglycæmic coma, on the other hand, the plantar responses are often of the extensor variety. There may be epileptiform convulsions, sometimes a status epilepticus. The patient may be restless, flushed and sweating. The blood sugar estimation and the examination of the urine will serve to establish the differentiation from diabetic coma.

(5) *Alcoholic Poisoning.*—It is perhaps trite to say that the smell of alcohol in the breath of the comatose subject is not necessarily an indication that the coma is alcoholic in origin. Yet mistakes in diagnosis based upon the assumption that it is are still made from time to time and with unfortunate results. No coma should be dismissed as alcoholic until a complete examination has excluded all other possible causes,

amongst which head injury with concussion, contusion, or intracranial
hæmorrhage should be considered, as well as all the other ætiological
varieties of coma already dealt with. There is a stale quality about the
breath of the chronic alcoholic that differs from that of the individual
who chances to have had a drink shortly before his lapse into coma—
from whatever cause. His tongue is coated, his conjunctivæ injected.
If he be not too deeply comatose, pressure on his calves may evoke from
him some sign of undue muscular tenderness—so common in chronic
alcoholics and indicating a low grade multiple neuritis. Even in the
presence of all these indications of addiction, it remains true that all
possible surgical and medical causes of coma must be excluded before
the subject is regarded simply as "dead drunk." In other words,
alcoholic coma is diagnosed most safely by a process of exclusion.
Despite these necessary cautions, it remains to be said that a recent
statistical analysis of 1,100 cases of coma admitted into the Boston
City Hospital revealed that 59 per cent. were alcoholic.

The Prognosis in Apoplexy.—It is a valid generalization that
the coma of intra-cerebral hæmorrhage is more often fatal than not,
and this within a matter of hours or a day or two. If the subject regain
consciousness the prognosis as to survival, until some further vascular
lesion occurs, is reasonably good. In subarachnoid hæmorrhage the
same holds true, though within the fortnight following the original
hæmorrhage there is a special danger of recurrent bleeding. If this
period be successfully passed, recovery, since there is no residual
paralysis, proceeds steadily and becomes complete and there may be
no further recurrence.

In embolism the prognosis depends upon the site of impaction of
the embolus and the extent of the brain rendered ischæmic. But here,
as in hæmorrhage, stability is reached relatively soon, that is, within a
period of days.

In cerebral softening, on the other hand, it may prove extremely
difficult to foretell the course of events. Stability may not be reached
for three or four weeks. An initial paralysis may clear up and later
return, extend and deepen, the subject lapsing gradually into a stupor,
then into a final coma. The prudent clinician will be very guarded
when called upon for a prognosis in the early course of a case of cerebral
softening. Daily blood pressure readings from the date of onset will
often reveal a fluctuation of systolic blood pressure from day to day of
30 or more mms. The patient cannot be considered out of danger while
this continues, and recovery of power in the hemiplegic often remains
negligible until the pressure settles to a steady level. This may not occur
for from two to four weeks.

In all cases of apoplexy associated with severe hemiplegia the
prolonged confinement of the subject to bed in the supine position

creates difficulties and dangers, especially in the case of elderly persons with the cardiovascular degenerative changes so commonly found in these circumstances. Bedsores develop readily over the sacrum and heels, and still more menacing are the œdema of the bases of the lungs and bronchopneumonia that may be called "the bedsore in the lung."

The Residual Paralysis of Apoplexy.—The vascular lesions, the onset of which is marked by loss of consciousness, almost invariably involve the middle cerebral artery, and, therefore, hemiplegia is the characteristic sequel. To this, if the sensory fibres which lie in the posterior genu of the internal capsule are involved, there may be added hemianæsthesia and hemianopia (see page 25). The clinical features of hemiplegia in its initial flaccid and its later spastic stages have already been described. The hemiplegia left by a cerebral hæmorrhage which the subject has survived is less likely to make a recovery than one resulting from thrombosis. In any event, the final measure of restoration may usually be gauged at the end of the third or fourth week. By this time, if a useful recovery is going to take place, it is already within sight, and subsequently recovery gradually slows down, and with the development of spasticity hope of further considerable restoration may be abandoned. The most severe disability remains in the hand. This may regain a measure of general strength, making a fairly strong grasp possible, but the isolated movements of the fingers, unless they are restored very rapidly after onset, do not return. The leg fares better, at least as far as its functions as a prop are concerned, but flexion may remain so weak that the limb is shuffled and circumducted in walking.

The same general laws are followed by disorders of speech function after left-sided cerebral lesions. If any degree of expressive or of receptive aphasia remains after four weeks, full command of language is not likely to return. When hemianæsthesia accompanies hemiplegia it often clears up, some degree of motor disability persisting. On the other hand, lesions involving the optic thalamus are characterized by relatively slight and transient hemiplegia, but by persisting sensory disturbances. Sensory ataxy of movement may be a feature of this loss, and to it may be added *after the lapse of a few weeks* the appearance of intractable pain on the affected side of the body. This combination of sensory loss, ataxy of movement, and pain together make up what is known as the thalamic syndrome.

ACUTE VASCULAR LESIONS WITHOUT INITIAL LOSS OF CONSCIOUSNESS

So far consideration has been given to vascular lesions with an apoplectic onset, yet the occurrence of hemiplegia without apoplexy in cases of cerebral softening has also been mentioned. In such cases it is the ingravescent nature of the pathological process that averts the "shock" produced by sudden vascular catastrophe. On the other hand, as has also been mentioned, when the region of the brain rendered ischæmic is relatively small, no general disturbance of cerebral function accompanies the onset of the local paralysis of function.

MEDULLARY THROMBOSIS.—Yet another factor may determine the absence of loss of consciousness, namely, the localization of the lesion.

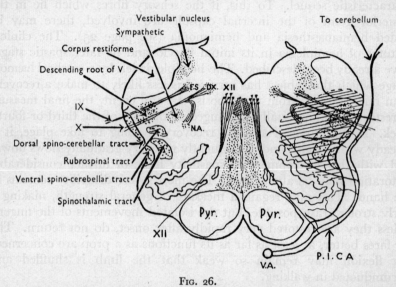

FIG. 26.

THROMBOSIS OF THE POSTERIOR INFERIOR CEREBELLAR ARTERY.

A cross section of the medulla at the level of the hypoglossal nucleus. The transverse extent of the thrombosed region is shaded. Its vertical extent cannot be represented but it extends from the middle of the seventh nerve nucleus above to that of the twelfth nerve nucleus below. F.S.—Fasciculus solitarius and nucleus gustatorius (IX). D.X.—Dorsal nucleus of Vagus. N.A.—Nucleus ambiguus of the Vagus. Pyr.—Pyramidal tract. M.F.—Mesial fillet. V.A.—Vertebral artery. P.I.C.A.—Posterior inferior cerebellar artery.

In syphilitic arterial disease as well as in the arterial degeneration of old age, the basilar artery or one of its branches may be the seat of the lesion. Such a branch is the posterior inferior cerebellar artery. This supplies the lateral region of the medulla as well as part of the cerebellar cortex. Occlusion of this branch has a dramatic mode of onset, consciousness being undisturbed. The patient is taken with intense giddiness and, if standing, tends to fall to one side. Dysphagia and dysarthria are present and there may be nausea. There is pain on one side of the face and subjective numbness over the entire half of the body on the opposite side. Diplopia is common, and there is gross ataxy of cerebellar type on the same side of the body as the lesion.

The resulting signs and symptoms are so interesting and straightforward an exercise in applied anatomy that they may be given in some detail. With the accompanying diagram (Fig. 26), which shows the anatomical structures involved and the extent of the region rendered ischæmic, the symptomatology may readily be followed.

The following table, read in conjunction with the figure, shows the symptoms and signs of this medullary thrombosis and correlates them with the anatomical elements involved.

Structure.	Signs and Symptoms. On the side of the Lesion.
Vth Nerve (descending root)	Pain and burning sensation on outer and inner aspect of cheek. Loss of sensation over face and cheek.
VIth Nerve.	Diplopia, External Rectus weakness, Squint.
VIIth Nerve.	Weakness of face.
VIIIth Nerve (Vestibular Nucleus) (Cochlear Nucleus)	Vertigo, Vomiting, Nystagmus. Deafness and Tinnitus.
IXth Nerve (F. Solitarius and N. Gustatorius)	Loss of taste.
Xth Nerve (Dorsal Nucleus, Nucleus Ambiguus)	Dysphagia, Paralysis of vocal cord and of palate. Tachycardia and nausea.
Sympathetic Centre	Smallness of pupil, slight ptosis. Dryness of face.
Cerebellar Tracts Cerebellar Cortex	Ataxy of limbs and gait.
	On the side opposite to the Lesion.
Spinothalamic Tract	Crossed sensory loss for pain and temperature over half of body, including face.
	Unaffected on both sides.
Mesial Fillet	Tactile sensibility, postural sensibility.
Pyramidal Tract	Voluntary power, tendon reflexes, plantar and abdominal reflexes.

These symptoms and disabilities tend to clear up, leaving as permanent sequels sensory loss over the face on the side of the lesion, a partial sympathetic syndrome (small pupil, slight ptosis), slight nystagmus, with loss of pain and temperature sense on the opposite half of the body. This measure of recovery is the rule, and patients rarely succumb to this lesion unless the occlusion of the artery spreads back to the parent trunk and a thrombosis of the vertebral artery ensues.

Other brain-stem thromboses are occasionally seen and they present a combination of cranial nerve palsies on the side of the lesion with motor or sensory symptoms on the crossed side according to the long tracts involved.

VASCULAR LESIONS PRODUCING SLOWLY PROGRESSIVE CHANGES IN CEREBRAL FUNCTION

When, from one of the forms of arterial disease, or from vasospasm, we get recurrent small regions of softening in the brain, we do not see apoplexy, but more commonly a condition of transient confusion, or the appearance of a localized paralysis such as a transient aphasia, hemianopia, or hemiparesis. These local symptoms clear up more or less completely, but after each episode the subject is slightly more feeble in mind and body. A form of senile decay thus ensues and may be characterized by loss of memory, of judgment, and of power of concentration.

There are accesses of disorientation as to time and place. The patient may be irritable and difficult to manage, insisting on conforming to a long-established regime of life for which he is no longer either mentally or physically fit. It is in such circumstances that testamentary capacity may become seriously impaired, with all the unpleasant consequences to which this disability may lead. A final bronchopneumonia or a massive cerebral softening or hæmorrhage brings this tedious and distressing illness to a close.

There are two relatively common variants on this picture: that of arterio-sclerotic muscular rigidity and that of pseudobulbar palsy.

ARTERIO-SCLEROTIC MUSCULAR RIGIDITY.—This refers to a slowly progressive disability in which a rigidity of Parkinsonian type invades the musculature. The patient's face tends to become set and "wooden," his movements slow, his stance one of flexion, while his steps are characteristically short and shuffling. As such a man makes his laboured progress along the street, the trained ear can recognize the shuffle of his feet on the pavement and the listener knows what he will see if he turns to look. Accompanying this growing disability are those mental changes already referred to. Numerous minute foci of softening and cell degeneration in the region of the corpora striata are the pathological basis of this state. On section numerous tiny holes can be seen in the affected region, from which the name "status lacunatus" has been given to it.

PSEUDOBULBAR PALSY.—This results from small bilateral softenings in the region of the internal capsules. There is usually a history of two or more mild apoplectiform seizures, neither of which has been followed by severe hemiplegia. In many respects the condition resembles bilateral hemiplegia of slight severity, but in addition to the loss of power in the limbs and the accompanying changes in the reflexes, certain bilaterally performed motor functions are gravely affected. Thus there is dysarthria, sometimes so gross as to render the patient's speech unintelligible. The tongue is small and spastic and usually cannot be protruded beyond the line of the teeth. Swallowing and mastication are laboured and imperfect, the lips hang apart and saliva trickles from between them. Emotional movements of the face are apt to be grotesquely exaggerated, the whole face being contorted into a smile or into an expression of woe. Spasmodic and uncontrollable laughter or weeping may occur from time to time upon what would for the normal person be quite inadequate stimuli. The limbs show some measure of spasticity with the clumsiness that always accompanies this. Added to this picture of physical disability and emotional instability is a progressive dementia.

Differential Diagnosis.—The clinical picture of arterio-sclerotic Parkinsonism may lead to a diagnosis of paralysis agitans without tremor, but the two states do not develop along the same lines. In the former the dementia is early and increasing, the blood pressure is commonly high, and there are the general indications of atheroma. In paralysis agitans, on the other hand, it is rare to find any appreciable dementia until the malady is in its terminal stages, while a level of systolic blood pressure much above the normal for the subject's age is excessively rare, nor does it terminate in massive cerebral lesions. In fact, it is very exceptional for cerebral hæmorrhage or thrombosis to occur during the long drawn-out course of paralysis agitans.

Pseudobulbar palsy may be confused with the spastic type of motor neurone disease (chronic bulbar palsy) in which the nervous lesion is a slow degeneration unconnected with vascular disease. In motor neurone disease the history of recurrent vascular episodes is lacking and the evolution of the clinical picture is essentially a gradual one. In the chronic, slowly developing state first described in this section there are certain features which may make differentiation from cerebral tumour difficult. In elderly persons the clinical picture of tumour, when this lesion is present, is always a blurred one. Papillœdema is rarely intense, headache not marked, and vomiting uncommon. If any error be made it is more likely to be in diagnosing tumour when arterial degeneration alone is present than the reverse. The retinal changes, the mental deterioration, the occasional presence of a hemiparesis all combine to suggest the presence of an expanding lesion. In other words, the differentiation of cerebral tumour from the vascular lesions that may resemble it clinically in elderly subjects calls for a sound working knowledge of general medicine.

The Treatment of Cerebral Arterial Degeneration.—Before considering details of treatment when cerebral lesions and paralyses arising therefrom have to be dealt with, a few generalizations upon the general management of the subject with hypertension and cerebral vascular disease may usefully be made.

In considering this we must bear in mind the very narrow limits within which we can hope to influence these states. They are essentially wearing-out processes in the arterial tree, and with them we necessarily fight a losing battle. Hypertension cannot be permanently reduced. Indeed, one of the consequences of unwise attempts to reduce it materially by dietary restrictions, purgation and other means may be to precipitate a cerebral thrombosis.

The "starvation" treatments so popular amongst certain classes of educated but gullible persons, and the extravagant notions entertained by them of the nutritive and health-giving properties of salads and fruit juices as substitutes for food, are not rarely followed in elderly hypertensive subjects by a too rapid fall in blood pressure, marked fatigue, and the development of cerebral softening. What this semi-starvation does not achieve unaided in the way of disaster, a commonly associated obsession about the action of the bowels and an addiction to saline purgatives may bring about.

If these foolish practices are usually indulged in at the behest of "healers" and cranks without medical training, it can hardly be denied that the ground has long been prepared for them by the dismal forebodings sometimes uttered to the subjects of hypertension by their duly qualified medical advisers, and by the excessive dietary and other restrictions imposed by them. Therefore, when a patient seeks advice for symptoms associated with, and probably caused by, developing cerebral arterial disease, such, for example, as accesses of dizziness, excessive fatigue, or frequent headaches, it is well to remember that there are limits beyond which it is neither justifiable nor useful to interfere with his life. If he be habitually gross in his feeding and drinking, if he works to excess or takes some form of exercise unsuited to his state, these habits must be corrected. On the other hand, it can rarely be necessary to forbid all alcohol or meat to such an individual, or to render his life a vegetative one by restrictions on his activities. More often than not the patient's regime of life is a moderate and reasonable one, and in these circumstances only minimal restrictions should be imposed.

There is a danger that drugs or other measures that cause a rapid fall in systolic pressure may precipitate a vascular disaster. For patients suffering from hypertension, with or without hypertensive retinitis, and complaining of headaches, vertigo or excessive fatigue, or sleep-lessness, theobromine and phenobarbitone (**B.P.C.** tablet night and morning) are useful, and 50 to 100 mgms. of nicotinic acid daily may also be given. Potassium iodide has the sanction of long usage, but is of uncertain efficacy. In no chronic and progressive malady are common sense in treatment, and an insight into the needs and weaknesses of human nature on the part of the doctor more essential. If he cannot increase his patient's expectation of life, he can at least refrain from being to him a bird of ill-omen and a cutter-off of those creature comforts and relatively harmless habits which have become part of life to the patient and are thus so much dearer to the old than to the young. It is probable that physical fatigue, especially when of long standing, is an important precipitating factor in cerebral thrombosis, in that it leads to a fall in blood pressure below the level at which an adequate arterial blood flow through the diseased cerebral arteries can be maintained. It is exceedingly common in the history of such a patient to find that a period of great fatigue preceded the "stroke." It is, therefore, essential that as far as possible the patient with hypertension and other indications of progressive cerebral arterial degeneration should be safeguarded by a regime of life well within his capacity for exertion, mental and physical. To ensure this is more likely to increase his expectation of useful life than are drastic changes in his long-standing dietary habits, or schemes of medication. Certainly, after a thrombotic seizure, however slight and rapidly recovered from, the patient should be persuaded to revise his way of life if this appears to be unduly strenuous.

The Treatment of Hæmorrhage and Softening.—It is probable that treatment has no influence upon the outcome of hæmorrhage into the cerebral hemisphere, but when the patient is stertorous, with a bounding pulse and a cyanotic flush, venesection may be tried. In softening the cerebral circulation is already gravely impeded and depletion by venesection can only add to the embarrassment. Steps should, therefore, be taken to support the circulation. The violent purgation that was formerly in favour is not indicated and the bowels should be moved during the initial period by enemata. The patient should be kept supine, with the head slightly raised and turned to one side when the respiration tends to be impeded by the tongue falling back against the fauces. The bladder must be watched, as retention and over-distension are not uncommon, and the development of rest-lessness in the semi-comatose patient is not rarely due to discomfort arising from this source. The intermittent passage of urine in the bed is not necessarily an indication that the bladder has been emptied, for no more than an overflow incontinence may be in question. When the patient is able to swallow, liquid food may be given.

The care of pressure points should be attended to from the outset. In heavily built subjects bedsores may develop early over sacrum or heels. Periodical changes in position may be necessary to facilitate movement of both sides of the chest, and to avert œdema of the bases of the lungs.

Once consciousness is restored the care of the paralysed limbs calls for attention. This question will be dealt with subsequently in Chapter XXV (pages 302 to 304).

CEREBRAL ANEURYSM AND SUBARACHNOID HÆMORRHAGE

Several references have been made in the present chapter to the ætiology, site, and symptomatology of cerebral aneurysms, but they are sufficiently important to call for further brief consideration. From what has been said of their varied causation it will be clear that aneurysms may be present at all ages from childhood onwards. They may never give rise to symptoms during life. They may reach such a size as to produce symptoms of pressure on adjacent nervous structures, or they may rupture with the production of hæmorrhage into the subarachnoid space.

(1) *Unruptured Cerebral Aneurysm.*—It is when situated on the internal carotid artery that pressure symptoms are most likely to arise, and the clinical picture is a fairly constant one. If the optic nerve be compressed there will be loss of vision and the development of primary optic atrophy. It is exceptional for general pressure signs within the skull to arise. The cranial nerves (3, 4, 5, 6) lying near the aneurysm and in the neighbourhood of the cavernous sinus may be pressed upon so that there is ptosis, diplopia, and squint. Pressure on the ophthalmic division of the fifth nerve gives rise to pain, sometimes severe and continuous, in the region of the eye and forehead. Finally, the eye on the side of the lesion may be proptosed. The onset of symptoms is sometimes sudden, owing either to a sudden increase in the size of the aneurysm, or to leakage of blood therefrom. The problems of differential diagnosis that may arise have already been discussed in the chapter on intracranial tumour (page 78).

(2) *Subarachnoid Hæmorrhage.*—This is most often seen before the middle period of life and may be called the apoplexy of young adults. Its clinical picture and course depend upon the severity of the hæmorrhage. When this is small in amount the onset, which is invariably heralded by sudden and intense headache, may not be followed by any loss of consciousness, but when abundant and unchecked, deep coma passing on to death within a few hours may be the result. It is when

there is also bleeding into the substance of the brain, sometimes even into the ventricles, that this last issue is most often seen.

In the ordinary case of moderate severity, the intense headache may be followed immediately by an epileptiform convulsion and coma. In cases that survive, this last is of short duration, a matter of a few hours, the patient gradually regaining consciousness. In this process he may pass through a period of restless delirium in which there are indications that the headache remains severe. Indeed, it may persist with waning intensity for two or three weeks. The temperature may rise after a few hours and remain swinging slightly round 99° F. to 100° F. for about a week when, in recovering cases, it finally drops to normal. The pulse may be slow, from 60 down to 55 or even 50 per minute. In fatal cases it tends to grow feeble and rapid towards the end. For about forty-eight hours, after which they disappear, there may be massive albuminuria and some glycosuria. Lumbar puncture reveals blood in the cerebrospinal fluid. With degress of hæmorrhage insufficient to produce unconsciousness, the picture from the outset is one of intense meningeal irritation, with headache, rigidity of neck and spine and Kernig's sign, but otherwise one not differing from that already described. Even in the comatose subject examination in the initial stages reveals these signs, and here as in the case of other varieties of meningeal irritation the tendon jerks may be diminished. The plantar responses are usually of the extensor type. Inconstant symptoms are squint and diplopia, œdema of the optic discs, retinal hæmorrhages, and smallness and sluggishness of reaction of the pupils to light. Finally, in the course of a few weeks all symptoms disappear. During the first fortnight there is always the possibility of fresh hæmorrhage, which may be fatal, and in the case of large aneurysms frequent headache may persist.

If there has been irruption of blood into the brain (meningo-cerebral hæmorrhage), hemiplegia is added to the symptom-complex and may remain as a spastic hemiparesis. When in what at first appears to be a cerebral vascular lesion associated with hemiplegia, there is added severe and persisting headache, stiffness of the neck with pain in the back, sometimes extending down into the legs, the intra-cerebral and subarachnoid rupture of a cerebral aneurysm on the middle cerebral artery—where this lies mesial to the Sylvian fossa in the posterior perforated space—should be suspected, and its presence verified by lumbar puncture.

Prognosis.—On the whole, recovery from the original attack is more common than a fatal issue. When recovery appears to be complete after the requisite period of convalescence is passed, no further trouble may be experienced and probably the majority of individuals thereafter lead lives of normal health and activity. Indeed it may well

H

be in some cases that the healing process in the wall of a small aneurysm may make it stronger than it was before the rupture. In some instances, however, one or more recurrences may occur at varying intervals of time.

Treatment.—When consciousness is not lost, or if with semi-coma the patient is restless, the administration of morphia is indicated (gr. $\frac{1}{6}$ to gr. $\frac{1}{3}$). This dose may have to be repeated when severe headache persists. It is an open question whether lumbar puncture is advisable in the initial stage when diagnosis is not in doubt. Of course if it be in doubt, lumbar puncture may be needed to confirm the presence of blood in the subarachnoid space. When this is the case, the fluid may be so abundantly mixed with blood as to look like venous blood. All degrees of admixture may be encountered, and in old cases the fluid may have a sherry or yellowish colour after the red cells have been centrifuged down. If the pulse remains slow or falls progressively in rate below about 65, repeated lumbar puncture may be resorted to to reduce intracranial pressure, of which the slow pulse is an indication. It is possible, too, that the relief of headache may be an indication for puncture. It has been argued, however, that this procedure may lead to recurrence of bleeding, and, therefore, *it should not be resorted to as a routine measure.*

During the first week it may be necessary to give analgesics to relieve headache. The patient must be kept absolutely at rest in bed, however favourable the progress of the case, for at least a month— preferably for six weeks—and thereafter the resumption of activity must be gradual and carefully supervised. A complete convalescence should never be less than six months, even if the patient be symptom-free. It is probably a counsel of safety to advise against violent exertion at all times in persons who have had subarachnoid hæmorrhage, but in view of the fact that most of them are relatively young the temptation to frighten them into permanent valetudinarianism should be avoided. If life is to be worth living, some risks must be taken.

SINUS THROMBOSIS : CORTICAL THROMBO-PHLEBITIS

Thrombosis of the cerebral venous sinuses may occur in marantic infants, as a terminal phenomenon, in association with middle ear suppuration and with infections of the face. Attention has recently been drawn to the occurrence of hydrocephalus as a result of superior longitudinal sinus thrombosis in children with middle ear disease, and the occurrence of hemiplegia and other cerebral symptoms in women during the lying-in period or after abortion has also been correlated with thrombosis of this sinus, with or without accompanying thrombosis of cortical veins. Gowers suggested that some cases of infantile hemiplegia with an onset with convulsions and coma might be due to thrombosis of the superior longitudinal sinus and cortical veins. Occasionally an adult case of what appears to be cerebral (arterial) thrombosis, ushered in by convulsions, focal or general, may, in fact, be one of cortical thrombo-phlebitis. Cerebral sinus thrombosis in women during the puerperium probably arises in the following way. The pelvic veins have long been known to anatomists to communicate with the vertebral system of veins, and this with the cerebral dural sinuses. If, as commonly happens in the circumstances named, the patient is wearing a tight binder and has thrombosis in the pelvic veins, any fragment of clot detached from the latter may find its way, not as commonly into the caval system of veins, but into the vertebral veins whence it may reach the superior longitudinal sinus. Here it may become attached to the sinus wall, or to the wall of one of the tributary cortical veins, where it forms the nucleus of a larger clot and may set up a local inflammation of the vessel wall (*cortical thrombo-phlebitis*). Thus, during the second week of the puerperium the signs and symptoms of this cerebral complication may develop.

Again, in middle ear disease in children, superior longitudinal sinus thrombosis may ensue, and may obstruct the re-absorption of cerebrospinal fluid, via the pacchionian bodies, into the venous system. A hydrocephalus may thus be produced. The carriage of infection by venous channels from the face may lead to cavernous sinus thrombosis.

Symptomatology.—The symptoms peculiar to thrombosis of the different sinuses were fully described by Gowers as long as fifty years ago, and may be summarized as follows:—

Superior longitudinal sinus.—A condition of stupor leading to coma may develop, and there are headache, sickness, and papillœdema. When the cortical veins become subsequently involved there ensue convulsions and hemiplegia. If, as may happen in the case of lying-in women and by the mechanism already described, the veins are involved earlier than the sinus, the onset is with convulsions, coma, and hemiplegia. Death may result, or recovery with residual hemiparesis or without any residual disability. Thrombosis of veins in the pelvis precede the cerebral complication. In children with middle ear disease, the development of superior longitudinal sinus thrombosis is indicated by headache and papillœdema and sometimes by stupor or coma.

Cavernous sinus.—This is commonly infective and the patient is clearly gravely ill and with a high temperature. There is proptosis, œdema of the eyelids, cranial nerve palsies (3, 4, 6) and some œdema of the optic disc.

Diagnosis.—It is hydrocephalus (otitic hydrocephalus) associated with middle ear disease and the sinus and cortical venous thrombosis of lying-in women that constitute the main neurological problems of sinus thrombosis. In the former, the development of headache and other symptoms of raised intracranial tension raise the question of abscess, meningitis, or hydrocephalus. In the last named, the cerebrospinal fluid is under increased pressure but remains normal in composition. In meningitis and abscess there is usually some meningeal reaction (lymphocytosis, etc.) in this fluid. The development of coma, hemiplegia, or convulsions during the puerperium should lead the observer to suspect sinus thrombosis and to look for evidence of pelvic or femoral vein thrombosis.

Treatment.—When there is reason to suspect thrombosis of pelvic veins after parturition or abortion the patient should be propped up in bed and the abdominal binder loosened. For raised intracranial tension the steps described on page 86 should be adopted, and for convulsions those described in connection with status epilepticus. For otitic hydrocephalus repeated lumbar puncture may suffice, it being assumed that the original focus of infection in the ear has been dealt with.

CHAPTER V

Epilepsy : Idiopathic and Symptomatic

INTRODUCTION

THE fit, which is the characteristic, indeed the only essential, feature of epilepsy varies so widely in character that a definition of it except in very general terms is not easy to give. It may be said, however, that it is the expression of a sudden and transient disturbance of cerebral function. If the disturbance be widespread there will be loss or alteration of consciousness. If the disturbance be localized, consciousness may be unimpaired. In either case sudden and transient symptoms, motor, sensory or purely mental, may be present, and they commonly take the form of "positive" symptoms; that is, motor spasm, abnormal sensations, or special sense phenomena. The "negative" symptom of transient weakness of a limb may also occur.

In what is called idiopathic epilepsy there is probably always some disturbance of consciousness, but in focal or Jacksonian fits only motor spasm or positive sensory symptoms may occur.

Ætiology.—Although epilepsy was amongst the first of all maladies to be recognized and described, and though for the best part of the past century it has been the subject of intensive research, its ætiology and nature remain incompletely elucidated. Its clinical features are, indeed, familiar, but its causation, the nature of the physiological disorder of function that shows itself as the fit, and the question of the heritable qualities of epilepsy are not yet matters of general agreement. It is known that recurrent epileptic fits may occur throughout life in otherwise healthy individuals, and this tendency is what we speak of as idiopathic epilepsy, but it is also known that fits indistinguishable from these may occur as symptoms of a wide range of pathological processes in the brain, and may be included in the symptomatology of diverse forms of intoxication. In consequence some maintain that epilepsy is a symptom pure and simple and not what has been called a clinical entity, and that it would be better to speak of "the epilepsies" according to the various known exciting factors than to keep the category of idiopathic epilepsy. Nevertheless, from the practical points of view of diagnosis and of treatment the two categories of "idiopathic" and "symptomatic" epilepsy remain useful and will be here employed.

Epilepsy has no morbid anatomy that has yet been discovered with the resources at our disposal. It consists in the recurrence of fits for a greater or less span of the individual's life, and the mental deterioration that may be found in some severe cases is no necessary part of the malady.

It has always been regarded as a heritable condition, though it obeys no known laws of inheritance, and it is probable that what is inherited—if anything be—is an instability of function in the cells of the cerebral cortex. Given contributory circumstances in the life of the individual thus defective, the instability may so increase as to overflow in a fit. In the idiopathic case nothing is known of what these exciting factors may be. In predisposed persons whose instability is less pronounced some gross disturbance is needed to provoke fits, such as a new growth in the brain, an inflammatory lesion, an injury, or an intoxication. In a sense, therefore, all epilepsy may be symptomatic.

Certainly the heritable qualities of epilepsy have been greatly exaggerated in the past, and in consequence severe restrictions upon the liberty of conduct of the epileptic have been imposed in the guise of medical advice; as, for example, in the matter of marriage and reproduction. The most recent statistical information indicates that direct transmission of epilepsy is exceptional, and the writer's experience is wholly in accord with this conclusion.

Of the physiological disturbance of nervous action that accompanies the fit, it has been shown that the normal rhythm of action currents (Berger rhythm) produced in the nerve cells of the cerebral cortex, which are regular in amplitude and frequency, undergoes characteristic changes during the course of epileptic fits. These changes, recorded by a suitable amplifying apparatus, constitute the electro-encephalogram (E.E.G.). Thus in the minor fit we may see alternating slow and fast spike-like waves, in the major fit a rapid rhythm of fast and large waves. Other characteristic patterns of cortical potential have also been described in epilepsy, and the most recent studies tend to stress the great difficulty in correlating the disorders of cortical rhythm revealed in the E.E.G. with clinical epilepsy. There can be no doubt, however, that upon occasion—though not invariably—the E.E.G. may provide confirmatory evidence of value in the recognition of doubtful epileptiform attacks and in the differentiation of epilepsy from hysterical fits. It will be seen, therefore, that the E.E.G. may provide information of essential importance in differentiating epileptic from hysterical fits—the cortical rhythm being undisturbed in the latter—and also in the recognition of clinically doubtful minor fits. It has also been claimed that the presence and site of such a local lesion as a tumour may be detected by changes in the rhythm of cortical potentials produced by it.

This diagnostic procedure has, however, certain limitations. Thus variations in cortical rhythm characteristic of epilepsy are to be found in some 10 per cent. of the population, while clinically recognizable epilepsy is found in no more than 0·5 per cent. Thus an abnormal E.E.G. may be found in a subject who has never had clinically discoverable fits: that is, who is not epileptic. Again, it has been estimated that as large a proportion of epileptics as 20 per cent. may show a normal E.E.G., while finally various pathological lesion of the brain and abnormal mental states may yield abnormal cortical rhythms.

The presence of abnormalities of cortical electrical activity cannot yet be accepted as a final elucidation of the essential process that underlies the epileptic fit, for all we can say of it is that it is a phenomenon accompanying the fit. That it stands in a causal relation to the fit is not yet established, and hence the recent definition of epilepsy as a "cortical dysrhythmia" makes an assumption that has still to be justified.

No constant or characteristic disorders of metabolism, or of endocrine functions, have ever been discovered in the epileptic subject, nor is there any macroscopic or histological lesion in the brain that can be correlated with the production of fits.

IDIOPATHIC EPILEPSY almost always makes its first appearance before adult life is reached; the age periods at which it is perhaps most prone to begin are infancy, the age of puberty and during the passing of adolescence into adult life. Whether infantile convulsions are necessarily to be regarded as the onset of epilepsy is not a matter upon which it is easy to pronounce definitely, but it can be said that these convulsions appear far more commonly in the early history of epileptic than of non-epileptic subjects. Its sex incidence is approximately equal. As has already been mentioned in the chapter on intracranial tumours, the appearance for the first time in middle life of epileptic fits often betokens the presence of some structural cerebral lesion; that is, such fits belong to the symptomatic category and not to the idiopathic.

Symptoms.—It is the recurrence of fits that constitutes what we call epilepsy, and in this respect there are the widest possible differences between individual cases. There are two main varieties of fits, the major and the minor, and their features will be subsequently described. Some subjects suffer from both forms, others from one or other only. The frequency of the attacks varies widely. They may be of almost daily occurrence or be separated by much longer periods of time—weeks or months. They may occur in small groups at short intervals separated by long intervals of freedom. They may have a special time incidence in the twenty-four-hour period. In some subjects the fits are wholly or almost wholly nocturnal, occurring within an hour or two of the change from waking to sleeping. In others they occur during the first hour or two after rising in the morning and at no other time, while in yet others they may occur at any time.

A patient may be subject to very frequent minor fits and to occasional major fits. Again, after several years of liability to minor attacks, major fits may make their appearance. A patient liable to major attacks may pass into status epilepticus, in which fit succeeds fit without intervening restoration of consciousness. In yet other subjects, slight localized twitchings of muscles without other disturbance may occur between fits, increasing in frequency as a fit approaches.

On the whole it may be said that there seems a greater liability to an attack in all epileptic subjects when they are at rest, mentally or physically. When free from attacks the subject may feel perfectly well and be mentally and emotionally normal, and many epileptics whose attacks are nocturnal only, or of a slight character (as may be the case with minor fits), lead physically and intellectually active and useful lives.

In others, however, the temperament may be altered. The child subject to frequent fits is apt to be intractable, untidy, destructive with his clothes and toys, and quarrelsome. It is, however, an exaggeration to say, as has been said, that there is a characteristic epileptic temperament which can be identified as such even when no fits are observed. In the most severe cases with an onset in childhood mental deterioration may set in, the general physical condition may fall off, the child may become dirty in habits, incoherent and almost inarticulate, and finally bedridden.

On the other hand, cases are known in which, after one or more fits, the affection disappears finally. It is not uncommon for a series of fits to occur at the critical periods of life, during the first year or two, at puberty, and at about the age of twenty. In girls and women the day before the menstrual period may show a special liability to an attack, though this is by no means invariable. It is common for fits to cease in a pregnant woman, recurring after parturition. The converse is known, but is exceptional.

Almost any disturbance of bodily function may lead to the appearance of attacks in the epileptic subject, such as indigestion or constipation. On the other hand, fits have been known to cease during the course of a febrile illness.

The Minor Fit: "Petit Mal."—This consists of a momentary disturbance of consciousness, ranging from a change so slight as to be scarcely perceptible, to complete loss, in which the patient falls to the ground. The infant seated in his nursery chair may suddenly let his head fall forward on to his mug or plate on the little shelf before him, and as quickly lift his head again. The older patient may drop what he is holding, stop for an instant in the flow of his speech and then resume where he left off. The observer looking at the patient will note, perhaps, a sudden lapse of fixation in his gaze, often described as "a vacant look," the eyes may turn up or to one side, the lids may flicker, a brief feeble convulsive movement of face or hand may be seen, a flushing or sudden pallor.

When consciousness is totally lost for two or more seconds, the subject may not be able to pick up his train of thought or action immediately and may have to be reminded of this. An essential feature of these phenomena is their transience. They have passed within a minute, but this is not to say that the patient is as quickly restored to *normal* consciousness. After minor attacks there is—in some subjects only—an intervening period of abnormal or incomplete consciousness before the normal state of mind is restored. In this period, which may last for a few minutes or for as long as an hour or more, the subject appears fully conscious, but he is not normally in touch with his environment or in full possession of his faculties. In these circumstances he may be seen to perform a number of simple or complicated acts that are inappropriate, and may upon occasion prove socially embarrassing or even bring the subject within the ambit of the law. The conduct so displayed is spoken of as "*post-epileptic automatism,*" and is a phenomenon with which the doctor should be familiar. The automatism of a given epileptic is often stereotyped. He may take off his collar and tie and put them in his pocket, he may proceed to undress himself more completely, he may empty his bladder deliberately, he may pick up and purloin any loose object within his reach, he may make a series of what appear irrelevant remarks, he may become pugnacious, or may walk from the room, or through a French window if one be handy.

Finally, normal consciousness is restored and the patient may be said to find himself again. This moment arrived, he is found to have no knowledge of any acts performed during his period of automatism, though he may see their consequences and thus deduce what has happened to him.

It will be readily understood that when so complex a train of events follow a transient blunting of consciousness that may not have been observed, in a person not known to be subject to minor epilepsy, the most erroneous deductions may be drawn, but the recurrence of such episodes and their more or less unvarying form in a given individual should put the medical adviser, when one is consulted, upon the scent. It is not intended to convey, however, that automatism is a common sequel of the minor fit. In some subjects it never occurs.

The Major Fit: "Grand Mal."—In this variety of fit there is a relatively constant sequence of events. About 50 per cent. of epileptics have an aura before consciousness is lost. This is commonly an indefinable sensation in the epigastrium, but it may consist in some special sense aura, *e.g.* flashes of light, a formed image, an unpleasant sense of smell or taste. It may be more complex and consist in the idea that the patient is somewhere familiar and is looking at a scene he has seen before. On the other hand a motor phenomenon may immediately precede the onset, such as a spasm of an arm, a turning of the head and eyes to one side. Some erroneously believe that this motor effect denotes that the fit is a true Jacksonian attack, and as such indicative of an underlying local cerebral lesion, and it is, therefore, necessary to emphasize that it is simply one of the known ways in which the onset of a major epileptic fit may be heralded.

After these momentary preliminaries, consciousness is suddenly lost, the patient sometimes uttering a guttural cry as this happens. He falls to the ground, the entire skeletal musculature enters into strong tonic spasm which arrests the respiratory movements. As a result the patient becomes cyanosed, "black in the face." If the strength of spasm is not equally distributed through the musculature the patient may turn over on his face, or perhaps only the head and eyes may be deviated, or one side of the face contorted. In a few seconds this tonic spasm intermits and a series of clonic jerking movements takes possession of the muscles. These persist for some seconds, becoming slower in rate, and finally, after a powerful jerk, they cease and the patient lapses into a flaccid coma. During this clonic phase the breath is forcibly expressed at each spasm, froth may be expelled from the mouth, and the tongue may be bitten if it be protruded between the teeth when the jaw goes into spasm. When this happens the froth may be blood-stained. Also during this phase there may be incontinence of urine, less often of fæces, and still more rarely a seminal emission. Some subjects almost invariably wet themselves and bite the tongue, while others convulsed with apparently equal violence never do so. The pulse may be rapid and forceful.

As the stage of flaccid coma arrives, the examination of the patient becomes practicable. The pupils are found dilated and the corneal reflexes absent. The tendon jerks may also be missing and the plantar responses are of the extensor type.

Rapidly the reflexes return to normal and consciousness begins to return, to be fully restored in a further minute or two. During this stage of returning consciousness the patient may be confused and disoriented. Vomiting, or more commonly headache, may then ensue, and in many cases the patient passes into a deep sleep.

After a severe fit a slight rise of temperature (half to one degree F.) may occur. In status epilepticus fit succeeds fit without intervening recovery of consciousness for one or more hours. In prolonged status there may be a progressive rise of temperature to 103 or even 105 degrees F. In these circumstances the issue may be fatal, the patient succumbing to heart failure. Again, in chronic epilepsy a bout of fits may be followed by a phase of "epileptic mania" lasting for periods ranging from an hour to several days.

Fits of all grades of severity between the minimal minor attack and the severe seizure above described may be encountered. There are also bizarre variants on both types, such as attacks in which the disturbance of consciousness consists in transient abnormal emotional states, in complex visual or auditory hallucinations. Such attacks are spoken of as psychic fits. Their recognition must depend upon their recurrence and constancy of form in a given patient.

Again, there are fits which appear to be precipitated by specific stimuli, such as the sound of music, a sudden movement from a state of rest, or some cutaneous stimulus. In what has been called laryngeal epilepsy, about of coughing may precipitate—and be the sole precipitant of—a major fit. The condition is uncommon, and the subject is usually a short, stoutly built man of middle age with chronic tracheitis, laryngitis, or bronchitis.

The Jacksonian or Focal Fit.—The essential feature of this is that the underlying cerebral disturbance begins in a circumscribed cortical region. It may remain confined to this, or it may spread to adjacent regions, in some instances becoming generalized so that consciousness is lost and the picture of a major epileptic fit is produced. From the fact that the onset of change in the brain is local, the initial manifestations of the fit correspond in character to the functions subserved by the discharging focus. Thus it may be motor, sensory, gustatory, auditory, or visual. If the change then spreads, other manifestations are added according to the direction of spread. The most familiar variety of Jacksonian fit is that which starts in the motor cortex. It begins with a localized clonic spasm, the usual regions of initial involvement being the angle of the mouth, the thumb and index finger, or the great toe. The convulsion may then spread in an ordered progress from the point of onset; thus, it may spread from the angle of the mouth to the remaining facial muscles, then to those of the neck and eyes, so that head and eyes deviate. Starting in the hand it may spread up the arm to the shoulder, trunk, thigh and leg muscles. Should convulsion spread to the muscles of the opposite side consciousness is commonly lost and the convulsion then becomes generalized.

When the uncinate gyrus is the focus of onset, the fit consists in a sensation of an unpleasant smell or taste, accompanied by a dreamy mental state in which the patient may lick or smack his lips.

Other varieties of attack corresponding to disturbance in the sensory or visual regions of the cortex may occur. It is widely believed that such fits invariably point to the presence of some local structural lesion in the cerebral cortex that might be amenable to surgical treatment. This may indeed be the case, but it must be emphasized that not infrequently exploratory craniotomy reveals no macroscopic change and none is present, and in some instances a Jacksonian fit may be no more than a variant of idiopathic epilepsy.

Diagnosis.—It is in the nature of things that diagnosis must very commonly be made upon the account of fits given by observers who, from unfamiliarity with epilepsy and from the stress of emotion which seeing the fit evokes in them, are not the most reliable of witnesses. Nevertheless, there is a degree of constancy about the major fit that rarely leaves considerable doubt when a reasonably good account is available. The story of the aura, of the guttural cry which betokens the onset, the cyanosis, convulsion, tongue-biting or other injury, frothing at the mouth, and incontinence of urine all go to make up an unequivocal picture. More difficulty may beset the recognition of minor fits. In both cases the fact of recurrence, the more or less stereotyped form of each attack, its relatively brief duration are all points of diagnostic importance. A negative physical examination is also of positive diagnostic value. Further, the general background of the case, the age of onset, and all the circumstances which mark the incidence of fits, as these have been already related usually make the diagnosis of epilepsy relatively simple. An experienced clinical judgment is still the most reliable diagnostic instrument in the case of epilepsy, but pressure of opinion, official, medical and lay, increasingly leads the clinician to seek the confirmation of his diagnosis by recourse to the electro-encephalograph. It cannot be claimed that this is infallible. The range of disorders of cortical electrical rhythm has proved to be wider than was at first thought, and other maladies than epilepsy may present one or other of these disorders, while, on the other hand, an unequivocal clinical case of epilepsy may yield a normal E.E.G., if not always, then at least sometimes.

In the case of infantile convulsions it is not always easy to decide whether they are to be dismissed as teething convulsions, or to be regarded—and treated—as epilepsy, and the matter will be dealt with under the heading of treatment.

The hysterical fit may also present diagnostic difficulties and the following generalizations as to its character may be made. There is no ordered sequence of events, there is no true loss of consciousness, there are no changes in the reflexes, no incontinence or tongue-biting, and the patient does not sustain injuries in her fall, nor fall in a dangerous place. The eyes are not passively closed as in true coma, but shut, and the attempt to open them with the finger is usually met with a tightening of the lids. The convulsion is not a matter of tonic and clonic stages but of wild struggling, which is aggravated by attempts at restraint. The greater the excitement aroused in those who flock to her succour, the more dramatic the fit. The patient who has to be "held down" by numerous persons and who "drags them across the floor" in her struggles is not having a major epileptic convulsion. The hysterical fit may appear to last for hours, phases of apparent unconscious swooning intermitting with phases of violent activity. Every hysteric is a law unto herself in the matter of fits as of other somatic symptoms. Here also, as in epilepsy, the general physical and mental background of the case must be taken into account. Originally coined by Charcot, the term "hystero-epilepsy" is still encountered from time to time. It has no place in clinical neurology, and its use betrays uncertainty in the mind of the observer as to what he is looking at, together with a natural desire to be right whatever the nature of the attack. A fit may be hysterical or it may be epileptic, or a minor fit may be followed by phenomena of automatism that suggest hysterical behaviour to the inexperienced observer, but there is not a hystero-epilepsy (see page 329).

THE FAINTING ATTACK (VASOVAGAL SYNCOPE).—While it is not rare for a minor or a mild major epileptic fit to be dismissed as a "faint," it is perhaps less common for the converse error to be made. Yet instances have occurred when this has been done, with serious consequences to the individual thus wrongly labelled as liable to fits.

The faint is a familiar example of sudden and transient cerebral anæmia, and though most frequently seen in the child or adolescent it may also occur in the adult. The factors which give rise to it are the fasting state, fatigue, unpleasant emotions, the debility that may follow illness, and confinement in a hot and ill-ventilated room. In weakly subjects the sudden assumption of the erect posture may suffice to induce a faint. A faint rarely occurs when the subject is lying down.

Symptoms.—The loss of consciousness which is the essential feature of the attack may be absolutely sudden, the subject falling precipitately, or it may be preceded by such warning symptoms as a sinking sensation in the abdomen, dryness of the mouth, nausea, sweating, a swimming feeling in the head, and a sensation of weakness and sagging of the legs. The face grows pale, the pulse feeble and almost imperceptible. Sometimes it becomes slightly irregular. The rate may fall as low as 50, but in some cases the pulse rate may rise. The blood pressure also falls to 60, 50, or even 40 mms. of mercury, and with this fall the subject loses consciousness. The muscles are flaccid, the pupils dilated and respiration sighing. With extreme fall of blood pressure there may be feeble convulsive movements of the face and limbs. These are never forceful and there is neither tongue-biting nor urinary incontinence.

In a few seconds the blood pressure begins to rise and the pulse to regain force and frequency. Complete consciousness returns rapidly, but the subject feels slack and inert for a few minutes and is then well again. A severe headache may then ensue.

The slowing or irregularity of the pulse betokens vagal inhibition, while the fall in blood pressure and the attendant loss of consciousness indicate splanchnic dilatation from vasomotor failure. Thus these attacks, and these alone, are entitled to the name of vasovagal syncope.*

Diagnosis.—In the majority of instances the circumstances leading to the attack and the general medical background of the patient render diagnosis simple. When, however, the loss of consciousness is sudden and convulsive movements are seen, the attack may be mistaken for an epileptic fit, and the ensuing headache may seem to confirm this view. In epilepsy the pulse remains full and normal, and does not react as in the true vasovagal attack.

Brief mention must be made of NARCOLEPSY, which may be confused with minor epilepsy by those unaware of its characters. The symptom-complex so named has two components: accesses of uncontrollable drowsiness only relieved by a short period of sleep, and transient accesses of muscular weakness. The latter are produced by sudden emotional stimuli, of which amusement with laughter is the one most commonly operative. Directly—to use a familiar phrase—the subject's fancy is tickled, he weakens, sags at the knees and cannot hold the arms elevated or extended if they chance to be in either of these positions.

Unless this symptom-complex is quite clearly described by the patient to an observer familiar with it, it is apt to be interpreted as epileptic in character. In the accesses of weakness—or cataplexy, as it is called—there is no diminution of consciousness. When present these symptoms are of daily occurrence.

SYMPTOMATIC EPILEPSY.—The considerations which lead to a diagnosis of symptomatic, as opposed to idiopathic, epilepsy are not questions of the form and features of the fits, but of all the circumstances in which they occur; such as the age of onset and their association with signs of bodily disease, injury, or intoxication. The fits of uræmia or of eclampsia differ in no essential clinical respect from those we have already described, and the same has already been said of the fits that may accompany the growth of an intracranial tumour. Thus in every case of fits in which the circumstances of their occurrence do not conform to what is usual in idiopathic epilepsy, or in which there are signs of organic disease of the brain or other organs, a diagnosis of

---

* This term, however, is widely used for a variety of ill-defined and ill-studied attacks Originally coined by Gowers, the term was applied by him to attacks characterized by a growing sense of præcordial and abdominal discomfort and a feeling of impending death. The extremities and face grow pale, but *consciousness is not lost*. The attack develops slowly and passes off slowly, lasting for as long as half an hour. Nothing is known of the heart's action in these attacks, and they were not personally observed by Gowers, but described to him by patients. As Gowers himself emphasized, the name of "vasovagal" attack cannot be strictly applied to them. Therefore the origins of the term are extremely unfortunate.

idiopathic epilepsy is safely made only by a process of exclusion. Fits may occur as a symptom in a wide range of diseases of the brain, but perhaps only as an exceptional symptom, and it may be suggested that in many instances of symptomatic epilepsy some congenital predisposition determines that a fit shall occur in a particular disease in a given individual. Head injuries provide an interesting commentary upon the multiplicity of factors that probably go to the production of a fit. Of such injuries fits are, on the whole, an exceptional sequel, yet when they occur it may be difficult to exculpate the injury as a precipitating factor. One source of fallacy besets the assessment of injury as a possible excitant of fits, namely, the not infrequent chance that in his first fit the patient may fall and sustain a head injury. He is thought to be concussed; the fact that he has had a fit is unnoticed, and all subsequent fits are attributed to the original fall and head injury, whereas these were but the sequels of a loss of consciousness. This possibility should always be borne in mind when a diagnosis of traumatic epilepsy is advanced.

One variety of symptomatic epilepsy, in which clinical examination may prove negative, should be briefly mentioned, namely the epilepsy of *cysticercosis* of the brain. The cysticercus stage of Tænia solium develops in the pig, and infestation of man by the adult tape worm comes from eating infected pork. If man accidentally ingests tape-worm eggs the resulting cysticercus tends to invade the brain, giving rise to recurrent generalized epileptic fits. Diagnosis depends upon the radiographic recognition of calcified cysts in the muscles, and these are also occasionally to be seen in radiograms of the head when they are situated in the brain. This infection accounts for a proportion of late cases of epilepsy in individuals who have lived abroad, particularly in the East.

Still another variety is that due to cortical venous angioma. Here, although the fits are commonly generalized, their mode of onset may be focal. The fits usually make their first appearance in the third or fourth decades of life, and for several years physical examination may be wholly negative. Finally, after a fit some residual symptoms are left: *e.g.* a hemiparesis, which is usually transient, but may in time become permanent. There are no indications of raised intracranial tension. A somewhat similar clinical course and picture are provided by certain cases of focal cortical atrophy of unknown origin. These are not rarely thought to be examples of a slow growing tumour, usually meningioma, and the history is one of recurrent epileptiform fits, focal or generalized, with focal paralytic signs: *e.g.* hemiparesis. Some degree of dementia may or may not be present, headache is common, but papillœdema is absent and the cerebrospinal fluid content and pressure are normal. Conclusive diagnosis calls for air studies (air encephalogram or ventriculogram) which reveal the degree and distribution of the atrophy. The age incidence of the condition is from 30 to 60.

Prognosis.—In idiopathic epilepsy it is virtually impossible to give a prognosis before a systematic course of treatment has been under trial for an adequate time, and this time is at least two or three years. It is a sound generalization that in the great majority of instances the liability to recurrence will not cease unless treatment be given. There are, of course, patients in whom fits cease spontaneously to occur, but the easy assumption that they will do so in any given instance is not one we have the right to make if doing so leads us to neglect treatment. When mental deterioration sets in, the prognosis as the recovery from the liability to continued fits is grave, but it is never prudent to give a bad prognosis to the patient or his relatives until treatment has had a fair trial. Yet there are few maladies in which doctors are more prone to wax gloomy when discussing prognosis, and the train of prohibitions which is often added by them may be a quite unnecessary addition to the patient's misfortune.

Treatment.—Certain guiding principles cannot be over-emphasized if success is to be achieved in the treatment of a case of epilepsy. These may be stated as follows:—

(1) There is no substitute for an absolutely regular medication maintained until the patient has been free from all indications of epilepsy *for a minimum period of three years*.

(2) When a given drug or combination of drugs proves unsuitable or inadequate for any reason it should be changed and not continued indefinitely.

(3) The patient's life should be interfered with as little as possible. This is especially the case with children, in whom the greatest care should be taken to avoid making the patient feel that he is different from other children.

Simple as these rules are, and long as they have been inculcated by those with most experience in the treatment of epilepsy, as often as not they are disregarded. In the case of children the unreasonable fear that continued medication will stunt the child's mental development, or in the case of adults that an addiction may be formed, too often leads, with the doctor's concurrence or not, to premature cessation of medication. Nothing could be more adverse to prognosis in the case of a child or adolescent who is developing recurrent fits than the too often given and fallacious counsel that he " will grow out of it" and, therefore, needs no treatment, or the equally unsound statement that nothing can be hoped for from treatment, which it is, therefore, futile to undertake. Far too many epileptic subjects of long standing are to be encountered who have been deprived of treatment in the early phases of their affliction on one or other of these specious pleas, both the expression of culpable ignorance. Also impatience may lead to its abandonment in favour of fantastic dietary habits that are at once so popular and so futile. These, together with carelessness, too often interfere with treatment, lead to failure, and produce a widespread despondency in patients and doctors alike. There is much to be said for allowing every patient under treatment always to carry a prescription, so that if his medicine runs short or his doctor is not readily available he can renew his supply and thus avoid those interruptions in treatment that militate so strongly against success. Whatever medicine is found to control fits should be continued in undiminished quantity for at least two years, lessening of the dose being carried out gradually throughout the third year. While this period of three years is the minimum safe period, in some cases special circumstances may indicate still more prolonged medication. If the fits are not completely controlled, treatment should be continued throughout life if necessary, for its cessation will allow the malady to increase in severity. Partial success may be all that is possible.

The substances of primary importance are the bromides and phenobarbitone.

It is probably wise when the case first comes under treatment to employ the bromides, preferably the sodium salt. A total of 30 grains in the 24-hour period is a reasonable initial dose, and it may be increased to 60 grains if necessary, but never higher. To avoid or to lessen the liability to the development of a bromide rash, liquor arsenicalis (m 2 to 3) may be given with each dose. Before raising the dose it is well to try the addition of tincture of belladonna (m 5 to m 10 t.d.s.) to the bromide. If bromide and belladonna prove inadequate, they may be combined with phenobarbitone in doses of from $\frac{1}{4}$ grain to 1 grain. Some patients tolerate bromide so badly that adequate doses cannot be given. Dark-complexioned subjects and those with greasy skins may develop bromism or acne, while a few others become dull and confused. In these circumstances a trial of phenobarbitone, alone or with tincture of belladonna, should be made. It is rarely necessary to give a total daily dosage of the former of more than $4\frac{1}{2}$ grains, but doses of from m 5 to m 15 of the tincture may be given according to effect and to tolerance.

In a few cases, the addition of phenazone ($2\frac{1}{2}$ to 5 grains) or of tincture of digitalis (m 5) may serve to improve the results obtained by the drugs of primary importance: namely, bromide and phenobarbitone. Borax and potassium borotartrate (10 grains to the dose) may be tried when other remedies fail, preferably in combination with these.

Recently, the attempt has been made to give larger doses of phenobarbitone than those mentioned, the narcotic effects being counteracted

I

by the additional administration of benzedrine sulphate (15 to 30 milligrams daily).

For some cases the best results are obtained by the use of sodium diphenyl hydantoinate (Epanutin, Dilantin, Solantoin), either alone or with phenobarbitone. The dose is from 1½ grains to 3 grains twice or thrice daily for an adult, or ½ grain for a child.

Occasionally toxic symptoms follow the use of this drug. In mild cases, ataxy of movement, dizziness, tremor, nausea and even diplopia may develop, while in more severe intolerance various forms of dermatitis, some of them purpuric, have appeared during the first week of administration. In patients who seemingly tolerate the drug well, marked hyperplasia of the gums may ensue upon prolonged administration. Its advantages are that it may control fits that have not responded to other forms of medication and that it has no sedative effect.

When a change-over from phenobarbitone to sodium diphenyl hydantoinate is being made, it should not be sudden, but the administration of the two should be dovetailed, as it were, the phenobarbitone being reduced gradually over a period of two weeks.

The distribution of the chosen drug or combination of drugs throughout the 24-hour period will depend upon the circumstances in each case. For example, when fits are wholly or mainly nocturnal the main dose is given in the evening, a smaller dose in the morning.

Before treatment is begun it is always impossible to say what drug or combination of drugs, and in what dosage, will yield the best results, and many changes may be necessary to achieve an optimum result. In short, a favourable result requires that all concerned should be ready to take trouble. Most difficult of all cases to treat successfully are those children who have very numerous daily attacks of petit mal. Often these fail completely to respond to the various remedies to be considered below. Such cases, however, frequently undergo marked spontaneous improvement after puberty is established, and then become amenable to treatment. In fact the years from about 9 to 13 are the most difficult ones in the matter of treatment in cases of the kind.

Status epilepticus is best dealt with by giving 4 to 6 drachms of paraldehyde by rectum, or three grains of soluble phenobarbitone hypodermically. These doses may have to be repeated, and in some cases large doses of bromide by nasal tube (30 grs.) repeated once or twice at hourly or two hourly intervals may prove the most effective. An enema may also be given. If, as sometimes happens, the patient shows signs of collapse, cardiac stimulants and easily assimilable liquid nourishment may be necessary. An infant who has two or more convulsions without any adequate exciting cause is probably best treated in the matter of medication as a potential epileptic and kept under treatment for at least two years.

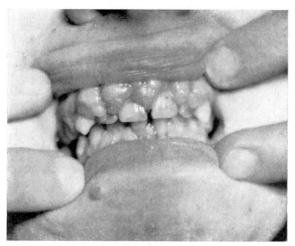

FIG. 27.

HYPERPLASIA OF THE GUMS AFTER PROLONGED ADMINISTRA-
TION OF SODIUM DIPHENYL HYDANTOINATE.

To face page 130.

In general, surgery has little place in the treatment of epilepsy, save when there is a history of a head injury and clinical indications of a focal onset of fits. In what has been referred to as laryngeal epilepsy, it appears that treatment of the chronic respiratory tract affection may suffice to prevent recurrence, but it is probably wise to "cover" the patient by at least a short period (*e.g.* six months) of medication on the lines already laid down.

Narcolepsy does not respond to any of the remedies of value in epilepsy, but does so remarkably to the administration of benzedrine sulphate in doses of from 10 to 20 milligrams twice daily. The second dose should not be given later than the early afternoon. Given at night it interferes with sleep. The signs of overdosage are excitability, restlessness, and dilatation of the pupils.

The general management of a case of epilepsy involves the regulation of the bowels, the taking of regular meals and the avoidance of eating between meals. A plain mixed diet is usually best. Abstinence from meat and fish presents no advantages. In children whose fits are refractory to treatment a trial may be made of a ketogenic diet, but unless this is strictly adhered to and the urine regularly tested for the presence of acetone bodies, it is not worth undertaking. Alcohol should be entirely debarred. Certain restrictions in activity are important. The epileptic subject should not drive a car, swim, or place himself in positions of obvious danger. On the other hand, physical exercises and games should never be forbidden, especially to a young person, except upon grave and quite definite reasons. It must often happen that some risks have to be taken if the patient's life is not to be made intolerable. Marriage of itself has no influence upon epilepsy, pregnancy may bring it temporarily to a stop, and—as has been said—the direct transmission of epilepsy from parent to child is exceptional.

The considerations which govern marriage and reproduction are rather personal and sociological than medical and can scarcely be said to be within the special province of the doctor to pronounce upon, and perhaps he is never on more unsafe ground than when he becomes an amateur exponent of eugenics and sociology. The most exaggerated notions are often held by doctor and layman upon the dire consequences of marriage, both to the epileptic subject and to his or her offspring. In few situations are a clear idea of what these consequences may be, and a scrupulous avoidance of overstatement or thoughtless generalization, more incumbent on the medical adviser. Epilepsy is a most distressing form of disability to an intelligent patient and debars him from so many of the satisfactions of a normally active life, including regular and gainful occupation in some cases, that the doctor should be careful not to add to his burdens in this respect. Indeed, the epileptic needs reasonable encouragement more than most sufferers from chronic nervous disease, and this encouragement is an essential part of treatment.

The treatment of symptomatic epilepsy is (1) that of the fits themselves by the methods of medication already described, and (2) when possible that of the underlying condition. When fits occur as manifestations of an acute illness; as in eclampsia, the necessity for treatment passes with recovery from the original illness, but when structural lesions of the brain are in question, the problem is less simple. Such lesions have been divided into atrophic (such as follow head and brain injury, or some vascular lesions) and expanding (tumours of the brain). In the former category we are dealing with scars left by disease processes now inactive, and it is sometimes possible and expedient to attempt to excise these when they are accurately localized and prove accessible. Yet surgical measures of this kind are not always effective, and whatever measure of success they may achieve must invariably be supplemented by medication on the principles laid down for idiopathic epilepsy. In other words, surgical intervention can never be a substitute for medication. In the case of expanding lesions, that is, tumours, the outlook is much more serious and treatment is governed by the factors discussed in Chapter III. If exploratory craniotomy reveals a cortical angioma recourse may be had to deep X-ray therapy, for this lesion is inoperable.

In addition to these strictly medical measures, the social care of the epileptics in the community, in which their proportion has been estimated to be over two per thousand, presents a special problem. Approximately 20 per cent. of all epileptics are mentally altered and of these, as well as of severe cases without mental derangement, a large proportion require institutional treatment. Their employment presents great difficulties, and the monotony of that aimless existence to which some of them are necessarily condemned tends to aggravate the severity of the malady. Therefore the provision of occupation, and where possible of gainful occupation, is as essential an element in the treatment as those measures here discussed. Public Health authorities must shoulder some responsibility in this regard, for the necessary steps are not often within the power of the medical adviser.

CHAPTER VI

Migraine (Paroxysmal Headache)

A PAROXYSMAL nervous disturbance of unknown nature of which the most constant feature is recurrent attacks of headache, but in the fully developed attack visual and sensory symptoms precede the onset of headache, while sickness accompanies it. This association of headache and vomiting has led to the terms "sick headache" and "bilious headache," by which migraine is also known.

Ætiology.—Migraine usually makes its first appearance at or about the age of puberty, and the subject thereafter remains liable to attacks until middle-age is past, or until in women the menopause is completed. In most instances there is a family history of migraine. It is common to say that there is an element of emotional or mental instability in the stock from which the migrainous subject derives and also in the subject himself. This factor is now so often and so loosely invoked that it has come to mean very little, but perhaps the situation in respect of the incidence of migraine is justly stated when we say that the migrainous subject is often a quick-witted and intelligent individual and as such more susceptible to fluctuations of mood, and also more likely to be found in positions and occupations involving responsibility and hard work, and, therefore, especially liable to fatigue and anxiety. If to be responsive to these is to be unstable there may be something in the thesis that migrainous subjects are inherently unstable, but common sense rebels against such a view. On the physiological side, it is probable that vasospasm underlies the visual and sensory prodromata of an attack of migraine, and that, for example, the transient scotoma, hemianopia or spectrum of an attack is due to spasm in cortical arterioles in the visual cortex. The very occasional persistence of a hemianopia after a severe attack of migraine—especially in an elderly subject—may thus be taken as indicative of a severe and more enduring spasm: one capable of producing some irreversible damage to the affected cortex. The ensuing headache has been attributed to vasodilatation following the initial spasm.

Symptoms.—On the day preceding an attack the subject may suffer from a vague malaise that warns him of its impending arrival. On the other hand, some declare that immediately prior to the onset they feel unusually well. In the complete attack there is a sudden onset of visual disturbance. This may take the form of a scotoma in

133

the field of vision or of a homonymous hemianopia, or on the other hand of what has come to be known as a "fortification spectrum": a curved zigzag of coloured light, in form like the chevron moulding of a Norman arch, that shimmers, enlarging and lessening in amplitude, or progressively enlarging until it almost fills the field of vision.

In some cases this figure is situated in the homonymous half-fields, left in some attacks, right in others. It persists for a period varying from five to fifteen minutes, as does a scotoma or hemianopia when present, and then rapidly passes off to be succeeded by the characteristic headache. Common, but less generally recognized, are other sensory phenomena. These include tingling in the hand and fingers, usually of one side—the side of the hemianopia—tingling in the lips and tongue, and a speech disturbance of aphasic type. The last-named may be very marked and render intelligible expression difficult if not impossible for some minutes. These symptoms cease with the passing of the visual symptoms.

The headache usually starts in one temple in a restricted area and gradually spreads in extent to the vertex and forehead, and then crossing the midline may become a bilateral frontal and bitemporal headache of a throbbing character, and often of great and disabling severity. Within an hour or two of its appearance, nausea, followed by vomiting, usually though not invariably, comes on and persists for several hours. The attack carries over to the following day in a few instances, sometimes ending on the day of onset, and in either case leaving the patient exhausted but often hungry.

The frequency of the attacks varies from time to time and from case to case. Under the influence of fatigue or anxiety they may be of almost daily occurrence for weeks at a time, but this is unusual, and the periodicity may vary from weeks to months. Between the attacks the subject enjoys normal health.

In some subjects the headache alone is present, while in a few— especially late in middle life—the sensory prodromata may occur alone without the ensuing headache and sickness.

While the headache is present, the eyeballs are tender to pressure and sometimes painful on movement, and the sufferer is unduly sensitive to strong light.

Diagnosis.—In most instances this presents no difficulties. Physical examination, both during and between the attacks, is negative, and the subject enjoys normal health between the attacks. When the sensory prodromata are striking and the ensuing headache relatively slight, a diagnosis of minor epilepsy is occasionally made in error, but in the latter case the attack is of the most transient character and does not endure for several minutes as do the sensory phenomena of migraine. Very rarely a cerebral tumour may produce attacks indistinguishable from those of migraine for months or years before objective physical signs are present. In such a case the headache and the sensory phenomena are constantly referred to the same side, and do not alternate from side to side as in migraine.

Treatment.—The avoidance of precipitating factors should be undertaken when possible. In cases showing great frequency of attacks, a preliminary holiday and change for two or three weeks may be essential. Whatever is required, or is done, in this respect, it can scarcely be over-stressed that an essential feature in the treatment of a case of migraine is *regular medication, day in day out, for a period of weeks at least*. The patient who is merely given some analgesic as each attack of headache appears cannot be said to be having treatment in the due sense, yet this is all that many migrainous subjects ever get. It is to cut short the sequence of attacks that we should try, and this requires the regular administration, either of phenobarbitone grs. $\frac{1}{2}$ twice or even thrice daily, or Gowers' mixture: viz. Liq. trinitrini ♏1, Liq. Strychninæ ♏3, Tinct. Gelsemii ♏15, Phenazone grs. 5, Sod. Bromidi grs. 5, Aq. chlorof. ad ʒi, t.d.s.

The addition to one or other of these of a morning dose of sodium bicarbonate (grs. 15) or of an alkaline powder may reinforce the effect. To cut short a developed migraine ergotamine tartrate may be given either orally or hypodermically (0·5 mgm.), and the dose repeated in an hour if necessary. However, this drug is not uniformly successful and appears to have no preventive value. A single or once repeated dose of Amidopyrin (grs. 5) may also serve to give relief, provided that the patient rests on or in bed. Occasionally, food or alcohol will serve to cut an attack short. Errors of refraction may act as a precipitating factor and when present should be corrected.

CHAPTER VII

Acute Infections of the Nervous System

INTRODUCTION

THE acute infections of the nervous system fall into two groups, the bacterial and the virus infections. The major incidence of the former is upon the leptomeninges in the form of an acute meningitis. This is more often secondary to infection elsewhere in the body than primary in the meninges. The virus infections, on the other hand, are essentially primary infections of the nervous system and not general systemic infections with secondary invasion of the nervous system.

In syphilis of the nervous system we have a protozoal infection the clinical manifestations of which may be acute or chronic, while its action is upon both meninges and parenchyma. For practical purposes it is convenient to consider neuro-syphilis separately.

In respect of bacterial infections a little more may be said in generalization. The brain may be secondarily affected when there is bacterial infection of the bones or sinuses of the skull. Less commonly we may see a pyæmic, blood-borne infection of the brain. In most instances such infections of the brain lead to abscess formation, but in very virulent infections there may be a spreading suppurative encephalitis clinically indistinguishable from acute meningitis. Further, bacterial infections which, when the meninges are involved, present a picture of acute infection give one of chronic illness when the brain is involved. Thus tuberculous meningitis is an acute or subacute illness, but tuberculoma in the brain behaves like other progressive expanding lesions, developing acutely only if the pia-arachnoid becomes infected.

ACUTE LEPTOMENINGITIS

The extent of the subarachnoid space and the feeble bactericidal powers of the contained cerebrospinal fluid make it inevitable that once a pyogenic organism, or the tubercle bacillus, gains access to the fluid, a rapidly generalized infection of the subarachnoid space must take place, and prior to the recent developments in chemotherapy such an infection was almost invariably quickly fatal. If death does not ensue, as in the case of meningococcal meningitis, inflammatory exudate may form in the basal cisterns, in the opening through the tentorium and over the foramina in the fourth ventricle through which the fluid leaves the ventricular system for the subarachnoid space. The formation of adhesions, by loculating fluid in the cisterns and by preventing escape of fluid from the ventricles and its absorption into the venous channels through the arachnoid villi, then leads to the development of internal hydrocephalus. With the advent of sulphonamide therapy, this distressing sequence of events is now rarely encountered.

Ætiology.—Save in the case of pneumococcal meningitis, acute leptomeningitis is secondary to a focus of infection elsewhere in the body. It was formerly believed that meningococcal meningitis was primary in the nervous system, the organism gaining access to the subarachnoid space from the nasopharynx through the filaments of the olfactory nerve. It is now known that the primary infection is nasopharyngeal, whence the blood stream is invaded by the organism. In other cases of secondary meningitis the organism may enter the subarachnoid space directly through the bone, or by the mechanism of septic thrombosis in a vein. Infection may invade the subarachnoid space by either of these mechanisms in the case of middle ear disease and by the latter in the case of cavernous sinus thrombosis.

The meningeal reaction to infection shows itself in three ways: by inflammatory changes in the meninges, by changes in the composition of the cerebrospinal fluid, and by a clinical reaction. In the presence of a pyogenic infection, whatever the organism, there is a certain constancy of character in these three aspects of the reaction and the common features may be considered before discussing the points of difference.

Pathology.—The pia-arachnoid becomes dull and opaque and at the same time intensely hyperæmic and œdematous, and as fibrinous exudate is poured out it becomes gelatinous in appearance and texture. This exudate soon becomes purulent, except in some intensely virulent streptococcal infections where hyperæmia may be the striking change. The exudate tends to spread from the base along the sylvian fossa to the convexity of the brain where it lies in the furrows between the convolutions. It is most abundant in the basal cisterns. The underlying cerebral cortex is congested. In tuberculous meningitis the exudate remains non-purulent, but tiny tubercles appear dotted over the pia-arachnoid in much the same distribution as the exudate of a purulent meningitis. The reaction also spreads down the spinal pia-arachnoid. In non-fatal cases of meningococcal meningitis the exudate may organize and form adhesions in the situations and with the consequences already mentioned.

The Cerebrospinal Fluid.—In pyogenic meningitis polymorpho-nuclear cells are poured into the subarachnoid space and cerebrospinal fluid by the inflamed meninges, while in tuberculous meningitis lymphocytes predominate in the fluid. The protein content is increased, while on the other hand the level of the chlorides present falls and the glucose diminishes and may disappear from the fluid. These changes in composition are dealt with in detail under the heading of the different ætiological varieties of meningitis.

The Clinical Reaction.—Each variety of meningitis presents its own characteristic clinical features, yet essentially in every case the picture is made up of the same components. It is in their severity and in their rate and sequence of development that the variations occur. The symptoms include intense headache which may be of such severity as to make the patient delirious or cry out, photophobia, an irritable drowsiness sometimes lapsing into a final coma, rigidity of the neck and back, with head retraction and opisthotonos in the meningococcal meningitis of infants, Kernig's sign, diminution of the tendon jerks, retention of urine, and sometimes cranial nerve palsies. The temperature is raised and the pulse rapid and sometimes irregular. A convulsion may be the initial symptom in a child, when it is followed by an immediate rise of temperature.

CEREBROSPINAL FEVER

This malady is not primarily an infection of the nervous system and is best thought of as a "meningococcal infection which in the case of carriers remains limited to the nasopharynx, but which may pass into the blood and proceed thence to many parts of the body, particularly the cerebrospinal axis. Similarly, the nervous complication is a continuous process, which may end in death at any point, but which can run from its beginning as an acute hæmorrhagic encephalomyelitis through the stage of acute or subacute leptomeningitis up to the final organization of inflammatory exudate" (Brinton). Clinically, therefore, cerebrospinal fever in its full development consists of a septicæmia with secondary nervous, and occasionally also joint and visceral involvement. Either the septicæmic or the nervous component may dominate the clinical course of the illness.

Epidemiology.—Cerebrospinal fever occurs sporadically, and then most often in infants, and also in epidemic form when its victims are predominantly young adults. Epidemics are seen in the winter and early spring months. They are essentially a war-time phenomenon and the factors leading to their appearance are a carrier epidemic, a young susceptible population and conditions of overcrowding and possibly also of strenuous physical activity. Therefore recruits housed under crowded conditions of living provide the soil for epidemic development. The carrier, who may or may not present catarrhal symptoms, carries the organism in his nasopharynx and disseminates it by the mechanism of droplet infection. Only a small proportion of those exposed to infection actually contact the disease. Preceding an epidemic the proportion of carriers in the susceptible population increases considerably.

Symptomatology.—From what has been said it will be appreciated that more than one sequence of events may be observed. In the acute fulminating cases the patient dies within a matter of hours from septicæmia before indications of meningeal involvement have made their appearance. In less severe cases the initial septicæmic phase is soon overlaid by the symptoms of acute meningitis which come to dominate the clinical picture. In a few cases the onset of meningitic symptoms may be delayed and not severe, while in the mildest cases the picture is one of a mild and short-lived meningeal reaction.

What Brinton speaks of as *the ordinary type* (90 per cent. of all cases) is ushered in by septicæmic symptoms: increasing fever, a petechial rash, rigors, pains in the limbs and trunk, and some drowsiness. This phase after about forty-eight hours passes into that of meningeal infection. The headache increases and may become intense. Vomiting may occur and the temperature is continuously raised, ranging from 100° to 103° or even 105° F. In children a convulsion may herald the onset of this phase, but in adults rigors are characteristic. The rash is hæmorrhagic and consists of tiny petechiæ, save in the fulminating cases when large ecchymoses, and hæmorrhages into mucous and serous membranes, may occur. A combination of drowsiness and delirium sets in, the headache is of great severity, and the patient lies on his side with head and spine extended and the legs curled up. It is in the sporadic cases of infancy (post-basic meningitis) only that marked head retraction and opisthotonos develop. Examination, however, shows that the neck and spine are rigid, and Kernig's sign is present. Cranial nerve palsies are occasionally seen, the sixth, eighth, third, and seventh nerves (in that order of frequency) being those affected. Signs of focal brain disturbance are exceptional, while the state of the reflexes is variable and affords no clear diagnostic information. If the patient be stuporose there may be incontinence of urine. When septicæmia is severe there is wasting and signs of dehydration.

Since sulphonamide therapy has come into general use relapses are not seen. In favourable cases improvement sets in during the second week and proceeds rapidly, the patient being left debilitated and usually wasted.

When inflammatory exudate organizes and occludes the foramina of exit from the ventricles or the space between the brain-stem and tentorium, hydrocephalus ensues. Headache then reappears, and there are sickness, progressive dementia and wasting and, usually, death in from two to four months.

The acute fulminating cases are characterized by intense septicæmia. We see a hæmorrhagic eruption and hæmorrhage into mucous and

serous membranes and into the suprarenal medulla. This last leads
to a rapid and severe fall in pressure, collapse, and death within a few
hours of onset. The blood culture is usually positive. Occasionally
an acute meningococcal arthritis of one or two joints may occur.

Post-basic meningitis differs from the "ordinary" type by the enlargement of the infant head from separation of the sutures consequent
upon hydrocephalus. The onset is sudden with convulsions and
accesses of screaming and the head retraction and opisthotonos already
mentioned. Progressive dementia and blindness (from primary optic
atrophy) follow, and death ensues in from six to twelve weeks.

Pathology.—The general pathology of acute leptomeningitis has
already been summarized. In cerebrospinal fever the following special
features may be mentioned. Blood cultures reveal the meningococcus in from 25 to 80 per cent. of cases, and under favourable
conditions and adequate technique the organism can also be identified
in the nasopharynx and its secretions. How long it may remain active
here in carriers and in convalescents is not certainly known, but
probably modern treatment has considerably shortened the period.
The organism passes from the nasopharyngeal mucosa into the blood
and thence, precisely how is not known, into the subarachnoid space.
Among the lesions due to the blood infection are hæmorrhages into the
skin, and occasionally also, as has been mentioned, into serous membranes. In the nervous system the lesions are not confined to the
leptomeninges. In the brain we may find areas of œdema, punctate
hæmorrhages, thromboses, and areas of cellular infiltration; degenerative
changes in nerve cells may also be found. All these lesions together
indicate that an encephalomyelitis is an essential element in the nervous
involvement. The meningeal lesions have already been described
(page 137).

The cerebrospinal fluid.—Lumbar puncture is now a diagnostic
procedure only, since repeated drainage of the theca has become
unnecessary as a mode of treatment. The cerebrospinal fluid pressure
may be considerably raised as measured by manometer (up to 300 mms.
of water). The fluid is found to be turbid early in the illness and then
becomes opaque and purulent later on, clearing as convalescence
develops. The cellular content is greatly increased, and from 500 to
15,000 per cubic mm. may be found, according to the stage of the
illness. These are polymorphonuclear, save in chronic cases in which
lymphocytes may predominate. The glucose content falls rapidly to
zero and the chloride content falls from its normal level of about
720 mgms. per 100 c.cm. to about 650 mgms. The total protein is
raised from the normal level of 10 to 20 mgms. per 100 c.cm. to as high
as 150 mgms. The meningococcus can be seen in a smear of the centrifuged fluid, both intracellularly and outside the cells. In early and

adequately treated cases the organism disappears from the fluid in most instances within forty-eight hours.

Treatment.—At the time of writing, current opinion regards combined sulphonamide and penicillin treatment as the method of choice in acute meningitis, and this general statement must be amplified as follows: (1) in no form of acute meningitis should penicillin be the sole form of chemotherapy. In meningococcal meningitis sulphonamides are still the drug of choice, and penicillin, if used, should be adjuvant or reserved for cases failing to respond satisfactorily to sulphonamides. For pneumococcal meningitis combined penicillin and sulphonamide should be used. (2) Both intrathecal and systemic penicillin must be used on account of the difficulty penicillin has in passing the blood-brain barrier. (3) Only the purest penicillin and that known to have a low irritant effect upon serous membranes should be used intrathecally. (4) The most scrupulous asepsis must be enjoined, and the danger of pyocyaneus infection, and the difficulty of countering it, borne in mind. (5) Cell reaction in the cerebrospinal fluid is not—at least in the early stages—a guide to progress.

The details are as follows: (*a*) Systemic penicillin, 120,000 units daily for four or five days, given either by continuous intramuscular drip, or divided into three-hourly intramuscular injections. (*b*) About 10,000 (8,000 to 16,000) units of penicillin for a maximum of five doses intrathecally. The second dose following from 12 to 18 hours after the first, and the remaining three doses at 24-hour intervals. In many cases the two initial intrathecal doses are sufficient. If there is evidence of block in the subarachnoid space the lumbar route must be reinforced by the ventricular. (*c*) Sulphadiazine is regarded as the sulphonamide of choice. A 4-gram loading dose is followed by 2 grams four-hourly, and after four to five days the dose is reduced to half. The customary duration of treatment is six to seven days, longer periods (up to nine days) being only rarely necessary. Relatively, children tolerate these drugs better than adults.

Banks gives the following dosage tables for the sulphonamides:—

Age . . .	0 to 3 years.	3 to 10 years.	10 to 15 years.	15 years onwards.
Initial dose.	I.V. ½ gm. Oral ½ gm.	I.V. 1 gm. Oral ¾ gm.	I.V. 1 gm. Oral 1 gm.	I.V. 2 gms. Oral 1½ gms.
1st period— (2 to 3 days).	½ gm. 4-hourly, oral.	¾ gm. 4-hourly, oral.	1 gm. 4-hourly, oral.	1½gm. 4-hourly, oral.
2nd period— (2 days).	½ gm. 4-hourly, oral.	¾ gm. 4-hourly, oral.	1 gm. 4-hourly, oral.	1 gm. 4-hourly, oral.
3rd period— (2 days).	¼ gm. 6-hourly, oral.	½ gm. 6-hourly, oral.	½ gm. 6-hourly, oral.	1 gm. 6-hourly, oral.

The initial loading dose (*I.V.*) is intravenous.

In all cases it is important to seek for a possible primary focus of infection in the cranal sinuses or elsewhere.

OTHER FORMS OF PYOGENIC MENINGITIS

Pneumococcal meningitis is said sometimes to be primary in the meninges, but streptococcal and staphylococcal meningitis are secondary to infections elsewhere in the body. The clinical signs are those already described, and associated with them are those of the original focus of infection, *e.g.* middle ear disease, cutaneous or wound infections, or erysipelas.

On lumbar puncture, the cerebrospinal fluid escapes under pressure, is turbid and may contain flocculent pus. There are very numerous polymorphonuclear cells, the protein is increased up to 0·05 per cent. or even higher. Glucose is diminished or absent, while the chlorides fall to 0·650, or 0·60 per cent. The causative organism is present.

BENIGN LYMPHOCYTIC MENINGITIS

This title has been given to a clinical condition in which the patient, usually a child, presents the signs and symptoms of an acute leptomeningitis of moderate severity, but of brief course and good prognosis. This may occur in association with middle ear disease, or sinusitis, or may develop in the absence of other illness or lesions. It probably represents a group of diverse ætiologies, despite its uniform behaviour. The typical findings in the cerebrospinal fluid are a count of from 100 to 200 lymphocytes to the c.cm., though in the initial stage of the illness there may be a considerable proportion of polynuclear cells in some cases. The protein content is slightly increased, but the glucose and chlorides are normal. The illness runs a favourable course, ending in recovery in about two weeks. In young children a convulsion, followed by a rise of temperature, may herald the onset.

It is possible that a proportion of the cases so grouped may be due to the virus of choriomeningitis, but not all cases are so caused, and it is useful to remember that this clinical picture and these cerebrospinal fluid findings are also those of the preparalytic stage of acute poliomyelitis. Thus, some cases diagnosed as benign lymphocytic meningitis may, in fact, be examples of an abortive poliomyelitis.

TUBERCULOUS MENINGITIS

This differs from the forms already considered in its commonly insidious onset. The infection reaches the meninges by the blood stream from a tuberculous focus, glandular or bony, elsewhere in the body, or the infection may be but a part of a generalized miliary tuberculosis. Its greatest incidence is in early childhood. The child develops vague symptoms of ill-health. He becomes apathetic and listless, is fretful, and sleeps restlessly. His appetite falls off and he is apt to be constipated. A slight irregular fever develops, with frequent headaches. These indeterminate symptoms persist for a varying period of weeks and then tend to become somewhat rapidly worse so that the meningeal source of the symptoms becomes clear. Examination at this stage may yield indecisive results, but sooner or later the picture of a meningeal reaction develops. There is some neck rigidity with headache, Kernig's sign may be present in mild degree, the tendon jerks are diminished or even absent. Retention of urine is frequently seen. One or more generalized convulsions may occur during the illness. Lumbar puncture at this early stage yields a clear fluid in which upon cooling a clot may form. If the cells be numerous (300 to 400 per c.cm.) the fluid may be faintly opalescent. These cells are found to be mainly lymphocytes, though up to 30 per cent. of polymorphonuclear cells may be present. The protein content is increased to the level of 0·03 per cent. The glucose is diminished and the chloride level falls to 0·650, or 0·60 per cent. If the clot be teased out on a slide and duly stained the tubercle bacillus may be found.

The child commonly lies curled up on his side, is fretful if disturbed and out of touch with his surroundings. The pupils may be dilated and various ocular palsies may be present. Rarely, ophthalmoscopic examination will reveal the presence of miliary tubercles on the choroid. There is slight and irregular fever, an irregular pulse, and periodic breathing in the final stage. This developed phase of the illness rarely lasts longer than two weeks. In the final stage the condition grows rapidly worse, but may appear to improve for from twelve to twenty-four hours before the child lapses into the final coma.

It is this variety of meningitis that presents the greatest difficulties in early diagnosis. Its differentiation from medulloblastoma of the cerebellum has already been discussed (page 74). During the first few days of definite meningeal reaction the possibility of acute polio-myelitis has to be considered, for this malady may present marked symptoms of meningeal irritation in the brief preparalytic phase. In these circumstances reliance must be placed upon the results of lumbar puncture, the composition of the cerebrospinal fluid in poliomyelitis differing from that in tuberculous meningitis in the maintenance of normal chloride and glucose levels in the former. The "meningism" that may accompany acute febrile illness in children, and occasionally in adults, may be distinguished from true meningitis by the examination of the cerebrospinal fluid, and by the clinical fact—long since put on record by Sir William Jenner—that headache ceases when delirium begins in the meningism of general infection, but persists in that of meningitis.

Tuberculous meningitis is invariably fatal and only symptomatic measures can be carried out. These include repeated lumbar puncture and drainage of the theca to relieve headache, and the use of drugs for this purpose.

VIRUS INFECTIONS OF THE NERVOUS SYSTEM

Our knowledge of these infections is far less perfect than that of the bacterial infections of the nervous system, and only in the case of acute poliomyelitis has much insight been gained into all the factors and processes involved. The viruses in question belong to the group of so-called "neurotropic" viruses. They appear to be obligatory intracellular organisms which multiply and exert their characteristic pathogenic effect only upon the cells for which they have an affinity. They then become inactive and die, so that virus-infections are said to be "self-limiting," save in the case of herpes labialis which may recur and persist.

By the term neurotropic we imply a virus that attacks primarily and directly the tissues of the nervous system, either the nerve cells or the glia cells, or both. In the case of the virus of poliomyelitis, an extreme of selectivity appears to be reached, for nerve cells only are attacked, and of these only certain groups. Thus we may call this virus "neuronotropic."

So far as is known neurotropic viruses do not attack white matter, and the so-called demyelinating diseases, such as disseminated sclerosis, are not due to virus action.

ACUTE POLIOMYELITIS

Ætiology—The virus is one of the smallest known and is, as has already been noted, neuronotropic. It can be isolated from the brain and cord of fatal cases. Outside the nervous system, it can be found in the naso-pharyngeal mucosa, in the wall of the gut and in the fæces. It is not found in the blood or cerebrospinal fluid.

Our knowledge of the reactions of the nervous system to the virus, and of virus distribution within this system, is steadily increasing, and within the past few years many previously accepted views have had to be discarded. The olfactory nerve endings, formerly thought to be the portal of entry of the virus into the central nervous system, are now found to be so only rarely, and new evidence points to the nasopharynx and the gastro-intestinal tract as the natural portals in man. How the virus crosses the barrier between these cavities and the nervous system is not known, but the incidence of the bulbar form of poliomyelitis in children recently subjected to tonsillectomy and adenoidectomy shows that in this region it may easily gain access to the nervous system if the barrier is destroyed.

It is probable that once the nasopharynx or gastro-intestinal tract is reached, the virus travels along the nerve fibres innervating these structures and gains, the bulb in the first case, and the spinal cord in the second.

It shows a characteristic distribution within the nervous system, being found in the ventral horn cells of the cord, the grey matter of the brain-stem, and the cerebral motor cortex, and it is in these regions alone that it appears to multiply and produce its characteristic lesions. Even—in the case of experimentally inoculated apes—in the so-called "abortive" or non-paralysed cases, there is invariably an encephalitis though spinal cord lesions may be absent, and this encephalitis, which may give rise to no symptoms, is an essential part of the nervous lesions of the disease. In the cerebral cortex the virus has a special affinity for the large pyramidal cells of the motor area, and it is here only that cortical lesions are found. From its point of access to the nervous system it travels along short neurones preferentially, but along long neurones such as the pyramidal tract when the spread becomes more general in the later stages of the process. The reaction of the glial elements is secondary to the virus-neurone reaction.

Pathology.—The nervous system may be widely congested, and lesions are found in the situations already named, being most severe in the ventral horn cells of the cord. These cells may undergo a rapid necrosis, a process followed by intense vascular congestion, by a phagocytosis of the dead cells by microglial cells and by a leucocytosis. In later stages lymphocytes replace the leucocytes in the perivascular sheaths of the neighbouring blood-vessels. These sheaths are distended by these cells which are poured out into the subarachnoid space, and reach the cerebrospinal fluid where they produce the changes characteristic of this fluid in the initial stages of the malady.

Epidemiology.—Poliomyelitis is a contagious disease. It is believed to be spread by healthy "carriers," by the subjects of "subclinical infection" and by sufferers in the incubation or early acute stage of the illness. Droplet infection is no longer believed to be the principle means of dissemination, and evidence points to the intestinal canal as the chief portal of entry of the virus into the body. What has been said, however, of bulbar poliomyelitis in children recently subjected to tonsillectomy, shows that the nasopharynx may yet be an important portal of infection.

The identification of carriers presents peculiar difficulties since the only available test of the presence of virus is the inoculation of

K

suspected material into the monkey and the development of the disease in the inoculated animal. Nevertheless, by this means it has been found that apparently healthy contacts may carry active virus in the fæces for at least one or two weeks before they develop symptoms of poliomyelitis, or even when they do not develop symptoms. Sufferers from the disease may also carry the virus in this way for some few weeks after they fall ill. The nasopharyngeal secretions do not contain virus so constantly, or for so long, as the fæces. In epidemic foci virus has been isolated from the sewage and also from the bodies of house flies. It is possible, therefore, that milk and other articles of food may act as vectors, and it is known that the virus may remain active for some time in milk and butter. Familiarity with the habits of the house fly will indicate the possibilities of dissemination here revealed. Thus, in its epidemic incidence poliomyelitis spreads along lines of human communication, and from places where susceptible subjects are gathered together, as in schools. Within an infected community, such as a village or a boarding school, the infection may smoulder for weeks, cases occurring singly or in small series at irregular intervals. It has been stated that in such a community all susceptible subjects fall victims to infection at the outset and that thereafter there is no further increase, but such a view is not wholly in accord with the recorded facts of epidemic occurrence.

The maximal incidence is during the first five-year-period of life. Thereafter susceptibility progressively wanes, but the disease may occur in adolescents and in adults up to middle age. This late incidence is most often encountered during epidemic outbreaks. The malady occurs sporadically at all times, showing its greatest incidence in the autumn. Large-scale outbreaks have occurred in Scandinavia and in the United States, but so far this country has been spared disastrous epidemics.

A further brief reference may be made to "abortive" and "subclinical" infections. During epidemics it has been observed that less than 50 per cent. of all subjects presenting the initial preparalytic symptoms of the disease subsequently develop paralysis. The majority recover after the brief opening phase, and it is now believed that although in these—as in paralysed cases—the virus has in fact gained the nerve cells, it is inactivated and destroyed before it has damaged the cells sufficiently to evoke disturbances of function. There is now evidence that there exists an additional category of "subclinical" infections in which the subject, while harbouring the virus, yet shows no clinical symptoms whatever. Probably such cases, together with the abortive cases, play the predominant role in the spread of the disease. An additional indication of the wide incidence of such infections is the presence in the serum of very many persons not known to have suffered from poliomyelitis, of protective antibodies such as are known to be present in all persons who have survived an attack of the malady. Nothing is known of the conditions governing the natural immunity some subjects appear to possess, or of the general immunity to second attacks.

Symptomatology.—The acute phase of the disease falls naturally into two stages: preparalytic and paralytic, the second stage being absent in a considerable proportion of cases.

The preparalytic stage develops after an incubation period which is believed to range from five to twelve days. It consists of a short-lived febrile illness of from one to four or five days that, except during the course of an epidemic outbreak, may pass unrecognized for what it is, being identified only in retrospect when paralysis has later appeared. The temperature may rise to 102° to 104° F. The child is nervous and fretful. Signs of meningeal irritation develop, namely, rigidity of the neck and back, irregular jerky muscular contractions, and Kernig's sign. The child cannot, when sitting or lying supine, flex his leg so as to touch his nose with his knee owing to this rigidity of the spine. In a day or so the temperature may drop to normal and the child appear to have recovered from his illness, when it rises again and paralysis suddenly sets in.

The paralytic stage.—As a rule the paralysis is sudden in appearance and maximal at onset. However, during epidemic outbreaks its behaviour is less predictable. There may be recurrent short bouts of slight fever during several days in each of which some new group of muscles becomes more or less severely paralysed. Occasionally, the mode of spread is a true ascending paralysis beginning in the legs and spreading to the abdominal and then the thoracic musculature until respiratory movements of the chest are lost and death ensues from asphyxia. This is, indeed, the common mode of death in fatal cases. Sometimes this ascent ceases before respiration is affected and the level then recedes, leaving a greater or less extent of the musculature more or less gravely paralysed.

The distribution of the paralysis is asymmetrical and inconstant, but the muscles most prone to be severely affected are those supplied by the lumbar enlargement, and in the upper limb the deltoid and adjacent muscles.

The paralysis is a true flaccid, lower motor neurone paralysis, with loss of tendon jerks in affected muscles. There is no sensory loss, but when the legs are severely paralysed there may be a short-lived (one or two days) retention of urine. In such cases there may be a bilateral Babinski response for the same period.

For the initial two to five weeks all affected muscles may be painful and tender to pressure, and when this passes off the case is said to have entered the convalescent stage.

The affected muscles may conveniently be divided into three categories: (1) those totally denervated and not capable of any degree of recovery; (2) those the motor nerve cells of which are extensively and severely damaged. In these, as in the former group, wasting soon develops, but they are capable of some measure of recovery during the ensuing three years; and (3) those the motor cells of which are but minimally affected. These recover rapidly and may never show any degree of wasting. It is only during the course of the first month or two of the convalescent stage that the affected muscles can be placed in their respective categories and an ultimate prognosis as to recovery of power be given. The recovery process, most striking at first, gradually slows down after the initial six months, by the expiration of which time, indeed, most of it has already occurred. In totally or severely paralysed muscles wasting does not become conspicuous for three or more weeks, and thereafter it steadily increases until, when no recovery takes place, there may be no contractile muscle fibre left. Thus a badly damaged limb may become extremely thin. When inadequately treated and not given due mechanical support, deformities due to fibrous shortening of muscles and to increased mobility in unprotected joints occur. Further, especially in the case of the lower limbs, the leg and foot may become reddened and œdematous and the seat of chilblains in cold weather. When the spinal muscles are involved, kyphoscoliosis develops unless mechanical support has been provided from the outset.

The Cerebrospinal Fluid.—During the preparalytic stage it is usual to find characteristic changes. There is an increase of cells, predominantly lymphocytes, of from a few above normal to a thousand or more to the c.cm. In a few cases up to 50 per cent. of these cells may be polymorphonuclear. The cell count commonly falls to normal in about two weeks. The protein shows a moderate increase, but this does not run parallel with the cellular increase, and it may not completely subside for six or seven weeks. The chloride and glucose contents remain normal. Colloidal gold curves regularly show a change in the lower dilutions (1122110000).

The blood count shows a leucocytosis (mainly polymorphonuclear) of moderate degree which subsides gradually over a period of some weeks.

Clinical Varieties of Poliomyelitis.—It was formerly the custom to speak of cerebral, cerebellar, brain-stem, spinal and neuritic varieties, the first-named being called polioencephalitis. It is probable, however, that only the spinal type and a few cases of brain-stem type really belong to this infection. Most cases of so-called polioencephalitis are probably due to other and unknown pathogenic agencies. Their clinical picture is that of an acute, brief febrile illness with convulsions, coma, and residual hemiplegia. The so-called neuritic type consists of spinal cases with widespread and slight paralysis and marked muscular tenderness.

Diagnosis.—In the preparalytic stage diagnosis is difficult unless an epidemic is in progress, when any febrile illness in a child or adolescent should be considered from this point of view. The examination of the cerebrospinal fluid is probably the most reliable method of diagnosis, but the presence of neck and back rigidity, of headache and of fever in a child is always suspicious. The changes in the cerebrospinal fluid characteristic of poliomyelitis, and differentiating it from an acute meningitis, have already been referred to. It should be borne in mind that in this country we are not in the habit of diagnosing poliomyelitis in its preparalytic stage, owing to the fortunate circumstance that we have had no widespread epidemics of the disease, and thus a diagnosis of abortive poliomyelitis is virtually never made. Yet cases of this order must occur from time to time, and it is probable that, if recognized as showing features of meningeal irritation, such a case might be regarded as one of *benign lymphocytic meningitis.*

Prognosis.—Unless the respiratory movements are paralysed the patient will survive, and the factors governing the degree of restoration of power have already been discussed. In cases where the initial paralysis is of but moderate degree, almost perfect recovery may ensue, but it is rare indeed for all weakness to clear up. In a greater or less number of muscles some degree of weakness and of loss of substance persists. Occasional cases are met with in which this residual defect is confined to one or two muscles only. Deltoid is apt to be such a muscle. In other cases there may be survival with extensive paralysis and wasting of all the limbs and of some trunk muscles, so that the patient is bedridden and helpless for the remainder of life. Between these two extremes are met cases in which with mechanical supports some measure of useful activity is possible. Probably all possible recovery has occurred within three years from the date of onset.

Treatment.—*Prophylactic.*—When the disease makes its appearance in a community the probable presence of healthy carriers and of infected persons with "subclinical" infections must be taken into account. No certain method of protecting susceptible contacts is known, and it is doubtful if gargles and nasal instillations are of any use now that the portal of entry has been found to be the alimentary canal. Regard must be had to the infectivity of the fæces of sufferers, and possibly also of those of contacts, and these excretions must be treated as potentially infective. Also, adult contacts, it has been urged, should not handle food or milk for distribution to the public for at least a fortnight after the development of a case of the disease in their households.

In village communities when multiple cases occur, children should be kept away from day schools and from congregating anywhere. In the case of boarding schools it is difficult to give a dogmatic ruling. It must be borne in mind that if we keep such institutions together, we are retaining an unknown number of susceptible subjects within an infected community in which the infection may smoulder for several weeks. Certain small village outbreaks have shown this feature, but it is right to say that in this country such boarding school outbreaks as have occurred have not behaved in this way, and most of them have been restricted to two or three cases as though due to common source infection and not case-to-case spread. That this will always be so we may not assume, and therefore, bearing in mind the natural anxiety of parents, it is probably best, when more than a single case has occurred, to give parents the option of removing their children. It should be made clear to those who take this option that they assume responsibility for segregating the child or children they remove from school, from other children and adolescents, for three weeks.

From what has been said earlier it is clear that when poliomyelitis is present in a district, children should not be subjected to removal of tonsils or adenoids.

It is not necessary to recapitulate the arguments given in earlier editions of this book as to the ineffectiveness of serum therapy, for this is now generally accepted.

Such trials as have been made of sulphonamide therapy, and of plasma transfusions have been unfavourable, and so far chemotherapy has yielded nothing in poliomyelitis.

In cases diagnosed during the preparalytic stage, it is probable that a minimum of movement and interference is advisable, and even lumbar puncture and the withdrawal of fluid may conceivably turn what might have been an abortive into a paralysed case. The doctor will, therefore, consider in such circumstances *precisely what he hopes to achieve by it for his patient* before he embarks upon it. Of course, in certain circumstances, the earliest possible identification of the disease may be important for other persons.

Treatment of the Paralysis.—During the acute stage the patient should be kept at rest in the supine position, with all affected muscles in the position of relaxation and shortening. This can be done by sandbags, light splints, or a double Thomas splint. Active local treatment to the muscles is strongly contra-indicated at this stage. Pain may require the administration of analgesics, and aspirin is adequate in most cases. Before the patient is allowed to move from this position an estimate of the extent and degree of paralysis should be made. When the erector spinæ is involved, prolonged immobilization in the supine position may be necessary, and this is best achieved in a well-made plaster boat.

If the respiratory muscles be involved and respiratory embarrassment present, the patient may be put into one or other of the respirator machines now available until an adequate degree of chest excursion is re-established. It should, however, be borne in mind that this procedure may allow the survival of persons who will remain permanently severely paralysed and helpless and requiring continued nursing care. This situation is apt to create grave psychological and other problems when the patient approaches or reaches adult life. The respirator is not a cure for the paralysis of poliomyelitis, and our hopes of it must be tempered with reason. Box respirators are now found in most hospitals. The Bragg-Paul type consists in an elongated rubber bag which is strapped round the chest and alternately inflated and deflated by a motor pump, and makes the nursing of the patient a much simpler affair than the box type in which all but the head and neck of the patient is enclosed. It may be hired from the Siebe-Gorman Co. of Westminster Bridge Road.

Active local treatment begins with the arrival at what has been called the convalescent stage, and consists in adequate orthopædic splinting and active muscular exercises. The patient must be trained to use weakened muscles, and this use is the most valuable element in treatment. Massage takes second place and serves to maintain the blood supply of muscles until a considerable degree of innervation is restored and voluntary movement is possible. The place of electrical treatment remains dubious, for there is no clear evidence that it averts wasting or promotes recovery. When employed as the main or only method of treatment it is harmful in that it involves the neglect of more useful methods. It is possible that for the patient to be able to see paralysed muscles contract under galvanic stimulation may have some psychological value. For such patients as have the necessary power, exercises in a warm swimming pool are of great value.

EPIDEMIC ENCEPHALITIS (LETHARGIC ENCEPHALITIS)

Ætiology.—Although this is believed to be a virus infection of the nervous system, nothing precise is known of the causative organism. A malady that assumed considerable epidemic proportions some twenty years ago, it has of late years rarely been encountered, though it is not rarely diagnosed. It has to be admitted that this view does not accord with the returns of the Registrar-General, according to which the annual deaths from this malady have not fallen below 600 in England and Wales since 1924. It has to be remembered in this connection that the diagnosis is one tempting to apply to cases of acute nervous disease that defy ready identification, and many and diverse are the maladies of the nervous system that we find erroneously labelled epidemic encephalitis. Within the author's experience these include subdural hæmatoma, intracranial tumour and abscess, hypertensive encephalopathy and tuberculous meningitis, as well as vascular lesions.

Therefore, in the absence of pathological confirmation of the clinical diagnosis, all cases so labelled may be regarded with the greatest reserve as far as the past decade is concerned.

What we do frequently encounter, however, is the organic affection known as *post-encephalitic Parkinsonism* from its resemblance to paralysis agitans (Parkinson's disease). This is a common sequel to an attack of epidemic encephalitis, and the numerous cases still to be seen are a legacy of the decade following the last war.

Epidemiology.—During the period of its epidemic occurrence the malady was widespread, involving both the old and the new world. The maximum recorded incidence in this country was in the period 1921–1929, and the winter and early spring months witnessed the peak of this incidence. The mortality was high, estimates ranging from 27 to 50 per cent. Case-to-case and familial infections appear exceptional. Nothing certain is known of its incubation period, but ten days has been suggested.

Pathology.—To the naked-eye the brain may appear very red and congested. On section petechial hæmorrhages may be seen. Microscopically, vascular engorgement and perivascular infiltration with mononuclear cells are always found. There is widespread neuronal degeneration with the microglial reaction described on page 59. The brain-stem and basal ganglia bear the brunt of the process in most cases and the substantia nigra seems constantly affected. In old cases, calcification of vessels may be seen.

The Cerebrospinal Fluid.—This is clear and colourless. There is often, but not constantly, an increase of lymphocytes ranging from 10 to 200 per c.cm. When the normal range of variation in the glucose content of the fluid was not fully appreciated, it was said that this might be raised in epidemic encephalitis, but it is doubtful if there is an actual rise. There is no increase in the protein content. Finally, the fluid may be normal.

Symptoms.—The clinical course and the components of the illness vary in the widest possible manner from case to case. At one extreme we have a brief and somewhat featureless febrile illness during which the patient may remain ambulant. In this form it is rarely recognized, and it is only the subsequent development of Parkinsonism that leads to a reconsideration of the original and perhaps long past onset. In such cases it may sometimes be possible to elicit a story of nocturnal delirium, or of great restlessness at night combined with drowsiness by day, perhaps also of a transient diplopia. At the other extreme we may find evidence of a grave febrile illness lasting some two or three weeks with symptoms indicating local nervous involvement. In its initially recognized form these symptoms consisted of a peculiar light somnolence by day with nocturnal delirium, accompanied by ocular palsies (squint, diplopia, and ptosis). Another group consisted of violent delirium and sleeplessness with involuntary movements, either choreiform or "myoclonic," that is, repeated coarse muscular jerkings and twitchings. In some cases the one syndrome succeeded the other. Most grave were the choreiform cases, in which the patient not rarely died of exhaustion. In the somnolent cases recovery was the rule, though full restoration to health was apt to be slow.

Sequels.—Either during the phase of convalescence, or two or three years later, the slow development of the Parkinsonian syndrome occurs in over 50 per cent. of cases. Gradually and very insiduously an extrapyramidal type of muscular rigidity invades the musculature, producing the Parkinsonian mask, the slow and restricted movements, and occasionally the tremor of paralysis agitans. This state may at first be confined to a single limb, spreading later to the others and becoming generalized. It runs a progressive course and finally, after a variable period of years, disables the sufferer, who becomes emaciated and finally succumbs. In a very few cases it undergoes arrest at some stage short of grave disability.

The early stage of this condition is commonly undiagnosed, for the syndrome is made up of such slight deviations from the normal that unless the general inspection of the patient as he moves and performs his natural actions reveals the typical slowness and limitation of range of movement, routine examination may fail to detect the disorder. Perhaps the earliest symptom is a failure of an affected arm to swing as the patient walks. If it be the right arm that is affected, the handwriting becomes slow and laboured, and the script progressively smaller as the months go by. The gait becomes slow and gliding in character, the figure slightly bowed and the face fixed. Close examination will reveal a fine flutter of the closed eyelids, a defect of convergence, a "cogwheel" rigidity of the limb musculature, or less commonly a visible tremor. The patient salivates freely by night, if not also by day.

In the initial phase, the patient's complaints are apt to seem out of proportion to anything that examination reveals, and many of the sufferers labour for many months or even longer under a diagnosis of "neurasthenia." If the condition develop unilaterally, a progressive hemiplegia may be diagnosed and an intracranial neoplasm suspected. Yet despite all this, once this syndrome has been seen and duly noted, it should never fail to be recognized.

One other common, though not invariable, feature of post-encephalitic Parkinsonism may be mentioned. It goes by the name of *oculogyric crisis*, and consists of a forced upward deviation of the eyes, with head retraction, lasting for from thirty minutes to an hour and causing some distress.

In children another post-encephalitic sequel is mental and moral deterioration, leading to refractoriness and sometimes to delinquency.

Diagnosis.—The somnolence, commonly a prominent feature of the acute stage of the illness, may be mistaken for the stupor of intracranial tumour or abscess, yet it differs from this in quality. It is peculiarly light and the patient is easily aroused and can take part in conversation, lapsing rapidly into light sleep when left. At night this state is apt to be replaced by a quiet muttering delirium in which the patient's utterances commonly refer to his ordinary daytime tasks (occupational delirium). The association of this picture with paresis of ocular muscles (squint, diplopia, or ptosis) is very suggestive of encephalitis. Papillœdema is characteristically absent, as also are headache, sickness, and a slow pulse. The intracranial pressure on lumbar puncture is not raised. The composition of the cerebrospinal fluid in encephalitis has already been mentioned. The opening stage of an acute leptomeningitis may present clinical difficulties for a brief initial period, but the examination of the cerebrospinal fluid (see page 140) should make diagnosis clear. Occasionally, barbiturate poisoning in virtue of the stupor and squints that may be present may raise a suspicion of encephalitis, but what has been said of the nature of the somnolence should enable differentiation to be made. Finally, here as elsewhere in neurological diagnosis, the careful taking of the history will avert many errors. The Parkinsonian sequel has been adequately described. It differs from true paralysis agitans, a degenerative disease of elderly persons, in that it may be seen at any period of life from adolescence to old age, in the presence of eyelid flutter, and defect of convergence, in the predominance of rigidity and the frequent absence of tremor.

Treatment.—For the acute illness no specific treatment is known, though favourable results have been claimed for the intravenous administration of 2·5 per cent. to 5 per cent. solutions of sodium salicylate in normal saline, given in doses of 10 c.cs. daily for a week. For the rest, the treatment is that of any febrile illness, with care to ensure a due convalescence and to avoid a premature resumption of full physical activity. It is necessary to secure a minimum period of three months' convalescence after any recognized attack of encephalitis, however mild it may appear to be. During the period of its epidemic occurrence (1918–1930) the mildest cases of the malady seemed as prone to disabling Parkinsonian and other sequels as those that were manifestly severe in the acute stage, and it is possible that the almost immediate return of patients who were but slightly and briefly ill to full physical activity may have had its influence in this result. This at any rate became the present writer's firm conviction during the later years of this period: a conviction for which, of course, the quality of proof cannot be claimed. The treatment of Parkinsonism is purely symptomatic and consists in the administration of increasing doses of the tincture of belladonna or stramonium, of hyoscine hydrobromide, or of atropine sulphate. The response to these cannot be foretold in the individual case. Sometimes there is none, at other times there is no objective change, but the patient professes himself as better and less disabled, while in a few cases a striking objective diminution of muscular rigidity may be seen. Tolerance also varies widely from patient to patient for these drugs. Full details are given in the chapter on paralysis agitans (page 192).

POST-INFECTIVE ENCEPHALITIS

An acute encephalomyelitis may follow certain of the acute specific fevers and also vaccination. Although it is associated with a virus disease (smallpox, chicken-pox, vaccinia, measles), it is not certain that post-infective encephalitis is itself a virus disease. Vaccinial encephalitis, during the few years in which it was encountered, usually followed a primary vaccination in late childhood or adult life. A similar encephalitis has been known to complicate anti-rabic treatment, and to follow infective hepatitis.

Pathology.—Post-infective encephalitis differs from the known virus diseases of the nervous system in that the essential lesion appears to be a focal demyelination (loss of myelin sheaths) and not a primary attack upon the nerve cell, and this in itself is a reason for doubting its origin in a virus infection. Strictly speaking, therefore, it does not belong to the category described in this chapter, though it is most conveniently dealt with here.

As a rule post-infective encephalitis develops during the second week of the original illness, and the severity of the latter seems to have no influence upon the occurrence or non-occurrence of this complication.

Two types are noticed, a predominantly encephalitic and a predominantly spinal or myelitic. Usually the fever of the original exanthem has fallen. It then rises again, the patient becomes somnolent, headache, rigidity of the neck and spine, Kernig's sign, and convulsions may be present, and drowsiness and coma ensue. In the myelitic form there is a flaccid paraplegia with sphincter paralysis and the signs of an acute upper motor lesion. Many apparently moribund patients then make a rapid recovery, while others remain comatose or semi-comatose for weeks. In these, as consciousness returns, the signs of focal cerebral disease become more obvious: hemiplegia, aphasia, choreiform movements, an extrapyramidal syndrome, etc. No specific treatment is known.

HERPES ZOSTER (SHINGLES)

This is believed on general and on epidemiological grounds to be a virus disease of the nervous system, though this is not yet finally proved. Clinically, it consists in an acute vesicular eruption within the cutaneous distribution of one or two adjacent dorsal nerve roots, or within those of the sensory roots of the fifth and seventh nerves.

Ætiology.—On the whole, perhaps, males are more frequently affected than females. It may occur at any age from childhood upwards, though herpes of the ophthalmic division of the fifth nerve is more common in the second half of life. It has a close relationship with chicken-pox, and not rarely the latter appears in a household in which some two weeks earlier a case of herpes has developed. Herpes and a generalized chicken-pox eruption may occur in the same person.

In most instances herpes zoster develops without any discoverable cause, and we may regard it as an acute infection, probably by a virus, of the sensory root ganglia.

Pathology.—The lesion consists in (1) necrosis of one or more adjacent ganglia with intense lymphocytic infiltration and hæmorrhage; (2) a localized poliomyelitis confined to the same side of the cord and to the same segments as the affected ganglia, and more marked in the dorsal than in the ventral horn; (3) a mild localized leptomeningitis of the involved segments and nerve roots; and (4) a true neuritis of the dorsal and ventral roots and of the nerve roots immediately distal to the ganglion.

The eruption corresponds to the cutaneous distribution of the root of the ganglion most severely affected, and the nerve root lesion probably underlies the neuralgic pains and the motor paralyses sometimes encountered in cases of herpes zoster.

Symptoms.—There may be a brief febrile illness, the temperature rising to 100° or 102° F. There is a variable degree of general malaise. Pain of some severity then appears in what is to be the site of the future eruption. The latter develops on or about the fourth day, where the cutaneous twigs of the affected root reach the skin. There is an erythema, followed by a crop of vesicles containing clear fluid. From the fifth day after their appearance these begin to dry and scab. Much erythema and some œdema of the skin may surround them. In so-called geniculate herpes the entire pinna may swell and redden. The degree of scarring varies, and some weeks may pass before the reddening surrounding the scar disappears. Ultimately, the scars are anæsthetic and analgesic. Pain dwindles as scar formation proceeds, but in some elderly persons it may persist and intensify so as to become almost intolerable. It may continue as a *"post-herpetic neuralgia"* for one or more years and prove an exhausting and quite intractable symptom. Occasionally muscles innervated from the cord segment corresponding to the infected ganglion are paralysed: *e.g.* in a thoracic herpes a unilateral paralysis of the abdominal wall may be seen, while a third nerve palsy may accompany an ophthalmic herpes. Sometimes a facial palsy may accompany a herpetic eruption in the external auditory meatus, behind the pinna and on the soft palate. It has been usual to attribute this palsy and eruption to herpes of the geniculate ganglion, and they may be accompanied by an eruption on the side of the neck and in the occipital region (herpes occipito-collaris). It is possible, however, in some instances that such cases do not betoken involvement of the geniculate ganglion, but a neuritis of the seventh nerve associated with cervical herpes. The third nerve palsy of some cases of ophthalmic herpes provides a similar example of herpes and a neuritis of a motor nerve not corresponding to the herpetic ganglion.

Treatment.—If the patient be elderly, or there is a febrile onset, he should be kept in bed for at least a week. When its situation allows, the affected area should at once be covered by a collodion dressing. This of itself seems to have some analgesic quality, while it protects the lesions from the friction inseparable from the use of loose dressings, and also from infection. When this is impracticable, the eruption may be dusted with a boric or zinc oxide powder. In ophthalmic herpes the cornea may be involved, so that bathing of the eye, the instillation of castor oil, or even of atropine ointment, and the use of a pad and eyeshade may be expedient. Aspirin or a combination of aspirin and codeine (gr. $\frac{1}{8}$ to $\frac{1}{4}$) may suffice to relieve pain. Post-herpetic neuralgia may be difficult to relieve in those patients in whom it does not gradually wane during the year following the acute attack, and may in severe cases considerably impair the subject's general health and state of nutrition. Occasionally, the local application of a 1 per cent. novocain ointment may afford some relief, while other cases seem to derive benefit from local warmth. X-ray therapy, the details of which need not here be given, is probably more effective than any other measure, and this in proportion to the shortness of the period between the acute attack and the start of treatment. In long-standing cases its results are uncertain.

In a few old and frail patients whose lives are rendered quite wretched by pain, it may be justifiable to give heroin by mouth (gr. $\frac{1}{12}$ to $\frac{1}{8}$). Such cases must be carefully selected and should exclude those whose general condition remains so good as to belie their expressed assessment of the severity of their sufferings.

CHAPTER VIII

Syphilis of the Nervous System

INTRODUCTION

THE belief that syphilis is the commonest single cause of organic nervous disease dies hard. It is a legacy from the text-books of the end of the last century in virtue of which syphilis of the nervous system still occupies the place of honour, as though "by merit raised to that bad eminence," in most accounts of diseases of the nervous system. While in some countries it may yet deserve that place, to-day and in this country intracranial tumour and disseminated sclerosis certainly take numerical precedence of it amongst chronic nervous diseases, while if we take into account nervous diseases of vascular origin and such an ambulant malady as epilepsy, neuro-syphilis falls into the fifth place in the matter of relative incidence.

It is of greater importance than might at first sight appear that we should have a due sense of proportion on this question, for the tendency still exists in the case of organic nervous disease to diagnose syphilis until it can be positively excluded. As a result innumerable unnecessary Wassermann reactions in the blood are tested, and many unwarranted lumbar punctures and examinations of cerebrospinal fluid performed. There arises also from this tendency the still more unhappy consequence that the clinical observer too often and prematurely passes his diagnostic problems to the clinical pathologist, when it is his primary function to exhaust the possibilities of clinical observation before he asks the pathologist to carry him on his back.

There is still much that remains unexplained in the *pathogenesis and morbid anatomy* of syphilis of the nervous system, but the following statements embody what is most generally believed as to its pathogenesis and as to the essential lesion of neuro-syphilis.

THE INVASION OF THE NERVOUS SYSTEM.—To gain the nervous system the spirochæte has to penetrate the meningeal barrier, and therefore the first attack of the organism is upon the pia-arachnoid. This attack takes place early in the evolution of syphilis, and if penetration and invasion take place it is during the secondary stage and not at any later period. Neuro-syphilis begins from this invasion, and since throughout its course from this point the pia-arachnoid is involved to a greater or less degree in the syphilitic process, we may form a fairly accurate impression of this process from the study of the cerebrospinal fluid. As was pointed out when discussing acute meningitis, the reaction of the pia-arachnoid to infection is mirrored by changes in the composition of the cerebrospinal fluid as well as by clinical signs. In syphilis this is equally true, and the original attack of the organism upon the meningeal barrier and the subsequent development of neuro-syphilis may be traced in the changes which examination reveals in the cerebrospinal fluid. It may be emphasized, however, that the initial attack upon the meninges during the secondary stage of syphilis while it leads to changes in the cerebrospinal fluid does not necessarily indicate penetration of the barrier by the spirochæte. Whether this has occurred cannot be determined at the time, but only when, perhaps years later, clinical symptoms and cerebrospinal fluid changes reveal that neuro-syphilis is in fact established.

We may now briefly trace the meningeal reaction to the syphilitic infection from the primary stage onwards to the final development of what is called parenchymatous neuro-syphilis.

In the early primary stage before the Wassermann reaction (W.R.) in the blood has become positive, the cerebrospinal fluid in a small proportion of cases shows a slight rise in the lymphocyte count (from 5 to 10 cells per c.cm.). This pleocytosis is the initial reaction of the fluid, and in this case is the sole change.

During the late primary and the secondary stages, about 20 per cent. of all cases of syphilis show changes in the cerebrospinal fluid. The lymphocyte count per c.cm. ranges from 10 to 50. In a smaller percentage there is also an increase in the globulin content, and in a still smaller percentage there may be a positive W.R. Usually this reaction is negative in the fluid at this stage.

The cutaneous eruptions of secondary syphilis are not necessarily accompanied by changes in the fluid, while on the other hand there may be clinical signs of meningeal irritation and changes in the fluid in the absence of cutaneous eruptions.

If adequate treatment be undertaken both clinical and cerebrospinal fluid indications of meningeal irritation pass off.

A latent period now ensues which in untreated cases may last from one and a half to three or four years. During this period a certain proportion of cases show a recurrent meningeal reaction. They are spoken of as "meningo-recidives," and if clinical symptoms be also present (headache, cranial nerve palsies, etc.) as "neuro-recidives." In the latter circumstances the lymphocyte count per c.c. of fluid may rise to several hundreds, with the addition of some plasma, mono-nuclear and polymorphonuclear cells. Both the total protein and the globulin fraction are increased and the W.R. is positive.

With adequate treatment the fluid returns to normal again in some 60 per cent. of these cases, but in the remaining 40 per cent. some changes persist and it is this residue of cases from which the future incidence of cases of neuro-syphilis is derived.

Should the fluid remain consistently normal throughout this latent period we may assume that, although attacked, the meningeal barrier has not been penetrated and the future development of neuro-syphilis need not be feared. Even to this generalization, however, a few exceptions have been recorded.

Any later indications in the fluid or clinically of nervous involvement may be taken to indicate that penetration has occurred and that neuro-syphilis is already established.

When the tertiary stage of syphilis arrives, the fluid will be found normal in every respect unless there are clinical indications of syphilitic meningitis. Such a meningitis may be acute or slowly developing and chronic. If acute, the lymphocyte count per c.cm. will range from 50 to 500, with the addition of the other types of cell already mentioned. The total protein ranges from 50 to 100 mgm. per 100 c.c. The globulin reaction is strongly positive and so also is the W.R. In chronic meningitis and in the different forms of meningo-vascular syphilis—cerebral and spinal—the reaction in the fluid resembles that just described but is less intense: lymphocytes from 10 to 50; protein from 30 to 50 mgm. and a relatively weak W.R.

Finally, we come to the so-called parenchymatous syphilis, namely: tabes dorsalis, dementia paralytica, and optic atrophy. In tabes dorsalis the changes in the fluid are of slight or moderate severity: a slight excess of cells, weakly positive globulin reaction, a positive W.R. in the blood but not invariably in the fluid. These changes are less readily responsive to treatment than those of the varieties of neuro-syphilis already mentioned, and this is particularly true of the W.R. Rarely, a normal fluid is found.

In dementia paralytica, the lymphocyte count varies from 50 to 500 per c.cm. The protein level is from 40 to 100 mgm. per 100 c.c. and the W.R. is invariably positive. These changes also are refractory to anti-syphilitic treatment, and a fall in the cell count may be no more than that due to successive lumbar punctures.

There remains another reaction in the cerebrospinal fluid in neuro-syphilis to be briefly considered, namely, *the colloidal gold reaction of Lange*. This reaction is based upon the following observations:

The protein content of the cerebrospinal fluid consists of albumin and globulin fractions, of which the former is always the larger whenever there is an increase in the total protein. Such an increase takes place in numerous diseases of the nervous system. In two of these, namely, neuro-syphilis and disseminated sclerosis, the globulin increases disproportionately and may almost equal the albumin fraction.

This high globulin content imparts to the cerebrospinal fluid the property of precipitating colloidal particles from suspension, and colloidal gold is especially sensitive in this way. This fact is made use of not only for the recognition of neuro-syphilis but also for the differential diagnosis of the various forms thereof. Thus, if cerebrospinal fluid be added to a colloidal gold suspension in various dilutions, the dilutions in which precipitation is maximal vary according to the form of syphilis present. Thus, in dementia paralytica the gold is precipitated in the first six dilutions, giving what is known as the paretic curve when the results are plotted on paper.

In tabes and meningo-vascular syphilis precipitation is maximal from the third and fourth dilutions, while in pyogenic meningitis it is greatest from the sixth to eighth dilutions. Thus we have "paretic," "luetic," and "meningitic" curves. Disseminated sclerosis is characterized by a paretic curve associated with a negative W.R. This reaction has its greatest value, not in the diagnosis of disseminated sclerosis, but in the differentiation from dementia paralytica of the forms of meningo-vascular syphilis.

THE ESSENTIAL LESIONS OF NEURO-SYPHILIS.—The invasion of the nervous system which takes place in the late secondary stage may give rise to no pathological signs for five or more years. The course of events within the nervous system during this long latent period is not known. Speaking broadly, there are two main types of lesion in the nervous system, a *meningo-vascular syphilis* in which we find active pathological change in meningeal and vascular elements with minimal damage to the nervous elements themselves, and a *central or parenchy-matous syphilis* in which degenerative changes in nerve cells and fibres predominate, meningo-vascular lesions being minimal and not always active. Yet these two types of lesion do not represent fundamentally distinct processes. It is probable that there is a single type of essential initial lesion, namely an arteritis with an associated perivascular lymphangitis in the pia-arachnoid. The latter consists of a proliferation of lymphocytes and plasma cells which fill the perivascular spaces. There is intimal thickening in the arteries and these two processes tend secondarily to affect the neighbouring nervous tissues by pressure and by interference with their blood supply and nutrition. The peri-vascular lymphangitis may be a diffuse granulomatous process or may lead to local gumma formation. A gummatous meningitis may occur in any region, but is most common in the interpeduncular space where it involves the meningeal sheaths of the optic and other cranial nerves. When it occurs on the surface of the cord, the underlying spinal cord becomes infiltrated and the seat of gumma formation.

In tabes dorsalis the conspicuous lesion is a degeneration of the intramedullary prolongations of the dorsal root ganglion fibres as they lie in the root entry zone in the dorsal columns (Figs. 28 and 29). There is also an associated secondary glial proliferation and arterial thickening. It was formerly believed that this fibre degeneration was

L

secondary to a meningitis of the root just external to the cord and proximal to the ganglion, but the genesis of the lesion remains obscure. In optic atrophy we find a combination of interstitial infiltration and of nerve fibre degeneration. Dementia paralytica is essentially a chronic meningo-encephalitis of syphilitic origin, affecting mainly the

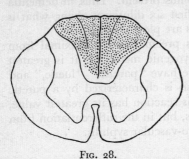

FIG. 28.

THE SITUATION OF THE CORD LESION IN TABES DORSALIS.

Tabes Dorsalis, showing the situation of the essential lesion in the dorsal columns. The lesion is marked by dots.

frontal lobes. To the naked eye, the pia-arachnoid is seen to be thickened and to be firmly attached to the subjacent brain substance. The cerebral fissures are abnormally wide owing to shrinking of the convolutions, this change being most marked at the frontal poles. There is some dilatation of the ventricles, and the ependyma covering their walls has a granular appearance. Microscopically both dura and leptomeninges are thickened and infiltrated by plasma cells and lymphocytes. The nerve cells show the chronic cell change mentioned already (page 59). The normal arrangement of the cortical cells is markedly disturbed and there is a diminution in the number of nerve cells seen. Those that remain show various grades of degeneration. There is a proliferation of blood-vessels and a marked astrocytic reaction (numerous spider cells) as well as a microglial reaction.

CLINICAL FORMS

MENINGO-VASCULAR OR CEREBROSPINAL SYPHILIS

The manifestations of neuro-syphilis included under these headings vary according to the site of the disease process and also according to whether the arteries or the meninges are predominantly involved, and it is clear, therefore, that numerous and varied clinical pictures may result. It is often the practice to describe these in separate categories of cerebral and spinal syphilis, but it will be understood that this can be no more than a rough working classification and that, except in the case of purely vascular syphilis (endarteritis), all cases of meningo-vascular syphilis are cerebrospinal. The frequency with which the Argyll Robertson pupil is found in what is called spinal syphilis is an apt illustration of this fact.

SYPHILITIC MENINGITIS.—We have seen that an acute meningitis may arise in the secondary or in the tertiary stages of syphilis, but it is a relatively rare form most often encountered in young adult males.

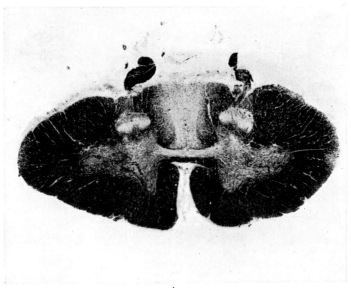

A

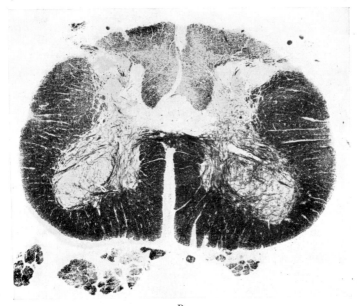

B

FIG. 29.

TABES DORSALIS.

Two transverse sections of the spinal cord (A from the cervical and B from the lumbar region). A shows the degeneration of the exogenous posterior column fibres derived from the lumbar posterior roots, and at this level occupying the columns of Goll. B shows the more widespread degeneration in the posterior columns in the lower lumbar segments.

To face page 162.

The onset may be sudden with intense headache and high fever (103°) with delirium, rigidity of neck and spine and other indications of an acute meningeal reaction. The cerebrospinal fluid reaction has already been described. There may be a slight œdema of the optic discs, cranial nerve palsies, and diminished tendon jerks. With adequate treatment recovery is the rule.

More common is a chronic form of gummatous meningitis at the base of the brain, giving rise to preliminary headache which may occur over an initial period of some weeks before ocular palsies develop. These palsies vary greatly in incidence and severity. Most commonly affected are the third, fourth, and sixth nerves, but the fifth, seventh, and the optic nerves and chiasma may also be involved. Although the inflammatory process in the meninges is bilateral the clinical signs (palsies) may be unilateral.

The Argyll Robertson pupil reaction is not constant, but is more often seen than in acute syphilitic meningitis. It was formerly held that this form of neuro-syphilis accounted for the majority of all cases of ocular palsies, but it is doubtful if this is any longer true.

Associated with these focal signs it is common to find symptoms of slight general impairment of cerebral function: emotional instability revealed by irritability, mental deterioration shown by defects in judgment and in memory, persistent headache, and less commonly slight œdema of the optic discs. When the optic nerves or chiasma are involved there may be defects in the visual fields and some primary optic atrophy, and when the neighbouring hypothalamic region is affected we may find polyuria, obesity, and somnolence. If the exudates organize, hydrocephalus may ensue.

The condition tends to run a chronic and fluctuating course, and even with rigorous treatment complete recovery may not be achieved.

Differential Diagnosis.—Ocular palsies and headache being the common manifestation of the process we have been considering, it is clear that difficult problems of differential diagnosis may arise. While examination of the cerebrospinal fluid may be essential to con-clusive diagnosis, and the state of this fluid in neuro-syphilis has already been described, it is well to consider the purely clinical points in diagnosis.

In young adults perhaps the commonest cause of ocular paresis and diplopia is disseminated sclerosis. In this malady the paresis is rarely severe enough to produce visible squint, and it is always transient, enduring for a period of hours or days at most. Ptosis is not seen and the pupil reactions are normal. In middle-aged and elderly persons ocular palsies of sudden onset, usually unilateral, and involving one or more of the third, fourth, and sixth nerves, may develop suddenly, associated with severe pain in the distribution of the ophthalmic division of the fifth nerve. Nothing is known of the ætiology of this syndrome, though it has been attributed, without pathological confirmation, to periostitis of the superior orbital fissure leading to compression of the nerves as they enter the orbit. It may develop subacutely, one nerve being affected after another over a period of some days. The pain may persist for two or three weeks, and two or three months or even longer may be required before recovery, which is the rule, is complete. This syndrome has nothing to do with syphilis. A similar syndrome of more gradual development may, as described in the chapter on space-occupying lesions, indicate the presence of an enlarging and unruptured aneurysm of the internal carotid artery. It is in these circumstances unilateral and accompanied by some degree of exophthalmos of the affected eye. The pain is very severe, and if the optic nerve be compressed loss of vision and primary optic atrophy may ensue. The subject is usually of middle age. There remain occasional cases of isolated unilateral ocular palsy for which no ætiology can be discovered. In the case of orbital cellulitis and cavernous sinus thrombosis the general symptomatology makes diagnosis a matter of comparative simplicity.

CEREBRAL SYPHILITIC VASCULAR DISEASE.—The cerebral thrombosis associated with syphilitic endarteritis has already been described in the chapter on vascular diseases. While the blood W.R. is positive, the cerebrospinal fluid may be wholly normal unless there is an associated syphilitic meningitis or meningo-encephalitis. Cerebral thrombosis occurring in young adults should always suggest syphilis as a possible cause.

SYPHILITIC MENINGO-MYELITIS.—Paraplegia is the common expression of this incidence of the syphilitic process, but the clinical picture and course vary greatly from case to case. Thus a chronic meningo-myelitis affecting the cervical region of the cord may give rise to a condition somewhat resembling motor neurone disease. This is the so-called amyotrophic meningo-myelitis. In the thoracic segments we may have an acute or subacute transverse meningo-myelitis leading to paraplegia, or a chronic process leading to what is known as Erb's syphilitic paraplegia. These forms may now be briefly described.

(1) *Amyotrophic meningo-myelitis.*—There is an atonic atrophy, with loss of tendon jerks, of the muscles of the upper limbs and shoulder girdles. It is bilateral but not bilaterally symmetrical, may advance rapidly to profound wasting of all the limb muscles, or may suddenly cease to progress while some muscles remain untouched or but relatively weak. During the active wasting process fibrillation may be seen in the affected muscles, but this disappears when the condition becomes stationary. In the lower limbs we may find increased tendon jerks, extensor plantar responses, or, alternatively, a complete loss of knee and

ankle jerks, the legs being otherwise unaffected. Root pains often precede and accompany the early stages of the affection. Sensory loss is absent or minimal. As a rule, though not constantly, the pupils show a complete or an incomplete Argyll Robertson reaction. In the cerebrospinal fluid the changes are those of a relatively mild meningeal reaction, already described, with a feebly positive W.R. and a luetic curve to colloidal gold.

(2) *Erb's syphilitic paraplegia.*—The clinical condition known by this name is simply a relatively mild and chronic form of syphilitic meningo-myelitis. The patient gradually develops a spastic and shuffling gait, with severe impairment of control over the vesical sphincter, and with sensory loss of posterior column type, namely, impaired postural and vibration sensibility. Although the gait suggests that the legs are very spastic, passive movement as the patient lies on his back does not reveal much spasticity, nor is there a severe degree of weakness. So insidiously does this clinical type develop that the patient may be able to shuffle along for many years after the initial appearance of symptoms. The disability fluctuates from year to year, but does not respond to anti-syphilitic treatment nor is its progress arrested. The arms are usually unaffected. The pupils show a complete or incomplete Argyll Robertson reaction. The cerebrospinal fluid changes are those of a mild meningeal reaction.

(3) *Acute and subacute syphilitic meningo-myelitis.*—Paraplegia in association with this lesion may develop rapidly. After a few days of root pains, usually in the mid-thoracic region, the legs weaken, sensation is impaired, there are retention or incontinence of urine and all the signs of a diffuse transverse lesion of the cord. In time a spastic paraplegia-in-extension is established, and if the condition be untreated or does not respond to treatment it may progress to paraplegia-in-flexion. In such a case the pathological diagnosis requires a blood and cerebrospinal fluid examination, though the Argyll Robertson pupil, if it be present, will reveal the syphilitic nature of the lesion.

Prognosis.—In all forms of meningo-vascular syphilis prognosis depends upon early and adequate treatment. If severe damage to the cord ensues before response to treatment develops, only imperfect recovery can be looked for. In the chronic varieties, as has already been stated in connection with Erb's paraplegia, the outlook as to recovery or material improvement is bad.

Treatment.—The substances at our disposal are arsenic, mercury, bismuth, and the iodides. The arsenical preparations in use are neo-salvarsan (914, novarsenobillon) and silver salvarsan. Tryparsamide is used in the post-pyrexial treatment of dementia paralytica. In acute syphilitic meningitis it is prudent to refrain from using arsenic until a week's preliminary treatment with mercury and iodides has been given, otherwise an acute exacerbation of symptoms may ensue. A course of six intravenous injections of the arsenical preparation chosen may then be given, the dosage of neosalvarsan rising from an initial dose of 0·3 gram to a final dose of 0·6 or 0·9 gram if no untoward reaction develop.

Bismuth has to some extent superseded mercury and is given intramuscularly in doses containing 2 or 3 grains of bismuth, a course consisting of twelve injections.

The iodides have their chief use in neuro-syphilis in chronic meningeal lesions, and as large doses as can be tolerated should be employed.

Treatment, by whatever combination of drugs, must be continued over a period of years in meningo-vascular syphilis. Courses of arsenic or of bismuth may be needed twice yearly, or the two may be used alternately. The intensity of treatment should not be wholly determined by the blood and cerebrospinal fluid reactions, but also by the clinical response. For reference to the penicillin treatment of neuro-syphilis see page 174.

TABES DORSALIS (LOCOMOTOR ATAXY)

There can be few senior medical students unable to recite the components in the symptom-complex of this familiar syphilitic affection of the nervous system, and still fewer who have a clear or accurate notion of the natural history of this common malady. Tabes is an apt example of the importance, stressed in the opening chapter of this book, of regarding an illness as a sequence of events, during the course of which it develops successively the features by which it may be known. Clinical skill consists in making this recognition as early as possible, that is, before the sum of its signs and symptoms have appeared.

The development of tabes is notoriously a slow process, spread over many years in most cases, and not rarely prone to arrest before its full development. Thus it is that those who regard it as a malady character-ized by the Argyll Robertson pupil, loss of knee and ankle jerks and ataxy of gait, necessarily fail to diagnose it in a large proportion of early cases, and when they achieve diagnosis do so after prolonged and avoidable delay.

It may be called a characteristic of tabes that although from case to case there is no *essential* variation in the neurological signs found on examination, the symptoms which first bring the patient under observation present the greatest diversity. Any one of the following may thus bring a case of tabes to light: a sudden painless effusion into a knee joint, an attack of abdominal pain and vomiting, a chronic ulcer on the sole of the foot, pains in the legs, failing vision, or imperfect control of the vesical sphincter. This diversity and the apparently non-neurological nature of some of these symptoms are factors in the not uncommon failure to recognize tabes in its early stages or in its incomplete forms.

Ætiology.—It is no longer necessary to labour the syphilitic origin of tabes dorsalis, and its morbid anatomy has already been summarized (page 161). It makes its appearance from five to twenty years after the primary infection, more commonly in men than in women. Unlike dementia paralytica, which has shown a steadily falling incidence during the past twenty years in this country, tabes still occurs with but slightly diminished frequency. It may result from congenital syphilis, when it manifests its presence in childhood, adolescence or early adult life.

Symptoms.—It is essential to bear in mind the extremely slow unfolding of the clinical picture of tabes, and the undoubted fact that it can be diagnosed long before this unfolding is complete. Indeed, in a considerable proportion of cases it never is complete, for the malady often undergoes arrest at some stage short of its full possible development, and this quite irrespective of any question of treatment.

It is an affection of the afferent neurones, sensory and non-sensory, and subjective sensory symptoms commonly usher in its clinical course and may remain its sole manifestation for a period of several years. Lightning pains are commonly the earliest symptoms, though they are not necessarily the symptom first complained of when the sufferer seeks medical advice. Frequently, he has satisfied himself that his pains are due to rheumatism and does not present himself for observation until some more disabling manifestation of the disease has developed.

The difficulties that may beset any enquiry as to the occurrence of these pains has already been referred to, and repeated and variously worded questions may be required before the long existence of lightning pains is admitted (page 4).

Lightning pains commonly occur in paroxysms which vary in frequency, duration, and severity from time to time and from case to case. Most patients complain that they are worse in wet weather or immediately before rain. The pains are sudden and lancinating, seeming to strike into the limb from outside rather than coursing along its length. Occasionally numerous tiny punctate ecchymoses appear on the skin over the shins after a severe bout of the pains. A paroxysm may consist in frequently repeated stabs of pain in the same place; e.g. the heel or knee, or of stabs of pain ranging from knee to ankle. They may be present in the trunk—lower thorax and abdomen—when they are often accompanied by considerable cutaneous hyperæsthesia. They may also occur in the distribution of the cervical segments, or of that of the trigeminal nerve.

While in some patients these pains tend to diminish in frequency and severity with the passage of years, in others they remain prominent and distressing throughout life, and it is in such cases that perforating ulcers, Charcot joints, and gastric crises seem also to figure largely, ataxy and other manifestations of postural sensory loss being minimal or absent.

Paræsthesiæ do not always trouble the tabetic subject, and the areas of sensory loss to be described may only be revealed by examination; but numbness of the feet, a sensation described as the feeling of walking on cotton wool, numbness of the face—often most obvious when the patient is shaving—and a sensation of "stiffness" of the legs (in striking contrast to the actual flaccidity of these members) are often complained of.

Next in sequence is the appearance of sensory loss. Perhaps earliest of these manifestations of loss is diminution and disappearance of pain sense in the tendo achillis on pressure. A feature of this abnormality is the delay in perception of painful sensation when the tendon is pinched between finger and thumb, and two or more seconds may elapse before pain is felt, and once evoked it tends to persist unduly. Evidence has recently been produced suggesting that this very characteristic delay may not be due to a slowing of impulses as they pass along degenerated fibres, but to a loss of function in the more rapidly conducting pain fibres.

During the evolution of the malady and while the symptoms described are present, others gradually develop. An early loss of libido and of sexual potency in male patients, and minor abnormalities of micturition are among the most characteristic of these. Micturition becomes hesitant, the passage of urine is held up before the bladder is emptied, and a fresh effort is needed to start it anew. Later a tendency to dribbling of urine after the apparent completion of the act may develop, though none of these sphincter disturbances is invariable. When they are present, catheterization usually reveals the presence of some residual urine after voluntary micturition, and in long-standing cases of tabes there is generally some degree of chronic cystitis. This may become acute from time to time, and as it does so all the patient's symptoms and disabilities tend to increase and he becomes progressively more thin and pale. Indeed, the cachexia and pallor so common in tabetics are probably in large measure due to chronic vesical infection —and not to the progress of the tabetic affection. A plump, fresh-coloured tabetic is the exception, and when he is found, it will usually be discovered that he has no impairment of sphincter control and no residual urine.

Physical examination in the early stages of the malady reveals some or all of the following signs. In the matter of *sensation* delay or loss of pain sense in the tendo achillis is constant and a diagnosis of tabes can rarely be made in the absence of this early sign. Over the front of the chest, from about the level of the second rib down to the xipnisternum, there is commonly, though not invariably, loss of painful sensation to pin-prick, sensibility to light touch being preserved (Fig. 30). The abdominal wall may appear unduly sensitive to pin-prick, and this is especially likely to be the case in subjects who have recurrent gastric crises. Great stress has also been laid upon an area of cutaneous analgesia (light touch being intact) over the nose and immediately surrounding skin. This sign is not constantly present, is indeed usually absent as long as some light reaction is retained by the pupils, though what the connection between these two phenomena may be cannot even be surmised. Analgesia may overflow, as it were, from the upper level of loss on the chest down the mesial aspects of the upper limbs to the fingers, including the little and ring fingers, and the ulnar nerve at the elbow may be insensitive to pain when rolled under the observer's finger.

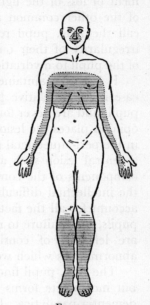

Fig. 30.

The Distribution of
Cutaneous Sensory Loss
in Tabes Dorsalis.

Some loss of cutaneous pain sense may also exist over the feet, legs, and—if sphincter disturbances be marked—over the perineum.

Examination will also reveal loss of one or both ankle jerks, and—later in the evolution of the disease—of the knee jerks, though many obvious cases of tabes retain the latter jerks for many years. At some stage of the illness postural sensibility will become impaired in the legs, less often in the arms. This defect will show itself as swaying when the eyes are closed (Rombergism), and then as ataxy of gait, and by error of projection in the heel-knee and finger-nose tests (see page 37).

A characteristic distribution of cutaneous analgesia in a case of tabes dorsalis. The segmental regions involved include the lower cervical and upper thoracic segments, and there is also analgesia round the tip of the nose and the lips.

The arm jerks may be permanently retained if, as often happens, the tabetic process does not invade the cervical region of the cord.

Finally we come to the characteristic abnormalities of pupillary reaction that are so constant in tabes, namely, to the consideration of the Argyll Robertson pupil.

The Pupil in Neuro-syphilis: Argyll Robertson Reaction

The sign that goes by the name of the Argyll Robertson pupil is one of the most familiar in clinical medicine, yet there are few signs about which there are more misconceptions. In 1869 Argyll Robertson described four cases of loss of the pupillary light reaction *associated with miosis*, but this latter component of the condition is now usually regarded as a non-essential, inconstant, and adventitious accompaniment of loss of the light reaction. Further, the same view is adopted of the other common accompaniments of what, for brevity, we may call the A.R. pupil reaction, namely, inequality of the two pupils, irregularity of their outline, atrophy of the iris, and irresponsiveness of the pupil to mydriatics.

It is here maintained that these components, varying from case to case in their relative prominence, are essential elements in the A.R. pupil, and are never found together apart from neuro-syphilis. Current opinion places the lesion underlying loss of the pupillary light reaction in the peri-aqueductal grey matter of the mid-brain, but it is clear that a central lesion such as this cannot adequately account for the other components of the complete A.R. pupil, and it may be partly due to the intellectual difficulty created by the inability of the hypothesis to account for all the facts, that miosis, inequality and irregularity of the pupils, their failure to respond to mydriatics and the atrophy of the iris are left out of consideration and regarded as separately caused abnormalities which we are not called upon to account for.

The A.R. pupil finds its most complete expression in tabes dorsalis, but incomplete forms are found in meningo-vascular syphilis and in dementia paralytica. In a fully developed case of tabes we commonly find complete loss of the light reaction in both pupils to direct and to consensual illumination. The pupil is small (1·5 to 2·5 mm. in diameter) in the great majority of cases, but except in extreme miosis the loss of circularity of outline and the inequality of the two pupils are readily visible. The instillation of mydriatics results in very slight dilatation which does not abolish the irregularity of outline, or in complete failure to dilate. In the blue-eyed tabetic, in whom the iris stroma is not hidden by the pigment that colours the iris of brown-eyed persons, this stroma is seen to be thinned and atrophic, the concentric fibres may have disappeared, and the blue has become discoloured to a washed-out greenish tint. In short, loss of light reaction is never found as an isolated anomaly. In incomplete forms the pupil is larger, but still non-circular in outline.

In dementia paralytica, miosis is not the rule and iris atrophy may be inconspicuous. In tabes with optic atrophy large pupils are found, but irregularity, inequality, and iris atrophy are usually present in greater or less degree.

Finally, though these pupil anomalies of neuro-syphilis cannot be explained by a central lesion, it has to be stated that so far no satisfactory alternative pathological explanation is available, and the genesis of the phenomenon and the seat—or seats—of the underlying disease process remain unknown, though speculations on the subject abound.

In advanced cases of tabes of many years' standing, the pupil is usually extremely small and often becomes completely immobile both to light and to convergence.

DIFFERENTIAL DIAGNOSIS OF THE A.R. PUPIL.—In very rare cases of post-encephalitic Parkinsonism, and also in rare examples of focal mid-brain lesion, the light reaction may be lost in an individual who is not syphilitic. If this loss be unilateral, the affected pupil is larger than its fellow, contrary to what is the case in the A.R. pupil of syphilis. When bilateral, both pupils are large, circular, and equal. The iris is normal.

Under the name of the *myotonic pupil* is described a rare condition, most often encountered in young women, in which with a pupil of normal size and contour the light reaction is abolished, while the reaction to convergence (constriction and subsequent dilatation) are markedly slow, each taking several seconds to complete. This anomaly is not related to syphilis, may give rise to no symptoms, but may upon occasion be found in association with loss of the knee and ankle jerks. In these circumstances a diagnosis of tabes may be erroneously made. The points of difference already enumerated indicate that a true Argyll Robertson pupil is not in question, while the absence of any form of sensory loss and the complete absence of clinical or serological signs of tabes or of syphilis make a differential diagnosis possible. If the myotonic pupil be unilateral, its defective reaction to convergence may lead to a complaint of blurring of near vision, but the condition is often symptomless, being accidentally discovered during the course of a routine ophthalmic examination. It calls for no treatment.

From what has been said, it will be apparent that, like the general clinical picture of tabes, the Argyll Robertson pupil takes time to reach its full expression, and a diagnosis of tabes may often be possible in a subject in whom some light reaction still persists and in whom miosis has not yet supervened. It is for this reason that the description of the condition just given is of importance. The early stages of development of the A.R. pupil should be appreciated if delay or error in diagnosis is to be avoided.

In a proportion of tabetics progressive primary *optic atrophy* develops and invariably leads to blindness. The onset is not usually simultaneous in the two eyes, and thus atrophy with blindness develops in one eye earlier than in its fellow. The optic disc has the characteristic appearance of primary optic atrophy. Its margins are clear-cut and distinct, it is very pale, the lamina cribrosa is extremely distinct, the vessels are normal. In those cases in which optic atrophy develops, the tabetic process in the spinal cord may cease to progress early and the fibres carrying impulses underlying postural sensibility commonly escape damage. Ataxy, therefore, does not develop. It is as though the brunt of the process falls upon the optic nerves rather than upon the posterior root fibres.

Amongst the other common but inconstant features of tabes are the following:

Cranial Nerve Palsies.—Of these a partial, and frequently bilaterally unequal degree of ptosis is perhaps the most often seen. With the thinness, pallor, and miosis of the tabetic this drooping of the eyelids completes the facies so typical of the advanced tabetic. Squint and diplopia may also be present. These palsies are in part due to nuclear degeneration and possibly in part to chronic syphilitic meningitis.

Charcot Joints.—The so-called trophic changes in bone, cartilage, and ligaments are usually precipitated by injury. The joint cartilage is eroded, and a combination of loss of bone and of new bone formation together with effusion give the characteristic picture of a painless, swollen joint in which there is a grossly abnormal degree and direction of mobility. Following a strain to a joint ensuing upon a fall, there is a rapid painless effusion with swelling, and the train of changes enumerated then develop. The knee, ankle and hip joints, and less commonly wrist and elbow and lumbar (spinal) joints may be affected.

Perforating Ulcer.—The formation of a callosity under the great toe or ball of the foot is common in normal persons, and when this becomes thick and raised above the general level of the skin it becomes painful and is dealt with. The loss of pain sense in the tabetic foot leads to a neglect of this precaution, and finally, the callosity separates from the underlying dermis, fluid collects in the intervening space, and escapes from a split at the periphery of the callosity. The space then becomes infected, and the callosity separates leaving a chronic painless septic ulcer which does not heal. If neglected, it may deepen until bone or joint is reached and infection spreads into them, leading to the necessity of amputation of the toe and sometimes of the metatarsal bone.

Crises.—Several varieties of tabetic crisis are described, laryngeal, gastric, and rectal. Of these the gastric is by far the most common. It consists in an acute attack of abdominal pain with (usually) or without vomiting. It may last for several days and during its persistence there is marked cutaneous hyperæsthesia of the abdominal wall, but no rigidity such as is seen when a local abdominal lesion is present. Some tabetics are subject to recurrent gastric crises, while others never present this symptom at any time. The vomiting is incessant and continues when the stomach is emptied, the vomit then consisting of clear liquid, then of bile, and in the severest cases of blood. Hiccough may accompany the crisis. Nausea is inconspicuous or absent.

Paroxysms of rectal pain (rectal crises) with severe tenesmus may recur from time to time, and the laryngeal crisis may also be observed. This consists in an attack of noisy respiration, with cough and dyspnœa, and lasts for an hour or less.

Finally, a chronic syphilitic meningo-myelitis may accompany tabes, leading to a wasting of the upper limb muscles that resembles that seen in motor neurone disease, but is characterized by total loss of all tendon jerks.

Among the other less striking symptoms of tabes are flat foot, and loss of pain on pressure on the testicles.

Prognosis.—It has been already mentioned that tabes not uncommonly undergoes arrest. It may be questioned whether this can be said to be the case where lightning pains persist, yet these may be the only indication of its activity in patients who never become ataxic, who retain good general health and lead lives of approximately or wholly normal activity until old age or an intercurrent illness carries them off. Treatment cannot claim credit for these arrested cases, for many of them have never been treated save for some perfunctory steps taken during the stage of the primary infection.

In other cases the malady progresses, either steadily or by sudden increase in disability. The latter may occur when a severe intercurrent illness or an injury impairs the subject's general condition and necessitates his confinement to bed. On getting up again he is found to be grossly ataxic and the malady seems to take a fresh lease of life and to advance more rapidly.

In some long-standing and progressive cases the patient becomes emaciated and very anæmic. He endures a constant dribbling from an over-distended bladder that he can empty only by pressure on the abdominal wall. Prolapse of the rectum and bleeding piles are common. There may be recurrent gastric crises, accesses of severe lightning pains, osteoarthropathy with flail joints, and in some cases blindness from optic atrophy. The loss of postural sensibility may be so great that the patient is bedridden, can make no co-ordinated movements, and when his eyes are closed—or in the dark—has no notion of the position of his body or limbs in space. In short, the final stages of the malady may be the most distressing that can be encountered. In a proportion of long-standing cases, some of the signs and symptoms of dementia paralytica appear.

Treatment.—This may be considered from two aspects: the treatment of the syphilitic tabetic degeneration, and that of symptoms and disabilities. Despite the disillusioning experience of the past, few will be found to admit that anti-syphilitic measures are valueless in tabes, but even of those who are most enthusiastic in recommending them, none would venture to promise any result from their employment in the individual case. The present writer cannot claim ever to have been satisfied that anti-syphilitic treatment influences the course of tabes. The most intensively treated cases may be seen to deteriorate ruthlessly, while many of the arrested cases have never been treated since the malady was recognized in them. Nevertheless, various considerations may make some measure of anti-syphilitic treatment expedient, with the proviso that if anything of the kind be undertaken it is not in the patient's interest that his life should be made a mere appendage to treatment and that he should be subjected to endlessly reiterated courses of arsenical or other injections, and to repeated blood Wassermann tests and lumbar punctures. Unwise zeal of this order may make the patient's life wretched, and do more damage to his personality than tabes does to his physique. Further, this form of treatment cannot be wholly determined by the results of serological tests, but only by giving due weight to the clinical condition.

Intramuscular injections of bismuth, in courses of twelve injections twice yearly repeated not for longer than two or three years, are probably the method of choice. Between these courses mercury and iodides may be given by mouth (liq. hydrarg. perchlor. $\mathfrak{z}\frac{1}{2}$, pot. iodide grs. 10. Inf. quass. ad $\mathfrak{z}\frac{1}{2}$, t.d.s.). The arsenical preparations are not indicated, save in early cases.

Optic atrophy is certainly not arrested by any of these measures, and lightning pains are rarely, if ever, relieved by them. It has recently been claimed that optic atrophy may be arrested and vision saved by malarial or other form of pyrexial therapy. It is not yet possible to assess the value of penicillin in the treatment of neuro-syphilis. There is some evidence that it is of value in meningovascular, but of no yet ascertained value in parenchymatous syphilis. Early dementia paralytica is apparently uninfluenced by it.

The improvements noted in the cerebrospinal fluid after penicillin administration are not necessarily accompanied by clinical improvement.

Symptomatic Treatment.—(1) *Ataxy.*—It is often found that the confinement to bed of a tabetic subject who may have little or no disturbance of co-ordination precipitates severe ataxy of gait, and for this reason no tabetic should be confined to bed for longer than is necessary should any intercurrent illness develop or should he sustain some injury. Whenever possible, the patient should be allowed up for some period each day. The re-education exercises devised by Frænkel are the only useful measures to overcome ataxy of movement. The patient unable to stand or walk can perform the simpler of these in bed, when they consist in the active performance of simple movements on boards in which are cut holes into which he plants his heels. The ambulant tabetic walks along a floor or a strip of canvas painted with footprints in which he endeavours as accurately as possible to place his feet, a hand-rail being provided if necessary. In cases of acutely developing ataxy in relatively early cases, the most striking improvement may be achieved in this way.

(2) *The bladder.*—Any infection of the bladder, a common complication when there is residual urine, should be carefully watched and treated by the ordinary methods for the treatment of cystitis. All varieties of spinal cord disease tend to deteriorate when an infected bladder is neglected.

(3) *Charcot joints.*—When an osteo-arthropathy develops acutely with effusion, a Scott's dressing should be applied and the joint immobilized until the effusion has subsided. In the case of the knee, perhaps the joint most commonly affected, a splint should then be worn to protect it from the development of hyper-extension and of genu recurvatum. The patient should not be kept in bed longer than is imperative, for reasons already given.

(4) *Perforating ulcer.*—A simple ulcer with no infection of underlying bone or joint should first be cleaned by fomentations, and a stimulating lotion then applied to promote healing. It may be necessary to keep the foot off the ground or otherwise to avoid pressure upon it.

(5) *Lightning pains.*—These present one of the most difficult problems in treatment, and in some patients no really effective relief can be given. For obvious reasons the use of morphia or heroin are contra-indicated, and reliance has to be placed upon such drugs, singly or in combination, as aspirin, phenacetin, amidopyrin, and codeine. The last-named in small doses (gr. ⅛ to ¼) combined with aspirin is most generally useful. In a few cases where the patient is not old, is in good general health and suffers no disability from his tabes but very severe and disabling lightning pains in the legs, permanent relief from these may be obtained by cordotomy. This operation consists in the bilateral section of the lateral spinothalamic tract in the thoracic region. It is clear that cases must be carefully selected for this procedure.

(6) *Gastric crises.*—The patient may be given ice to suck and small doses of tincture of iodine. A hypodermic injection of phenobarbitone (1 cc. of a 20 per cent. solution) may be tried once or twice daily, and chloretone (grs. 5 to 10) has also been recommended. In debilitated patients in whom the vomiting proves intractable a hypodermic injection of morphia may upon occasion be necessary. It should always be borne in mind that the subject of gastric crises is not immune from acute abdominal disease or from renal colic, and renewed physical examination should always precede the treatment of a gastric crisis even in a known tabetic subject.

DEMENTIA PARALYTICA (GENERAL PARALYSIS)

Ætiology.—The syphilitic origin of dementia paralytica is now established. The subjects are more often males than females, the onset occurs from ten to twenty years after infection, that is, in middle age, not later. The morbid anatomy of the malady has already been described (page 158).

Symptoms.—These consist essentially in progressive mental deterioration, the indications of this varying from person to person according to his mental constitution, and in a progressive development of signs of organic disease of the brain. When unmodified by treatment the malady runs its course to a fatal termination, though sometimes with marked remissions, in a period of from three to five years. Since the introduction of pyrexial therapy the remissions may be more striking and longer lasting, and the subject survives by a variable period of years the normal course of the disease. The initial symptoms, or at least those which first attract attention, consist in manifestations of mental deterioration and emotional change. Judgment, the power of attention, and memory are insidiously impaired. The patient's standards, both ethical and social, become lowered. He is apt to be irritable and suspicious, and his family circle receives the brunt of this debasement. In some instances he becomes euphoric and boastful, extravagant and overbearing. This boastfulness is not necessarily extreme, but it is rather more obtrusive than one would consider becoming in oneself or in one's friends. It may be concerned with his intellectual capacity, his social standing, his means, or simply his health. Commonly, such a patient will assure the doctor that he never felt better in his life. In its more extreme degrees this change leads the patient into reckless and futile expenditure. This picture is, however, by no means invariable, for the patient may become silent, morose, and unsociable. In these circumstances his condition is often diagnosed as neurasthenia or anxiety neurosis, and if in the patient's past history the material of psychological stress be found, this view receives a fictitious confirmation, as though such stress could prevent its subject from developing the ordinary physical ills.

This steady downhill course is accompanied by certain characteristic physical signs. The articulation becomes affected, the terminal syllables of polysyllabic words are slurred, as may be seen when the patient attempts to pronounce such words as "constabulary," "artillery," and the like. As he talks there may be seen an irregular wavy tremor of the lips. The pupils show some components of the Argyll Robertson syndrome: inequality, irregularity of outline, a defective light reaction. There may be tremor of the extended hands, the tendon jerks are increased, and sooner or later the plantar responses become of the Babinski type.

From time to time brief epileptiform seizures may occur, sometimes generalized with loss of consciousness, sometimes consisting of localized convulsive movements without such loss. Transient paralysis of hemiplegic type or an aphasic speech disturbance may ensue upon these attacks.

Gradually, a widespread paralysis of upper motor neurone type, incontinence of urine and profound dementia make their appearance. During this course, partial remissions of some weeks' or months' duration may ensue. Optic atrophy with blindness is not uncommon. The patient's last year is one of bedridden and helpless dementia.

The variations that may be seen in this grim picture are mainly in the matter of the mental state during the earlier stages. Pure dementia, depression with delusions of persecution, exaltation with megalomania, or even maniacal excitement may be encountered.

In a few subjects the signs of tabes dorsalis are also present. In these circumstances the malady, *tabo-paresis* as it is called, runs a much quieter and greatly prolonged course, and even in untreated cases life and a large measure of physical capacity may endure for ten or more years.

Under the influence of pyrexial therapy (malarial or other) the course of the disease has been greatly modified. Striking remissions lasting for years may be seen, and during these the patient may, to superficial inspection, seem almost normal, though it is rare indeed for a patient previously engaged in work of any intellectual quality to regain anything like his former capacity. Yet he remains ambulant, reasonably normal emotionally, and often capable of simple regular work.

Such somatic physical signs as may be present never completely disappear. The articulation may improve and the tremor of the lips almost disappear, but the pupil reactions do not become normal, nor do changes in the reflexes disappear. It is, of course, in cases treated early and before severe dementia has ensued that the best results are obtained, but even in these a useful measure of restoration is not to be confidently predicted. Cure cannot be spoken of.

Diagnosis.—Usually the early clinical picture of dementia paralytica is readily recognizable by whomsoever has once seen it. The obvious dementia, the wavy tremor of the lips, and the slovenly articulation and the slight but manifest tremor of the hands together make up a characteristic picture, and when this has commanded diagnostic recognition the other signs can then be systematically sought for.

It is important to obtain corroboration of the history from some member of the patient's family, for the subject himself is commonly lacking in insight and may be wholly unaware that there is anything the matter with his health, mental or physical. The patient's wife or husband is commonly the best source of information.

M

Certain rare forms of what are called pre-senile dementia may closely resemble dementia paralytica, and only examination of the blood and cerebrospinal fluid may render differential diagnosis possible. The blood W.R. is almost always positive, that in the fluid invariably so. The other changes in the fluid have already been enumerated.

Treatment.—Anti-syphilitic measures alone have no influence upon the course of the malady, and only pyrexial therapy followed by anti-syphilitic measures is effective. Pyrexial therapy, whether by means of giving malarial infection, or by chemical or electrical agencies, should only be carried out under hospital or institutional conditions by those experienced in its use, and it is not necessary here to describe it in detail. Not every patient survives it, and in some it has to be terminated prematurely. Yet there is no alternative to its employment save to allow the patient to progress to an inevitable death, and therefore risks are justifiable.

Following ten or twelve malarial rigors the patient is allowed to regain strength and energetic anti-syphilitic treatment, preferably with tryparsamide, is undertaken. A second course may sometimes be necessary in the case of relapses.

In early cases and whenever pyrexial therapy is contra-indicated, or not practicable for any reason, a course of injections of tryparsamide may be tried: 2 grams are given intravenously at weekly intervals for as long as twelve weeks. Some authorities prefer to precede pyrexial therapy by this measure.

CONGENITAL NEURO-SYPHILIS

The subjects of the inherited forms of neuro-syphilis do not necessarily show the ordinary stigmata of congenital syphilis; nor do they commonly develop tertiary syphilitic lesions in bones or viscera. Perhaps the signs of an old interstitial keratitis provide the indication of congenital syphilis most commonly encountered.

The mortality of congenital neuro-syphilitic infants is high, and hence the majority do not live long enough to develop tabes or dementia paralytica. It is said that some 30 per cent. of congenital syphilitic infants show a positive W.R. in the cerebrospinal fluid, but only a small proportion of these later develop clinical signs of neuro-syphilis.

Syphilitic meningitis may occur in infancy, usually as an insidiously developing and chronic affection. The customary signs of a lepto-meningitis are present and hydrocephalus may ensue, with secondary optic atrophy, blindness, and dementia. Unless treated very early and energetically recovery is rare. Hydrocephalus may be the first indication of this process, and the development of this in an infant should always give rise to a suspicion of congenital syphilis. Cerebral vascular lesions (thrombosis) may also occur during infancy.

More commonly encountered than these manifestations of inherited syphilis is *juvenile dementia paralytica* (juvenile or congenital paresis). Slowly progressive mental deterioration is the striking clinical feature, with slurring articulation, tremor, and pupil changes as in the acquired type. The blood and cerebrospinal fluid reactions are those characteristic for dementia paralytica. Optic atrophy is not uncommon. Pyrexial therapy modifies the course of the malady, but rarely so markedly as in the acquired disease of adults. Juvenile tabes dorsalis and tabo-paresis are relatively rarely seen. Optic atrophy is common, but on the whole the malady tends to run a slow and quiet course; that is to say, lightning pains, visceral crises, and trophic lesions in skin, bones, and joints are uncommon.

Congenital neuro-syphilis may be asymptomatic, the patient being healthy but showing signs of syphilis in blood and cerebrospinal fluid.

Other manifestations of congenital neuro-syphilis are deafness, epileptiform fits, and choroido-retinitis. For all these treatment follows the same general lines as in the acquired disease.

CHAPTER IX

Disseminated Sclerosis (Multiple Sclerosis)

DISSEMINATED sclerosis is a disease developing in early adult life in otherwise healthy individuals and characterized by a fluctuating course that is "punctuated" at irregular intervals by acute exacerbations with intervening periods of improvement and quiescence. Its development may extend over many years and it ultimately becomes completely disabling in the majority of cases, though not in all. The lesions underlying this characteristic sequence of events are multiple inflammatory foci disseminated irregularly throughout the cerebrospinal axis and occurring in successive crops over a period of years. It is one of the commonest of all chronic organic nervous affections in these islands and in Western Europe.

Ætiology.—The onset in most cases is during the third decade of life, but occasional cases arise during late adolescence and in middle age. Women are more frequently affected than men, in the proportion of 3 to 2. The malady is found in persons of widely varying occupations and in all strata of society.

Pathology.—The pathological process is essentially a focal demyelination and the appearance and distribution of the lesions suggest that some myelin-destroying agent is present in them. Whether this agent is of organismal origin, or is an enzyme or other chemical substance, is unknown, and nothing is known of its mode of access to the nervous system. We know of no virus that acts upon white matter and the malady does not behave like any known infection.

The characters of the lesions are that they are sharply defined (Fig. 27) as though cut out with a punch, they are irregular in form and vary widely in size, they do not destroy the axis cylinders but strip their myelin sheaths from them, leaving them deformed as they pass through the focus. A secondary gliosis develops in old foci, and in fresh lesions there is some perivascular infiltration. They are found most thickly in the brain beneath the ventricles, where the white and grey matter of the cerebral cortex meet, round small blood-vessels, in the optic chiasma and scattered throughout the spinal cord (see page 59). (Figs. 31 and 32.)

Symptoms.—The fluctuating course and diverse symptomatology of disseminated sclerosis make it difficult to give a clear or concise clinical description of the malady, yet in fact these features are of the very essence of the clinical picture and lend the malady its striking

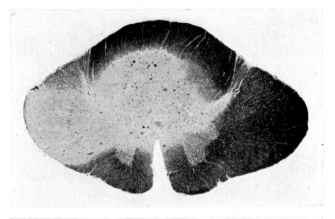

A

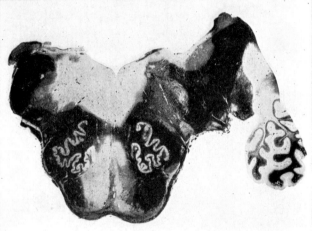

B

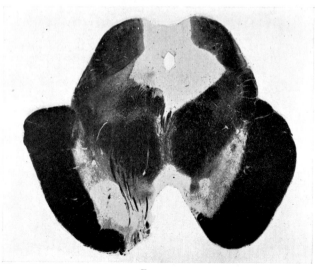

C

FIG. 31.

DISSEMINATED SCLEROSIS.

Three transverse sections, stained by the Weigert-Pal method, showing
the characteristic appearances of the areas of demyelination with their
clear-cut borders and irregular form. A, cervical region of the spinal
cord. B, upper part of the medulla. C, midbrain.

To face page 180.

individuality. It cannot always be safely recognized by its physical signs alone but, as has already been emphasized, by its behaviour in time; that is, by the sequence of events which have led to the condition found on examination.

A common though not invariable sequence of events in its evolution is as follows. A healthy young adult, more often a woman than a man, suddenly develops a mistiness of vision in one eye. This may be painless or accompanied by some aching in the globe on pressure or on lateral deviation of the eyes. It rarely amounts to blindness, but to a blurring of vision rendering the affected eye useless. This persists for a period varying from a few days to two or three weeks when it clears up. It often happens that the patient has not sought medical advice, but when she does so there is always the probability that a diagnosis of retro-bulbar neuritis from sinus infection is made. Ophthalmoscopic examination is usually negative and a central scotoma is found.

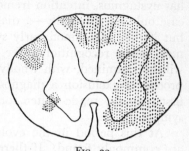

Fig. 32.

FORM OF THE LESIONS IN DIS-SEMINATED SCLEROSIS.

A transverse section of the cord, showing the typical form and sharp outlines of the lesions in disseminated sclerosis, and their transgression of the border between grey and white matter. Within the shaded areas the essential change is a destruction of myelin sheaths.

Following the recovery from this disturbance the patient may remain apparently healthy and symptom-free for a period varying from a few months to fifteen or more years when the malady again manifests its presence, perhaps by a similar affection of the other eye, or by symptoms indicative of a lesion of the spinal cord. Yet another possibility is that a short-lived diplopia without visible squint may be the symptom complained of.

At any rate, sooner or later, spinal cord symptoms do develop, and commonly very insidiously.

The subject begins to complain of unduly ready fatigue in one or both legs on exertion. By the end of the morning's work the housewife finds one leg "heavy," and inclined to drag. After a rest it feels stronger but soon tires again. In time she notices that this dragging wears out the toe of the shoe on the affected foot. Some subjective numbness is usually experienced in the leg, and not unnaturally continued use of a weak limb tends to make it ache. The patient therefore persuades herself that she has rheumatism or neuritis or flat foot; she seeks medical advice, proffers her own diagnosis, runs considerable risk of having it accepted, and is given a foot support, a tonic, or some form of electro-therapy or "ray" treatment. As the months pass the disability increases, may spread to the other leg, and one or both arms are noticed to be unsteady and clumsy. A little precipitancy of micturition develops. Finally, after some mild intercurrent illness or a confinement she gets up to find herself alarmingly weak and unsteady on her feet; she is at last methodically examined and the signs of an organic nervous affection are detected. If in the course of this examination it is found that she has nystagmus, intention tremor, and scanning speech—and this is the case only exceptionally—a diagnosis of disseminated sclerosis is made, but if this uncommon early symptom-complex is absent, the malady may escape recognition. Her blood W.R. and her cerebrospinal fluid will be examined, with wholly negative results, and thus by a tedious process of exclusion a diagnosis that should have leapt to the eye at first is finally made—often some two or three years after the onset of symptoms.

At this period in the evolution of the disease the following signs are commonly found. If there has been a retrobulbar neuritis in the past there will be temporal pallor of the optic disc or discs, but visual acuity may be quite or almost normal. Usually the cranial nerves show no abnormality of function, but sometimes when ordinary tests reveal no nystagmus, the fundus of the eye is seen through the ophthalmoscope to be in constant fine and rapid nystagmus. More often than not examination of the upper limbs reveals no abnormality other than a marked increase in the tendon jerks. The abdominal reflexes are absent. The knee and ankle jerks are exaggerated and there may be ankle clonus on one or both sides. The plantar responses on both sides are of the extensor type. There is no impairment of cutaneous sensibility, but there will almost certainly be loss of vibration sensation at the malleoli and possibly some impairment of postural sensibility in the toes.* In early cases there may be little or no weakness evident on examination, but if the patient be made to take a walk and re-examined some paresis may be detected. This makes its first appearance in the movement of dorsiflexion of the foot, then in flexion movements, and not in plantarflexion or extension of the leg until there is very evident weakness on walking. The gait will vary in character according to whether there is postural sensory loss in the legs, or involvement of the cerebellar mechanisms. In many cases there is a simple paresis which, owing to the predominant weakness of dorsiflexion, shows itself by a tendency of the foot to drag, and by an inability of the patient to lift the front of the foot or feet when asked to walk on her heels. In other cases there may be a slight measure of ataxy with Rombergism. Perhaps most characteristic is the gait of the patient in whom there is weakness, and both sensory and cerebellar defects. This gait has a characteristic

* The perception of the vibrations of a tuning fork is a mode of sensibility, the impulses underlying which travel up in the uncrossed sensory path in the posterior columns. It is tested by placing the foot of a vibrating fork (C 128) on the malleoli or other bony points.

tottery, stiff appearance and the patient holds her hands and arms out so as to be ready to grasp at the furniture when she feels herself reeling or about to fall.

In short, the essential objective signs in the initial stage of the malady comprise some or all of the following: pallor of the temporal half of one or both optic discs, increased arm jerks, loss of abdominal reflexes, increased knee and ankle jerks with or without clonus, extensor plantar responses, loss of vibration sense at the ankles.

These signs, especially if there be a history of fluctuations in the course of the illness, occurring in an otherwise healthy young adult are almost invariably the expression of disseminated sclerosis.

In other cases the onset is more acute. Numbness and tingling develop in one or more limbs, associated with the fairly rapid development of weakness in them. These symptoms may be heralded by an attack of giddiness and vomiting lasting for several days, during the course of which the symptoms mentioned above make their appearance. In these circumstances, recovery is also apt to be rapid, and within two or three weeks of onset, even if some paræsthesiæ still remain, normal power may have been regained and the reflexes may have returned to normal. It is in such cases, not systematically examined while organic signs are still present, that a diagnosis of hysterical disability is apt to be made.

Occasionally, the first lesions develop in the dorsal columns of the spinal cord, on one or on both sides. When this is the case sensory ataxy (page 37) is the striking initial symptom. Sometimes a single upper limb may thus develop ataxy. There is no weakness, but all movements of the arm and fingers are clumsy, and the patient describes the limb as "useless." There is gross error of projection in the finger-nose test with the eyes closed and objects held in the hand cannot be identified, or their shape and size appreciated.

This state of affairs may be associated with signs of an upper motor neurone lesion in the lower limbs, but is known to occur by itself. Recovery, complete or almost so, within a few weeks is the rule when the malady makes its first appearance in this way.

Other cases are known in which the limbs of one side become weak, and this picture has been spoken of as representing a "hemiplegic type" of disseminated sclerosis, but this is a misleading term since the reflexes (especially the plantar responses) are always abnormal on both sides, and usually the limbs regarded by the patient as normal will show some degree of paresis upon systematic examination.

In yet other patients, symptoms of cerebellar ataxy dominate the clinical picture from the outset. There is nystagmus, scanning speech, the feature of which is that each syllable of a word tends to be articulated slowly and deliberately as though it were a separate word. This defect is well seen when the patient is asked to pronounce such words as "constabulary," and the like. Signs of upper motor neurone lesion usually accompany these various signs, while intention tremor and unsteadiness of gait are marked.

Another variant is the slowly progressive spastic paresis of the legs, without cutaneous sensory loss, but with vibration loss and increased arm jerks.

In all clinical variants there may be recurrent diplopia, usually transient and without visible squint. From time to time there is precipitancy of micturition with occasional slight incontinence. The emotional tone is usually altered, the patient being euphoric, seeming to have little insight into the gravity of her condition and sometimes prone to attacks of unduly facile laughter. This prevailing mood is not, of course, seen in all patients.

Retrobulbar neuritis is not constant, nor invariably the initial symptom.

Course and Prognosis.—It is simple to generalize, for the malady, despite its wide fluctuations, tends to progress and ultimately to become completely disabling. The patient usually ends with paraplegia-in-flexion, incontinence, tremor of the hands, nystagmus, and scanning speech. Yet nothing can be more difficult than to forecast the future of the individual case when this is seen at the outset of the illness, and the general tendency is to be far too gloomy in discussing the situation with the patient's relatives. When an apparently healthy young adult develops a retrobulbar neuritis it is highly probable that disseminated sclerosis is in question, yet no one can say with any measure of accuracy how many weeks, months, or even years may pass before any fresh manifestations of the disease will appear, or even if they do appear, how many years will pass before grave disability will ensue. It is true that the period of freedom is more likely to be one of months than of years, but there is no certainty on this point. The difficulties which arise from this cause when discussing the situation with patient and relatives will be discussed under the subject of treatment.

Once a measure of residual weakness is established, though there still remains the possibility of later disappearance of signs, the balance of probability is that some disability will persist, and that only a carefully restricted life will, for the time, check further deterioration. When cerebellar symptoms are early and prominent no improvement can be looked for, and the same holds true of the slowly progressive non-remitting case. The full evolution of the malady may take many years, and the later in life the disease appears the more likely is it to run a mild course. In most cases final disablement is not reached earlier than ten to fifteen years from the initial manifestations. Permanent cure or recovery is probably unknown, but a few cases undergo arrest short of complete disability, reach old age and die from other causes.

Diagnosis.—As has already been implied, disseminated sclerosis should be recognized by what it is, and not by a routine process of exclusion in the course of which many unnecessary biochemical and serological investigations and much expensive and equally futile radiography are indulged in. Its age of incidence, its characteristic behaviour and its not less characteristic constellation of early objective signs, give it an individuality facilitating recognition in all but anomalous cases. Charcot's triad of nystagmus, intention tremor and scanning speech which is still commonly regarded as an early and constant feature of disseminated sclerosis, though Charcot explicitly described it as inconstant and late in appearance, is not a criterion upon which reliance should be placed. The appearance of unilateral retrobulbar neuritis in a healthy young adult is more commonly due to disseminated sclerosis than to any other cause, and sinus infection is rarely if ever responsible for this lesion. While vision is still blurred ophthalmoscopic examination is commonly negative, though rarely slight œdema of the optic disc may be seen. The residual temporal pallor does not develop for some two or three months after the invariable restoration of vision. It would be misleading to imply that compression of the cord by a ruptured intervertebral disc is a common lesion, but it does occur from time to time, and then presents a clinical picture that may be mistaken for one of disseminated sclerosis of what it has been the custom to speak of as the "spinal type." Yet, in view of all that follows a diagnosis of disseminated sclerosis such an error is at all costs to be avoided. Therefore, the presence of a history of injury to the back, an insidious onset and development of spastic weakness of the legs, indications of sensory impairment with an upper level, focal signs such as are enumerated on page 209, and, on the other hand, the absence of remissions and exacerbations, of past or present visual disturbance, or of recurrent phases of sphincter weakness, should lead the observer at least to consider the possibility of cord compression by a herniated disc, or indeed by any other local lesion.

Treatment.—Few maladies of the nervous system fill the doctor with a more humiliating sense of helplessness than this. There is no form of medication that has any certain influence upon the course of the malady, though its variable behaviour and its tendency to temporary remission have in the hands of those not familiar with it led to many unfounded claims for various remedies. These include protein shock therapy, pyrexial therapy, liver therapy, and the administration of various arsenical compounds. Arsenic is undoubtedly a useful tonic, but that it has any specific influence upon disseminated sclerosis can no longer be maintained. Recently quinine hydrochloride has come into use, a form of treatment based upon the belief that the serum of patients with disseminated sclerosis contains an excess of lipase, that such a lipase may be responsible for the demyelination which is the essential pathological process, and upon the fact that quinine inhibits the activity of lipases. Yet doubt has been cast upon the presence of this lipase excess in the serum, and it is becoming clear that in quinine we have no specific remedy. In short, medication offers nothing certain. Of pyrexial therapy we may say that it is not free from the danger of provoking an exacerbation—a result that can surprise no one who recalls that an intercurrent febrile illness often has the same sequel. There is no objection to the use of arsenic or of quinine, the latter either as the hydrochloride in doses of 5 grains once daily, or as a course of 12 weekly injections of iodo-bismuthate of quinine (1 c.cm.).

One oral method of arsenic administration is to give gradually increasing doses, beginning with ℳ3 of liquor arsenicalis thrice daily, and adding a further minim to each dose on every third day until a total dose of ℳ8 thrice daily is given. Once this level is attained, the dose is dropped to the original level again and the process repeated. Not every subject will tolerate this and the common initial symptoms of intolerance are looseness of the bowels with some griping pain. Even when well-tolerated, this method should not be too long continued, and it is best to prescribe it for alternate months over a period of six to twelve months.

The value of massage and active exercises for the spastic and paretic limbs is discussed in a subsequent chapter on treatment. Perhaps the most important measure, though one often quite impracticable, is to secure the patient from fatigue due to exertion. Overwork and fatigue are manifest and constant enemies to the subject of disseminated sclerosis. So also are intercurrent illnesses, injuries, surgical interventions, and the artificial termination of pregnancy designed to avert the exacerbation of symptoms that may follow delivery at full term. Pregnancy is not invariably deleterious to the course of events, and would probably be even less often so were the patient more carefully guarded from fatigue during pregnancy, given longer rest during the puerperium and afterwards, and not allowed to nurse her child. Yet it must be admitted that the malady may first come to notice after a confinement or may take a fresh lease of activity in these circumstances. There is, however, no evidence that the termination of pregnancy in the third month averts these consequences.

Perhaps the most difficult problem arises when a young person on the verge of matrimony develops a unilateral retrobulbar neuritis. In view of what has been said of the uncertainty of the future, and of the possibility of a long period of normal health, the greatest prudence should be observed in giving a prognosis, and this should be conveyed to a responsible relative and not to the patient. To cloud with gloomy apprehensions the life of a young subject who may yet have several years of normal health to come is to assume a responsibility that calls for careful thought, and something higher than a purely materialist view of life.

OTHER DEMYELINATING DISEASES

Disseminated sclerosis is not the only affection of the nervous system in which the essential pathological process is demyelination, though it is the only one encountered with any frequency. We have already seen (page 155) that post-infective encephalitis is an acute demyelinating disease that does not vary with the particular exanthem with which it may be associated. Apart from the exanthemata we may see an acute disseminated encephalo-myelitis with demyelination as its pathological basis, and a clinical picture and course like those of an acute disseminated sclerosis, though its relationship to the latter disease is not yet fully understood. In addition we may see the combination of bilateral retrobulbar neuritis, leading sometimes to permanent blindness, and of acute myelitis in which, again, the pathological process is a demyelination. The retrobulbar neuritis may precede the myelitis by a variable period, or alternatively the order of appearance of these two elements in the disease may be reversed. This syndrome goes by the name of *neuromyelitis optica*, and is to be distinguished from disseminated sclerosis by the simultaneous appearance of retrobulbar neuritis in both eyes, by the total and sometimes permanent blindness that may ensue, and by the severity and sometimes rapidly fatal nature of the myelitis. Finally, there is a comparatively rare disease of the brain in which a massive demyelination develops bilaterally, usually in the occipital lobes, and extends forwards throughout the cerebral hemispheres. It is a malady of childhood, is known as *encephalitis periaxialis*, and shows itself by blindness, progressive spastic paralysis, epileptiform fits and dementia. It runs an acute or subacute course to a fatal ending.

Nothing is known of the causation of any of these affections, and there is no specific treatment for them.

CHAPTER X

Paralysis Agitans (Parkinson's Disease)

IN 1817 James Parkinson, a London doctor, first described the malady which has since borne his name as consisting in "involuntary tremulous motion, with lessened muscular power, in parts not in action and even when supported; with a propensity to bend the trunk forwards, and to pass from a walking to a running pace, the senses and intellects being uninjured." It would be impossible to convey a clearer picture of the clinical features of paralysis agitans in so few words, and it remains but to say that it is a very slowly progressive affection of the degenerative period of life.

Ætiology.—Nothing is known of the factors leading to the development of paralysis agitans, but it is probable that it represents a local incidence in the brain of what is essentially a senile degeneration. It usually makes its appearance in the sixth and seventh decades of life, and on the whole more commonly in men than in women.

As in the case of other nervous affections of unknown origin, injury has been invoked as a precipitating cause and the sequence of injury and paralysis agitans has been several times recorded, but that this represents anything more than coincidence cannot be maintained on the evidence available.

A clinical picture closely resembling that to be described may follow the inflammatory lesions of epidemic encephalitis and less rarely those of vascular degeneration and of neuro-syphilis, so that it is probable that paralysis agitans owes its clinical individuality rather to the situation of the disease process than to its nature. Nevertheless, true paralysis agitans is a common malady, can be distinguished from these rarer symptomatic varieties by clinical examination, and, therefore, it is entitled to be considered in a category by itself.

Pathology.—There is not yet universal agreement about the essential lesion of paralysis agitans, and it may be recalled that a generation ago it was classed with the "functional" diseases on this account. Unquestionably, however, there are always degenerative changes of a senile order in the cells and fibre tracts of the corpus striatum and substantia nigra. There is considerable loss of ganglion cells in the affected area and many of those remaining are altered. There may also be visible in sections minute holes surrounding blood-vessels, as though necrotic tissue had fallen out. Generalized or even local cerebral atheromatous changes are not characteristic of the disease, and this absence is associated with certain negative features in the clinical picture to which reference will be made.

Symptoms.—The onset of the malady is insidious and one or two years may pass before the patient himself or even his relatives awake to the fact that he is becoming slowly disabled. This delayed recognition is the more likely when tremor is not an initial symptom, and at this point we break off the task of description to emphasize that, broadly speaking, there are two clinical types of paralysis agitans: a type in which muscular rigidity is the first and throughout the prominent symptom, tremor being inconstant and never troublesome, and a type in which tremor is the initial symptom and remains the obvious and disabling one throughout the illness. A less common form is that in which tremor is absent throughout.

The elderly man in whom the malady is developing is almost invariably in good general health, his arteries are soft and his blood pressure normal for his age. Hyperpiesis is excessively rare in the subjects of paralysis agitans and they do not succumb to cerebral hæmorrhage or softening.

Almost imperceptibly the natural mobility of facial expression wanes, the patient's face becomes a little "set," then more definitely "wooden." He becomes somewhat slower in all his movements. Gradually the characteristic Parkinsonian rigidity which has been described in the introductory chapter takes possession of his limb and trunk musculature, first on one side, then a year or so later on the other. The arm on the affected side ceases to swing as he walks. He may or may not notice this himself, but those patients who do discover it will say, on being questioned, that the arm won't swing "unless I swing it deliberately," adding that "it stops swinging directly I forget it."

The affected leg begins to feel heavy to the patient and won't clear the ground readily in walking unless—as with the arm—the subject deliberately lifts it. In the majority of patients intermittent tremor then makes its appearance, not when the limb is actually in motion but when the patient is holding up his newspaper to read, or when the arm is inadequately or uncomfortably supported as he sits in a chair. The tremor is usually a fine rhythmic movement of a rate of from 2 to 5 per second, and may appear in thumb and index finger ("pill-rolling movement") or at the wrist. The leg also, when inadequately supported, later begins to shake in the same way. Fatigue, emotional disturbance, physical discomfort or pain, or the knowledge that his tremor is being looked at will aggravate the shaking.

Within two or three years the presence of the malady is plainly written on the patient for the close observer to see, yet at this stage non-recognition or erroneous diagnosis is common enough. The onset being unilateral, and a sense of weakness in the affected limbs being quite commonly complained of, a diagnosis of progressive hemiplegia may be made, and the notion of slowly developing hemiplegia begets that of intracranial tumour, with results that may place the patient in great hazard.

During this developing period of the malady the clinical picture is made up of such relatively slight deviations from the normal that routine examination may, save in careful hands, fail to reveal its presence. Yet if the patient has been observed as he approaches the examiner, his face, stance and gait noted, the picture leaps to the eye. In no chronic malady of the nervous system is this preliminary inspection a more important and essential feature of the general examination. Many cases both of true paralysis agitans and of post-encephalitic Parkinsonism are missed for the want of it.

Examination reveals a greater or less degree of fixity of expression, the power of emotional expression is there, but requires greater stimulus to evoke it, and the smile when it comes dawns slowly, spreads, and then fades as slowly. The general attitude is a stooping one, the arms are held closely adducted to the sides, with the elbows slightly flexed and the fingers adducted ("main d'accoucheur"). The arms may tremble in the manner described as the patient stands. In more advanced cases the lower jaw may also show tremor, and sometimes there is a fine to-and-fro tremor of the head. The muscles of the arm on passive movement show a lead-pipe and sometimes a cog-wheel rigidity and the legs a similar state. While there is no severe paralysis it is clear that muscular power is somewhat lessened. Movements carried out to order are slow and restricted in range, and when they are complex they may cease in mid-course and require a fresh effort to restart them. Getting up out of a chair is difficult and the patient may subside again into it several times before, with a greater effort, he finally heaves himself into the erect position. When standing he has a curious difficulty in looking round and tends to turn his whole body in a succession of little steps so as to face the desired direction. Turning over in bed is equally arduous, and such movements as doing up a tie or buttons, brushing the hair or doffing the coat may be almost impossible without help. They ultimately do become impossible. Many cases show a tendency to break into a trot when they walk, or, when they look up, to step backwards uncontrollably.

The tendon jerks are normal, save perhaps for a measure of briskness, the abdominal reflexes are brisk and rapid and the plantar responses are flexor.

Aching pain in the shoulder and arms may be complained of, and also painful flexion cramps in the toes. Many patients become so restless that they cannot sit long and have to change position, or to be moved into a fresh posture when disability is extreme. The voice tends to lose its natural inflexions and to become weak and monotonous. Mental alertness remains unimpaired for many years, but finally it loses its edge and sustained thought or conversation becomes difficult, but the fixity of the patient's face is apt to convey a quite false impression of mental hebetude.

This process develops slowly over many years, and the patient who is well looked after and avoids intercurrent illness may live for twenty years, though in the later period of this his rigidity totally immobilizes him and renders him unable to perform the slightest purposive action for himself.

The final stage of failing health is commonly ushered in by a progressive loss of weight, the patient takes to his bed, to succumb ultimately to some infection of the respiratory tract. Before this happens he may from rigidity have become almost if not wholly inarticulate.

Commonly the ordinary degenerative tissue changes seem in abeyance. The blood pressure does not reach abnormal levels, and many a patient with paralysis agitans has outlived his generation.

What has so far been stated applies especially to those cases in whom rigidity is a prominent feature, and in whom tremor is but intermittent, or even absent throughout. In other cases the malady begins with tremor and this becomes in course of time virtually continuous save when the patient is asleep. There is always some rigidity in paralysis agitans, but the less marked this is the coarser is the tremor. The severely tremulous patient does not survive for so long as the predominantly rigid one. The cerebrospinal fluid presents no abnormality in this malady.

Diagnosis.—Little remains to be said on this matter. The features which distinguish post-encephalitic Parkinsonism from true degenerative paralysis agitans have already been described. It is important to bear in mind that the onset may be unilateral. Senile tremor may develop in elderly subjects, but is not accompanied by rigidity and does not run the characteristic course described. Arterio-sclerotic muscular rigidity may be distinguished by its association with the signs of cerebral or general arterio-sclerosis, by the shuffling gait and the dementia, and by the final development of gross cerebral vascular lesions. Tremor does not occur.

Amongst the states that may occasionally be erroneously diagnosed as paralysis agitans or Parkinsonism is myxœdema. This condition develops very slowly and until fully developed may not present the skin and cutaneous tissue changes on which so much stress is laid in diagnosis. During the years of its evolution the patient tends to move more slowly, to complain of fatigue and of a sense of effort, and also of defect of memory and attention and of a general slowness of mental processes. On examination there is a certain fixity of facial expression as well as the pallor and malar flush. The hair is dry and thinned, the skin is dry, the pulse abnormally slow. There is no tremor nor true Parkinsonian rigidity, but the leg muscles may be abnormally rigid on passive movements, and the gait slow, short-stepped, or even unsteady. The patient is usually a middle-aged woman, and may have amenorrhœa before the normal age of the menopause is reached.

Prognosis.—Paralysis agitans is a slowly progressive disease, with no remissions or recoveries, yet it may not end life for many years.

Treatment.—Paralysis agitans being progressive, all that can be hoped for from treatment is the alleviation of symptoms. In its initial stage, and sometimes for two or more years, it produces relatively little disability. Of course the measure of this must depend upon the patient's occupation: for example, a musician or skilled craftsman will very soon lose his technical skill. When it is possible for the patient to continue at his work he should be encouraged to do so. When rendered idle the patient is very prone to depression, and for this reason also he should be kept usefully occupied, as long as this proves practicable. Even when the day of final retirement from regular work arrives, it is important to prevent the patient from retiring to his house and never emerging from it. Many subjects with paralysis agitans, especially the more tremulous cases, become sensitive to the notice they attract and tend to become sunk in a life of despondent inactivity. They should, therefore, be encouraged to take moderate exercise and to occupy themselves according to their taste and capacity.

While the drugs of the atropine group may appreciably diminish rigidity and thus render the patient more mobile, they are less effective in the case of tremor. Perhaps the most useful is stramonium which may be given in increasing doses of the tincture ($\mathfrak{m}$ 5 increasing to $\mathfrak{m}$ 30 as tolerance is established), or as Pil. Ext. Stramonium (U.S.P.) 0·0625 gram, from 2 to 6 daily. Hyoscine hydrobromide in doses of from gr. 1/200 to gr. 1/100 may also be tried, from twice to thrice daily. Better results may be obtained by combining one of these with benzedrine (amphetamine) sulphate in doses of from 5 to 10 or 15 mgms. The range of tolerance of the last-named varies greatly from subject to subject, and it is important to adjust the dosage with that of the stramonium or hyoscine. Sometimes it is best to give the benzedrine in small doses (half a tablet, *i.e.* 2·5 mgms.) hourly or two-hourly up to the afternoon. Doses given later in the day may interfere with sleep. A method of intramuscular injection of benzedrine sulphate in gelatin-saline solution has been recommended in America, so as to produce a longer-lasting and more slowly-acting result, but this method is not at present readily available. Apart from regular medication, it is often most useful to use these drugs whenever circumstances require some special effort from the patient—as for a meeting, social or business gathering.

The claim that vitamin B$_6$ is of value has proved unfounded.

Massage to the limbs affords some relief, especially in cold weather, but if this is to exert its maximal effect it should be given to the patient in his home. The exertion and ordeal of attendances at clinics for this purpose are often found to be exhausting. For those patients who are restless or sleepless small regular doses of phenobarbitone (gr. ¼ to ½ twice or thrice daily) are more useful than the bromides. If this be not adequate to deal with insomnia, there should be no hesitation in giving larger doses of a barbiturate. Electrotherapy has no place in this malady. In the final stages of profound immobility the patient can do nothing for himself and then requires nursing care.

N

CHAPTER XI

Rheumatic Chorea (Sydenham's Chorea)

CHOREA is an affection of the brain associated with rheumatic infection and characterized by irregular involuntary movements, by inco-ordination of voluntary movements, and by a varying degree of muscular weakness and of mental disturbance. It occurs chiefly in young persons and is of limited duration but subject to repeated relapses.

Ætiology.—Acute rheumatism and chorea are manifestations of a common pathogenic agent, and the subject of chorea very commonly presents other rheumatic signs and symptoms; for example, rheumatic nodules, rheumatic endocarditis, recurrent sore throats, erythema, or purpura. These various disorders may precede the first attack of chorea, or they may accompany it. Signs of endocarditis are more common in second and subsequent than in first attacks of chorea.

The age period of maximum incidence is between five and fifteen years; girls are more liable than boys, and in adults it is encountered chiefly in association with pregnancy when it may assume its most severe and grave form.

Pathology.—Of its morbid anatomy very little is known, but the clinical features of the illness indicate that the pathological process is in all probability in the cerebral cortex, and the nerve cells of the cortex in fatal cases show some degree of chromatolysis. In view of the fact that the symptoms are irritative rather than indicative of a destructive process, the absence of gross microscopical changes is perhaps not surprising.

Symptoms.—The mother who, unfamiliar with chorea, brings her child for advice in a first attack of the malady, usually opens her story with the statement that the child "can't keep still." Enquiry then elicits that for a week or two before definite movements were noticed the child has become somewhat fretful and excitable, eating badly and easily prone to tears and inclined to be restless and sleepless at night. By day she fidgets when not actively occupied, while at table she "dashes at" her spoon and fork and cup, is apt to drop things suddenly and to be clumsy. As she moves in the house she kicks the furniture with her feet. She is seen to grimace.

In past history probably one or more of the rheumatic manifestations already enumerated will have been noticed. On examination the patient is seen to make involuntary movements which are irregular in form, incidence, and rhythm. They are sudden and short-lived and consist in jerky movements of elevation of a shoulder, rotation of an arm, pronation-supination movements of the forearm, flexion and extension movements of wrist and fingers. There may be sudden jerky rotations of the head, or asymmetrical movements of the facial musculature. Articulation may be affected, and if the trunk muscles are involved there are quick movements of lateral flexion and rotation of the spine. In movements of the hands and arms made to order it is seen that these involuntary movements are superimposed upon the voluntary, rendering the latter inco-ordinate, sometimes cutting them short, sometimes prolonging or diverting them from their intended purpose.

Thus the hand grasping an object may be suddenly and prematurely relaxed, allowing the latter to drop. If the patient be asked to grasp the examiner's hand firmly an irregular waxing and waning of the muscular contraction can always and easily be felt, even in mild cases when the grasp appears to the eye to be smooth and evenly sustained. Adventitious involuntary movements may move the entire arm as the grasp is being performed. The legs, which have a relatively limited repertoire of normal movements, show these disorders less markedly, but irregular movements of feet and toes occur, and as the child walks the gait is clumsy.

If the arms be held vertically above the head, the wrists go irregularly into flexion and extension movements, a phenomenon which is conspicuous in unilateral cases by contrast with the immobility of the normal arm. There may also be a marked pronation of the forearm.

Muscular force is characteristically diminished, though in varying degree in different cases. In some weakness dominates the clinical picture, involuntary movements being relatively slight. These disturbances may be asymmetrically distributed in the two halves of the body, or they may be almost completely unilateral, though the face is never unilaterally involved. Ocular movements tend to escape completely. Gowers, whose clinical observations could always be implicitly relied upon, stated that he had seen transient diplopia in severe cases from choreiform movements of the eyes, but they must be excessively rare. The immunity that ocular movements enjoy in states of generalized motor disorder is quite remarkable and they seem to be a law unto themselves. Thus, they escape the tremor and slowness of movement typical of paralysis agitans, and the mobile spasm of athetosis, and even in cerebellar ataxy, nystagmus is sometimes lacking. It is interesting to recall in this connection that ocular movements have a separate topographical representation in the cerebral cortex anterior to the so-called motor cortex.

The limb muscles are hypotonic, the tendon jerks are sometimes diminished, especially in the cases in which weakness rather than

involuntary movement predominates. The so-called tonic or prolonged knee jerk of chorea obtains quite undue notice in accounts of
this malady. It owes its occasional appearance to the coincidence in
time of the knee jerk and a superimposed choreiform jerk of the knee
extensors. Free from this complication the choreic knee jerk is typically
short-lived and pendular. The plantar responses are normal. There is
no sensory loss.

In the more severe cases of chorea the involuntary movements may
be incessant and of great violence, rendering all voluntary movements
impossible of useful performance, and leading to grave and even fatal
exhaustion.

The last issue, extremely rare in children, may be encountered in
the chorea of pregnancy. In most cases there is some degree of emotional
instability, but in a few there is grave mental disorder, restlessness,
confusion, even maniacal excitement, with associated dementia, and
incontinence of urine and fæces.

Course and Prognosis.—Chorea runs a fairly constant course in
most instances, developing to its maximum over a period of about
two weeks, remaining there for a comparable time and then receding
to end in recovery about ten weeks from the onset. In a few cases it does
not completely subside and flares up again in a few weeks or months, or
recurrence may develop some months after an apparently complete
recovery. In severe cases the pulse rate is raised, there may be cardiac
murmurs, hæmic or associated with endocarditis and mitral lesions.
A slight fever may be present until improvement sets in. It is after
relapses that permanent cardiac damage is most often found. Fatal
cases in children are rare indeed.

Diagnosis.—For practical purposes we may say that the only
condition likely to be confused with chorea is the neurosis of multiple
tics, or habit spasm. It may be admitted that occasionally, to inspection, the involuntary movements of the latter affection do closely resemble those of chorea, and that this is so the not uncommon diagnosis
of chorea made in such cases clearly shows. Careful examination,
however, reveals significant points of difference. Facial grimaces are
more prominent in tics than in chorea, articulatory disturbance is
sometimes seen in chorea but not in multiple tics. Such repetitive
movements as blinking, smacking of the lips, clicking noises made by
the tongue are common with tics, but are not seen in chorea. Multiple
tics may persist for months undiminished, the predominant movement
changing from time to time and being replaced by another. There is no
muscular weakness. The child with tics does not drop things out of his
hand and his grasp is smoothly and evenly sustained—a useful point in
differential diagnosis. Finally, the indications of rheumatic infection
are lacking in children who suffer from tics.

Treatment.—(1) *General management of the case.*—Complete rest— physical and mental—is an essential preliminary to all other modes of treatment, and this may involve the child's removal from home to hospital or nursing home. Even in the mildest cases, an initial period of at least two weeks' rest in bed is necessary, and it is in these cases that especial care should be taken to keep the patient content and quietly interested. When the child is more seriously ill, either from the severity of the movements or from associated rheumatic affection of the heart, longer rest in bed and more complete quiet are required.

The child should be well clad in woollen night garments so as to avoid exposure and chilling from throwing off of bed-clothes. If, as is commonly the case, the child is poorly nourished and takes food badly, care must be taken to give a liberal and nourishing dietary. In the rare cases in which swallowing is difficult, recourse to nasal feeding may be necessary. Milk, Benger's food, glucose drinks and good soups should be given if the child is too ill to take solid food.

When the movements are violent, the sides of the bed or cot should be padded, and it may also be necessary to pad the limbs with cotton wool and bandages to prevent friction and injury. Sometimes it is necessary to place the mattress on the floor against a wall, pillows being arranged to form a soft protection on the free side.

When recovery sets in all these restrictions may be progressively removed and the child allowed more liberty of voluntary movement and of recreation.

(2) *Medicinal treatment.*—Aspirin is undoubtedly the drug of choice and it is commonly well tolerated by children. A child of from eight to twelve can take 10 grains thrice daily after food, an adolescent or adult 15-grain doses thrice or even four times in the twenty-four-hour period. Even more frequent dosage may be necessary. If the child be sleepless, bromides may also be given, but sedatives are not a substitute for aspirin, and in the writer's experience their use for this purpose is followed by recurrence immediately the dosage is diminished or the drug stopped. This applies to chloretone, phenobarbitone, and other sedatives. These, therefore, are useful only when employed in conjunction with aspirin. During convalescence cod-liver oil and malt may be given, and the writer is old-fashioned enough to believe that they are of greater value than pure vitamin preparations.

Unfortunately, in the children of the poorer classes in whom chorea is most often seen, it is not always possible to secure for the patient those conditions of adequate care and nourishment that protect against recurrence.

CHAPTER XII

Injuries of the Brain : Concussion and Contusion

THE heavy incidence of closed head injuries involving more or less damage to the brain, and the fact that the treatment of the latter is mainly conservative and medical when there is no external wound, make a brief account of injuries to the brain a necessary chapter in a text-book of neurology.

It is usual to classify brain injuries under the three headings of concussion, contusion, and laceration. While the last of these categories is clearly entitled to its own grouping, the distinctions between concussion and contusion have in the past been largely academic. However, recent experimental observations by Denny Brown and Ritchie Russell, which appear applicable to head injuries in man, indicate that the phenomena of concussion—with the important exception of loss of consciousness— are due to a direct traumatic paralysis of nervous function in the brain-stem, without vascular or other discoverable lesions in the nervous elements. The clinical signs of concussion are loss of consciousness, transient reflex loss of respiratory and vasomotor activity, loss of corneal reflex and of motor reflex reactions centred in the pons and medulla. Of the loss of consciousness we yet lack a satisfactory explanation, some regarding it as due to loss of hypothalamic function. Yet we cannot exclude the cerebral cortex from consideration in this connection. If there be a hypothalamic component of the complex state we name "consciousness" it must be a restricted one, probably akin to that shown by the decorticated dog which is concerned solely with response to internal stimuli (hunger, thirst, and a distended bladder or bowel). The consciousness which is related to adaptation to environmental stimuli must surely be cortical in respect of its anatomical and physiological substrata, and by what means the relevant cortical mechanisms come to be transiently inactivated in concussion we do not know.

Pathology.—In the brain of a person dying shortly after a brain injury we find, particularly at the frontal, temporal, and occipital poles, cortical bruises extending deeply in wedge-shaped areas into the subjacent white matter. These are most numerous beneath the site of injury and in the region of contrecoup. Small subarachnoid hæmorrhages overlie these lesions, being largest over the contrecoup region. There may also be small punctate hæmorrhages beneath the ventricular walls and in the brain-stem. Occasionally, however, in a fatal case, no naked-eye lesions may be seen. There is local œdema in the damaged regions, but not generalized œdema.

Microscopically, we find rupture of axis cylinders, necrotic changes in nerve cells, neuroglial reaction, hæmorrhages of various sizes, small hæmorrhagic infarcts, and in cases where long bones have been fractured areas of fat embolism.

In persons who have survived such injuries for long periods, dying ultimately of other causes, small areas of cortical atrophy at the summits of convolutions are found, with some demyelination of the subjacent white matter, and traces of blood pigment indicating the former presence of bruising. Thus, even in non-fatal cases the lesions are essentially the same as in the rapidly fatal cases.

Secondary glial proliferation and scarring may ensure upon these lesions, with the production of a small traction diverticulum of the ventricle. Such an atrophic lesion may, in a proportion of cases, come to be an epileptogenic focus.

Complicating these purely cerebral lesions we may find subdural hæmatoma, and, when the frontal sinus or cribriform plate is fractured, pneumocephalus and meningitis. Occasionally recurrent attacks of meningitis follow damage to the sinus walls.

Symptomatology.—The acute symptoms of head injury fall into two groups: those of general disturbance of cerebral function and those of local structural damage.

(1) *Symptoms of general cerebral disturbance.*—The most constant and invariable result of a head injury is a disturbance of consciousness. This may range from transient dazedness, followed by a brief phase of automatism in mild injuries, to profound and long-lasting coma in the most severe. In the latter case, the reflex paralyses already enumerated are also present. Between these extremes we find various grades of unconsciousness of varying duration. The return from coma to normal consciousness commonly occurs through a sequence of stages of incomplete consciousness: stupor, excitement or delirium, confusion and automatism. When full consciousness returns the patient is fully orientated, but has a period of retrograde amnesia dating from a few minutes to an hour or more prior to the injury and extending to the final return to normal. This gap in the stream of consciousness remains as a permanent record of the disorder of the conscious cerebral functions: that is, those functions by which we are aware of and respond to our environment.

The return from coma to normal consciousness by the stages enumerated may be compressed within a period of less than an hour, or may be prolonged over many days, being arrested at one or other stage. Thus a state of semi-coma or stupor may last for days. So also may a state of confusion in which the patient is capable of considerable motor activity and of some conversational exchange, but is disoriented and incapable of sustained thought or expression.

In mild injuries, such as may be sustained, for example, at football or boxing, the momentary dazedness is followed by an automatism like that described in the case of epilepsy (see page 121), in which the subject may continue his activities, and then on finally "coming to" may recall no part of them since the few moments prior to the injury. In an injury of this grade, then, amnesia and automatism are the striking features.

Another and occasional mode of reaction to mild injury without initial loss of consciousness is a form of delayed collapse after several hours. There may be intense vertigo, some confusion with or without automatism and a markedly slow pulse (60 to 40 per minute). This slowing of the pulse may persist for a period of hours or of several days, then finally clearing up. It has been suggested that it is due to contusion of the medulla.

In the most severe injuries the patient is profoundly comatose and shocked. For a few moments the entire nervous system may be paralysed, cardiac and respiratory movements ceasing. They are soon restored, but at first the pulse is fast and feeble, respiration shallow and rapid, and the temperature subnormal. In fatal cases death usually occurs during the first forty-eight hours, but in surviving cases the pulse gains gradually in force and slows down, and the temperature rises to or slightly above normal. Coma then lessens in depth gradually and the sequence of events already described begins. In such severe cases, signs of local damage are more likely to be found and recovery may be arrested short of complete restoration to normal.

In such injuries complete recovery does not invariably ensue, and the after-effects are described later. As a rule, however, recovery is complete, and we may, therefore, infer that no irreversible structural damage has been sustained by the brain. It is difficult to correlate persisting symptoms, in cases where recovery stops short of complete restitution of normal function, with the lesions described on page 199, since, as we have seen, such lesions may be present in the total absence of symptoms. Nothing is certainly known of the physical basis of persisting general symptoms of cerebral dysfunction after head injuries, but the fact that no macroscopic or microscopic lesions can be definitely associated with such symptoms does not mean that these symptoms are psychogenic. Disorders of cerebral function are not necessarily associated with lesions discoverable with the resources now available to us. Nevertheless, it is probable that in some cases psychogenic factors play a part in persisting after-effects. This sequence of events may be tabulated as on page 201.

Cerebrospinal fluid.—Now that lumbar puncture is being performed

GENERAL SYMPTOMS OF HEAD INJURY.

Disorder of Consciousness.	SEVERE.	MODERATE.	MILD.	MILDEST
Coma.	Transient paralysis of nervous system. Severe shock.	Flaccidity and loss of reflexes. Unconsciousness for several minutes, or longer.	Transient loss of consciousness.	
Stupor.	Profound stupor. Patient mute and inaccessible. Incontinence.	As in severer injury, but less profound and of less duration.	Short stage of stupor passing on to	Momentarily dazed.
Delirium.	Restlessness passing on to resistiveness, and sometimes violence. May respond to simple orders, otherwise non-co-operative.	As in severer injury, but less marked and briefer.	A short phase of elation or excitement. Very brief phase of confusion.	Very transient or absent.
Confusion.	Quiet confusional state. Can respond to simple orders and make simple answers. No power of sustained thought or speech.	As in severer injury, but less marked and briefer. As in severer injury, but probably briefer.	Active automatism for a period of from a few minutes to an hour or so.	Brief automatism.
Automatism.	Aware of environment. Elated or irritable. Capable of some purposive activity. Gross defect of memory and judgment.			
Recovery.	Full and correct orientation.		Amnesia for entire episode.	

SEQUENCE OF STAGES.

more as a routine measure of investigation and treatment, it is being found that the presence of blood in the cerebrospinal fluid is more common than was formerly supposed. Even in mild cases, clinically so considered, a small admixture of blood is not uncommon, while in the severer grades of injury it is the rule to find blood, though of course exceptions to this rule are found. A moderate degree of raised intracranial tension (up to 200 mm. of water) is frequently encountered when a manometric measurement is made at the time of lumbar puncture. In a few cases the intracranial pressure is subnormal. These pressure fluctuations bear no constant relation to the state of consciousness. In severe injuries with free hæmorrhage into the subarachnoid space, clinical indications of meningeal irritation may be present: *e.g.* rigidity of the neck and Kernig's sign.

(2) *Symptoms of local structural damage.*—These may consist of cranial nerve palsies from direct damage to the skull in the neighbourhood of foramina of exit from the skull. Thus, there may be anosmia from tearing of the olfactory filaments as they pierce the cribriform plate. This may occur in what are clinically mild injuries. Transient squint and diplopia from damage to the oculo-motor nerves, or occasionally unilateral blindness when there is a fracture through the orbit. Deafness, when it occurs, results from damage to the middle ear.

Local contusions or lacerations of the brain may also produce their characteristic localizing symptoms, but even in apparently mild injuries careful examination in the initial stages would probably reveal minor objective abnormal signs, such as changes in reflexes, slight degrees of paresis, and so on. Indeed, the frequency with which blood is found in the cerebrospinal fluid suggests that local physical damage within the skull may ensue even in apparently slight head injuries.

After-effects of head injury.—Apart from residual symptoms due to such local structural damage as has been mentioned, in some cases symptoms indicative of more general disturbance of cerebral function may persist for periods of varying length after head injury, and may even be permanent.

In elderly and arterio-sclerotic subjects some measure of mental defect may ensue. This is expressed as defect of memory and of judgment, impaired emotional control, unduly ready fatigue—both of attention and even of physical effort. Such symptoms do not stand in any close relation to the clinical severity of the original injury.

By far the commonest residual syndrome is that consisting of headache, dizziness, and emotional instability. This may persist for many months or for one or more years. The headache is paroxysmal and is described as throbbing or bursting. Accesses of dizziness are provoked by physical effort or by changes in posture, as on stooping or rising to the erect posture from stooping. The emotional traits are irascibility, an exaggerated response to noise or bright lights.

This syndrome lasts longer in middle-aged and elderly persons and also, it must be confessed, in patients whose injury comes within the scope of compensation legislation. Thus, Ritchie Russell found in a series of personally studied cases that after the lapse of eighteen months only 9 per cent. of "non-compensation" cases were still inactive, while no less than 30 per cent. of "compensation" cases were still idle and complaining.

This suggests that in this syndrome there is an interplay of physical and psychological factors. Unhappily, the clinical criteria by which we might hope to distinguish psychogenic from physical elements in this symptomatology are by no means as distinct as we could wish, but a few generalizations may be made. When the element of neurosis begins to dominate the clinical picture the symptoms as described by the patient begin to assume bizarre qualities, and to be complained of as totally disabling. Thus, the headache becomes continuous and is described in fantastic allegories and with a wealth of superlatives. The patient tends to become increasingly more aggrieved and querulous, and his whole family may be drawn into and subjected to the unhappy atmosphere he creates around him. In seeking to assess the role of psychological factors in this symptom-complex it is of value to enquire into the patient's past history. In some cases of persisting symptoms, this history will reveal indications of neurosis prior to the injury, though this is by no means invariable.

Immediate Treatment.—There can be few emergencies in which treatment and prognosis in the initial stages are more difficult to determine, and few in which complications are more likely to escape observation at a time when appropriate measures are necessary and of use. Skill and experience are of paramount importance, and the patient should be given the fullest opportunities of obtaining these at the earliest possible moment: this is to say that in all but the slightest cases removal to a hospital is desirable. Subject to these considerations the following emergency steps may be summarized. When the patient is comatose or shocked, as is frequently the case, he should be put in bed and kept warm, and examined, and moved no more than is imperative for at least twenty-four hours. Intravenous saline or serum injections may be necessary, and such a stimulant as camphor. Careful two-hourly pulse and temperature records are of great value in prognosis. Over-distension of the bladder should be guarded against.

With the passing of shock, radiographic examination of the skull *and of the cervical spine (which may be injured in association with head injuries)* may be made. In most cases, especially if the patient be still in coma, lumbar puncture is expedient to ascertain whether or not there has been bleeding into the subarachnoid space and to determine the intra-cranial pressure. If the pressure be over 200 mm. of water, some fluid may be withdrawn to reduce the pressure to normal. Thereafter, if necessary, a high pressure may be kept within safe limits by further withdrawals of cerebrospinal fluid and by dehydration. The last may be achieved by giving six ounces of a saturated solution of magnesium sulphate per rectum, or (and particularly if for any reason the patient is receiving a drug of the sulphonamide group) by intravenous glucose (up to 50 c.c of a 50 per cent. solution). Excessive dehydration must be avoided by seeing that the patient has an adequate fluid intake.

The head should be turned to one side on the pillow so as to prevent the swallowing by a comatose patient of blood or secretions. Restless-ness is best dealt with by the hypodermic injection of soluble pheno-barbitone (3 to 6 grains) or the oral administration of codein. It is probably best to avoid morphine when intracranial pressure is raised.

After-treatment.—Some prefer the supine and others the Fowler position when headache is severe and persistent after the recovery of consciousness. The duration of rest in bed is governed by the length of the initial period of coma and by the presence of headache, and as long as four or six weeks may be necessary in some cases. Other pallia-tives for headache are dehydration by saline aperients or enemata, and in severe cases lumbar puncture and withdrawal of cerebrospinal fluid. The sympathetic and tactful handling of the patient is of great importance, especially where it is likely that compensation factors will arise. The treatment of the "traumatic" neurosis is discussed in the chapter on the psychoneuroses (p. 332).

When coma persists or deepens and signs of rising intracranial pressure develop, the possibility that an extradural or subdural hæma-toma is present should be borne in mind. If the cribriform plate be fractured and the overlying dura torn there may be a flow of cerebro-spinal fluid from the nose. This is a serious complication since it commonly leads to a fatal meningitis. Its presence should be detected as early as possible, one of the sulphonamides preparation administered and surgical intervention invoked. Subdural or extradural hæmorrhage also calls for operation.

CHAPTER XIII

Compression and Injuries of the Spinal Cord

ÆTIOLOGY.—The spinal cord may be compressed as a result of narrowing of the spinal canal from injury or disease of the vertebræ, from the development of massive lesions upon meninges or nerve roots, or finally by the development within the cord itself of a new growth. Sudden compression is usually a result of trauma, but may occasionally follow the collapse of vertebral bodies invaded and eroded by disease.

VERTEBRAL INJURIES may follow direct or indirect violence. Direct violence ensues when the spine is actually struck or when in falling the subject lands on his feet or in a sitting posture. In these circumstances a crush fracture of one or more vertebral bodies may ensue. The spinal region commonly involved in accidents of this kind is the thoraco-lumbar junction. Indirect violence usually operates upon the mid-cervical region of the spine, and follows falls in which the head is first struck and the weight of the following body forcibly flexes the neck. The fifth and sixth cervical vertebræ are the common seat of such injuries, which may consist of fracture with or without dislocation, or of dislocation alone. The last may be transient and spontaneously reduced. It is important to remember that relatively slight violence may cause dislocation of the cervical spine.

Rupture and herniation of an intervertebral disc are considered on page 209. When this occurs at a higher level than the last thoracic vertebra the cord may suffer some compression.

VERTEBRAL DISEASE associated with cord compression includes tuberculous caries, primary and secondary malignant disease, osteo-myelitis, erosion by thoracic aneurysm and, even more rare, Paget's disease of the spine.

MENINGEAL LESIONS include syphilitic pachymeningitis, epidural abscess from osteomyelitis, arachnoiditis ("meningitis serosa circumscripta"), and new growths. Within the theca we may find diffuse sarcomatosis, and small neurofibromata, more often single than multiple, may grow from the sheaths of spinal nerve roots. A neurofibroma may grow out through an intervertebral foramen. Other forms of benign tumour may also be found within the dural coverings of the cord. The common *intramedullary tumour* is a glioma. It is central and may spread over several segments, producing an enlargement of the cord and a compression of its normal structures.

Pathology.—In gradual compression the cord is first displaced and then compressed. The compressed segments become anæmic and œdematous, nerve cell and myelin sheath degeneration follow. Ultimately some degree of ascending and descending degeneration of the long spinal tracts ensues. In sudden compression or contusion the lesions result from stretching, acute bending or compression of the nerve fibres; that is, the process is mechanical and consists of sudden deformation of nervous tissue. The lesions usually extend up and down the cord for several segments from the level of injury. In addition to the actual damage to nervous elements a spreading œdema results and this may cause an increase of symptoms for a period of time. Hæmorrhage plays no significant role in spinal cord injuries, and what has been called *hæmatomyelia* is not simply a result of injury, but an extremely rare lesion associated with some form of arterial abnormality. In arachnoiditis we find adhesions between pia-arachnoid, cord and theca, with the formation of loculi containing cerebrospinal fluid. The spinal roots are involved in adhesions. The degree of cord compression is relatively slight.

THE CEREBROSPINAL FLUID.—Once the compressing lesion blocks the subarachnoid space, the fluid in the distal isolated sac becomes changed and approximates in composition to blood plasma. Its protein content may rise as high as 1·0 per cent., and it becomes yellow from the transudation into it of blood pigment. The fluid may clot on standing. This combination of changes is known as the compression syndrome. Should the lesion be inflammatory the fluid will also contain an excess of lymphocytes. Compression of the jugular veins in the neck is not followed by a rise of pressure in the lumbar fluid as tested by a manometer (see page 57).

Symptoms of Gradual Compression.—These may be described as local (segmental) and general, the former indicating the segment actually compressed, the latter indicating interruption of conduction along spinal pathways below the level of compression. The latter group consists of progressive paraplegia with sensory loss and sphincter paralysis, and these have already been fully described in the introductory chapters of this book (see pages 25 and 40). We may, therefore, consider the segmental symptoms. These are due to damage to the grey matter and the spinal nerve roots of the compressed segment, and they serve to localize the vertical level of the cord lesion.

The compression of a dorsal root leads to the appearance of pain referred to the cutaneous distribution of that root. In the case of cervical, lumbar, and some sacral roots this pain is in the appropriate limb, but in the case of the thoracic roots the pain runs transversely round the trunk, and when both the dorsal roots of a segment are involved we get a "girdle pain." The pain varies in quality from case to case. It is commonly aggravated by active or passive movements of the spine, by coughing and sneezing. It may be continuous or inter-mittent, and in the case of nerve root tumours may precede the symptoms of cord compression by many months.

Compression of the grey matter and of ventral roots leads to muscular wasting and occasionally to muscular spasm. A third category of symptom results from interruption of the reflex arcs of spinal reflexes. This may lead to the abolition of a tendon jerk.

In Fig. 33 are given the levels of sensory loss corresponding to lesions of the segments indicated in the diagram. It is not strictly accurate to regard these sensory zones as representing the cutaneous distribution of a single spinal segment, for this is an overlapping dis-tribution covering at least three of the segmental zones therein repre-sented. For example, section of a single dorsal root is followed by no sensory loss, and no less than three adjacent roots must be divided to produce an area of sensory loss.

Other localizing symptoms include paralysis of the cervical sym-pathetic (miosis, slight ptosis with narrowing of the palpebral fissure and, according to some authorities, enophthalmos. The reality of the last-named symptom is doubtful).

In short, the vertical level of a focal or compressing lesion may be determined by the examination of the upper level of motor paralysis, specially noting any local wasting due to compression of ventral roots or of grey matter, the upper level of sensory loss, and the upper level and the nature of changes in the reflexes. This generalization applies equally to sudden compression or other local injuries of the spinal cord.

The clinical behaviour of a case of compression paraplegia may afford valuable information as to the nature of the compressing lesion. Thus in *tuberculous caries of the spine*, both lower limbs are equally or almost equally affected. The onset may be insidious or acute. It may precede all visible spinal deformity or may develop in a long-standing case of caries with deformity. It may respond to rest and immobilization of the spine and clear up completely, only to recur later once or more than once. If there be much associated pachymeningitis, root pains may precede the onset of paraplegia, and in most cases, even when there is no visible deformity, pressure or attempts to move the spine over the affected vertebræ are painful.

In *intrathecal spinal tumour* the asymmetrical situation of the growth often leads to marked asymmetry of paralysis in the limbs, even to the appearance of the Brown-Sequard syndrome (see page 39). Further, pressure on spinal roots may give rise to girdle pains or root pains of other distribution for months before any symptoms of cord compression develop. In venous angioma the same sequence of root and cord com-pression symptoms may be present, but the development of the symp-toms is apt to be very gradual and spread over several years.

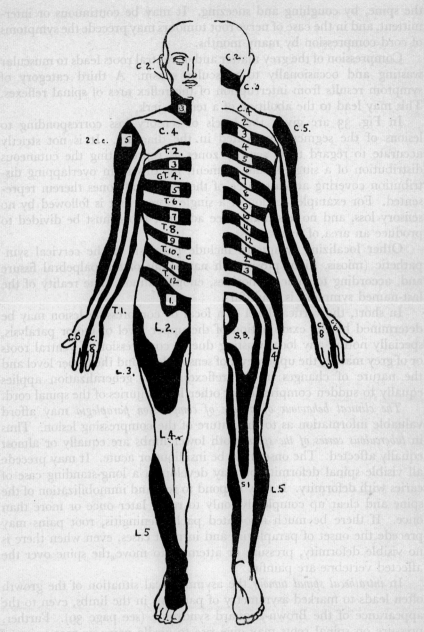

FIG. 33.
SENSORY SEGMENTAL LOCALIZATION IN THE SPINAL CORD.

The segmental representation of the tendon jerks is given on page 18.

The segmental representation of muscles is given in the following table:

SEGMENTAL REPRESENTATION OF MUSCLES

C. 4.   Scaleni, trapezius, levator anguli scapulæ, diaphragm.

C. 5.   Levator anguli scapulæ, scaleni, supraspinatus, rhomboids, infraspinatus, teres minor, biceps, brachialis anticus, deltoid, supinator longus, serratus magnus, pectoralis major (clavicular part).

C. 6.   Subscapularis, pronators, teres major, latissimus dorsi, serratus magnus, pectoralis major.

C. 7.   Triceps, extensors of wrists and digits.

C. 8.   Flexors of wrist and digits, small hand muscles.

Th. 1.   Interossei and small hand muscles.

Th. 2 to 12. Intercostals, abdominal muscles.

L. 1.   Quadratus lumborum.

L. 3.   Sartorius, adductors of hip, ilio-psoas.

L. 4.   Quadriceps extensor femoris, abductors of hip.

L. 5.   Flexors of knee.

S. 1.   Calf muscles.

S. 2.   Glutei, peronei, anterior tibial muscles, small foot muscles.

S. 3, 4.   Pelvic muscles.

In *herniation of an intervertebral disc* in the cervical or thoracic regions of the cord, symptoms of compression are likely to follow an injury. They may be evident immediately subsequent to this or develop within a short period. They may be very slowly progressive, or after a period of increase the signs and disability may become almost stationary. In the relatively few examples seen by the author, sensory loss was minimal. Such cases are very apt to be regarded as disseminated sclerosis unless the possibility of compression by a herniated intervertebral disc is borne in mind in cases where the characteristic manifestations of this malady are absent, *e.g.* visual disturbances, wide fluctuations and remissions of symptomatology.

In *arachnoiditis* ("meningitis serosa circumscripta"), a relatively rare condition of obscure causation, but sometimes a sequel to vertebral injury, root symptoms dominate the clinical picture, involve the territory of more than one root, and precede relatively slight symptoms of cord compression by long periods.

In *secondary carcinoma of the spine*, recurrent pains on movement, coughing or sneezing may precede all objective signs of cord or root

o

lesion. The presence of such sudden severe and transient pains in the back in the subject of visceral carcinoma (*e.g.* an old case of carcinoma of the breast) should always suggest the presence of secondary deposits in the spine, even if for a time examination reveals no clear indications of cord or root damage. Even radiography of the spine may for weeks fail to yield confirmatory evidence.

THE CLINICAL PICTURES OF INJURIES TO THE CERVICAL SPINE AND CORD.—Any accident in which the individual is pitched forwards or downwards striking his head first is liable to produce, with or without an accompanying concussion of the brain, an injury to the cervical spine with which there may or may not be a sudden compression of the cord. The fifth and sixth segments are those most commonly involved, and the degree of damage varies from the slightest to grave and irreversible crushing. Thus various clinical pictures of cord injury may result. Two will be briefly described, the slight and the severe.

Slight cervical cord injuries.—These are very frequently overlooked owing to the natural preoccupation with the concussion syndrome so commonly present. When, later, cord symptoms are noted, and this is often not until the patient resumes his normal activities and begins to be aware of certain disabilities he had not previously noticed, a diagnosis of disseminated sclerosis or of amyotrophic lateral sclerosis is apt to be made and the traumatic nature of the lesion overlooked or, when litigation arises, disputed. The patient commonly complains of pain in the neck on movements of the head, of stiff neck, and sometimes of pains and paræsthesiæ running down the arms and increased by flexion of the neck. Examination reveals some limitation of the range of movements of the neck. In the common case of spontaneously reduced dislocations an X-ray of the cervical spine often reveals no relevant abnormality. Symptoms of cervical sympathetic paralysis are usually absent, or if present minimal. A slight degree of weakness and clumsiness of hand movements is usual. The tendon jerks afford valuable evidence, for inversion of the radial reflex is almost invariably present, the biceps jerk may be normal or absent, while the triceps jerk is usually brisk (see page 18). Objective sensory loss is rare after the first two or three weeks. A slight degree of wasting of forearm or hand muscles may appear after an interval of some weeks. Recovery is slow, does not always occur, while occasionally a slow increase of symptoms is observed. The legs show a general increase of tendon jerks, slight spasticity, and usually unilateral or bilateral extensor plantar response. Sphincter disturbance is exceptional.

More severe injuries of the cervical cord lead to quadriplegia, the arms showing a combination of upper and of lower motor paralysis and the legs being spastic. If the deltoid muscles escape, as may happen in lesions of the two lower cervical segments, the arms take up a characteristic position: elevated and abducted at the shoulders, with the forearms and fingers flexed. There is sensory loss, pain and temperature being most severely impaired, retention of urine and intense priapism.

THE CLINICAL PICTURE OF THORACO-LUMBAR LEVEL INJURIES.— Here the lowest segments of the cord and the roots of the cauda equina are subject to damage. There is a flaccid weakness of the legs with muscular wasting most marked below the knees. The knee jerks may be preserved, or may be diminished or lost. The ankle jerks are characteristically absent and there is no plantar response. Sensory loss includes the territory of the sacral segments: that is, the skin region round the anus and over the genitalia, and when the second and first sacral segments are involved there is a strip of sensory loss down the back of the limbs to and including the heels. This loss, like the paralysis, may be greater in one limb than in its fellow. The feet are dropped. There may be severe pain from root damage. There may be an initial retention of urine, shortly followed by reflex incontinence, sometimes by continuous dribbling. In the least severe cases a transient retention may be followed by normal sphincter control. In its clinical picture this syndrome corresponds to that produced by other lesions at this level, *e.g.* tumour. Lesions within the lumbar enlargement of the cord present a very similar clinical picture, but pain is slight or absent, while loss of sphincter control is apt to be more severe.

Diagnosis.—It is in the case of gradual compression that difficulties of differential diagnosis are most apt to arise. The importance of the history has already been emphasized, and in this way the occasional case of disseminated sclerosis that presents an upper level of cutaneous sensory loss can usually be detected. In this malady the arm jerks are almost always exaggerated, and if there be a thoracic level of sensory loss this exaggeration of reflexes will show that the sensory level does not represent the uppermost limits of a focal process. Further, the signs of an old retrobulbar neuritis may be found. Syphilitic meningomyelitis may mimic spinal cord compression, but can be differentiated by the examination of blood and cerebrospinal fluid. In vertebral disease, the radiogram may reveal both the presence and the level of the bony lesion. Further, the compression syndrome in the cerebrospinal fluid, when present, is conclusive evidence of compression.

Radiography in Diagnosis.—As in the case of intracranial tumour, simple radiograms of the spine do not throw essential light upon diagnosis as commonly as is supposed. Yet radiography is a necessary procedure in every case of suspected compression of the cord. By its aid tuberculous caries and malignant deposits may be detected, though in the case of the latter clinical symptoms of cord or nerve root compression may precede the appearance of clearly recognizable changes in the bone. The rare cases of Paget's disease (osteitis deformans) of the spine leading to cord compression may also be identified in this way. In the ordinary case of intrathecal tumour, it is sometimes noticed that on one side—that of the tumour—the pedicle supporting the lamina at the level of the growth may be visibly rarefied, and thus provide a localizing indication of great value (Figs. 34 and 35).

Should simple radiography not give information, and when clinical investigation fails to confirm the presence of a suspected compressing lesion, or to indicate its precise segmental level, recourse may be had to the intrathecal injection by cisternal or by lumbar puncture of lipiodol. The former is effected through the atlanto-occipital ligament, and the lipiodol falls within the subarachnoid space until it is arrested by the compressing lesion and its situation revealed by the radiogram. After its introduction by lumbar puncture, the patient is so placed on the radiographic couch that the lipiodol runs upwards and thus indicates the lower level of the lesion.

As the retention of this substance within the subarachnoid space may lead to symptoms of nerve root irritation, its use should not be regarded as a matter of routine investigation, but should be reserved for cases that present diagnostic difficulties, or those in which a subsequent laminectomy is probable.

Prognosis and Treatment.—The former depends upon the nature of the lesion, as does the latter. When malignant disease is not in question the surgical removal of the lesion is generally indicated. In the case of severe back or nerve root pain when malignant deposits are present in the spine, deep X-ray therapy affords considerable relief in most cases. In all cases of compression paraplegia, the possibility that the bladder may be over-distended and that the passage of urine may be no more than an overflow incontinence should be borne in mind.

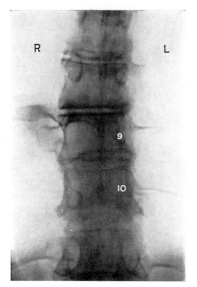
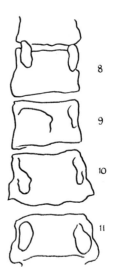

Fig. 34.

LOWER DORSAL SPINE.

On the right side of the body of the ninth vertebra there is erosion of the body
and of its pedicle. The lesion was a fibroma attached to a nerve root within
the theca.

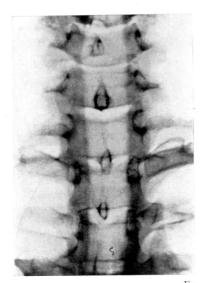
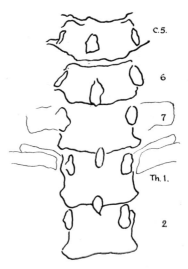

Fig. 35.

CERVICO-DORSAL REGION OF SPINE.

Showing erosion and separation of pedicles on the right side in the fifth cervical
to the first thoracic vertebra. The lesion was a fibroma attached to the seventh
cervical posterior nerve root within the theca. The diagram on the right shows
clearly the separation of the pedicles.

To face page 212.

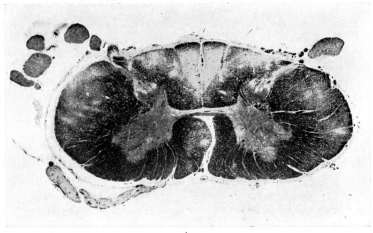

A

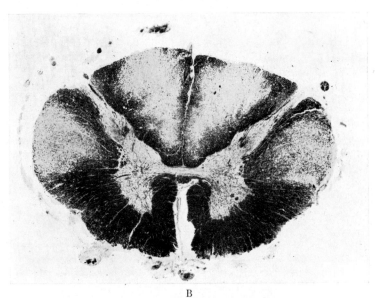

B

FIG. 36.

SUBACUTE COMBINED DEGENERATION OF THE SPINAL CORD.

Two transverse sections, stained by the Weigert-Pal method. A, the cervical and B, the thoracic region. The sections are from different cases. Both show the areas of degeneration in the posterior and lateral columns.

To face page 213.

CHAPTER XIV

Subacute Combined Degeneration of the Spinal Cord

A S the name implies, this is a progressive degeneration of the dorsal and lateral columns of the spinal cord. It is to be added that the peripheral nerves also undergo degenerative changes, and that the malady is associated with pernicious anæmia.

Ætiology.—It is a common nervous disease of middle and later life, affecting both sexes equally and, like pernicious anæmia, occasionally encountered in more than one member of a family. Its association with pernicious anæmia is constant, but since its severity does not necessarily or even usually run parallel with the degree of the blood change it is probable that not all the causative factors are common to both. It does not occur with other varieties of anæmia, though in some of them, as in the case of tropical sprue, there are signs of involvement of the nervous system; signs which are not identical with those encountered in pernicious anæmia.

The closeness of the association between the spinal cord and the blood disease is further indicated by the constancy of achlorhydria in both. There can be no doubt that an essential condition of its development is the absence from the circulating blood of a substance formed in the normal stomach and stored in the liver, but that this substance is identical with the hæmopoietic factor and not merely related to it cannot be positively stated.

The development of subacute combined degeneration of the cord may precede all clinical manifestations of pernicious anæmia, and when this is not the case it follows close upon the appearance of pernicious anæmia and not in the later stages of the latter.

Pathology.—In the spinal cord the characteristic changes consist in small areas of degeneration in the white matter of the dorsal columns and at the periphery of the lateral columns in the thoracic segments of the cord. The degeneration first affects the myelin sheaths which break down, and later the axis cylinders also degenerate. When the last-named change occurs we find both ascending and descending degeneration of the dorsal and lateral columns at all levels (Figs. 36 and 37).

Despite the title of the malady, peripheral nerve degeneration may be a prominent pathological feature and may, at least in the initial stages of the malady, dominate the clinical picture. Here also de-myelination is the primary lesion, axis-cylinder breakdown expressing a later and more severe stage of the process (Figs. 36 and 37).

The cerebrospinal fluid is normal. The blood shows in varying degree the changes characteristic of pernicious anæmia, the minimal changes being a high colour index and the presence of megalocytes. Achlor-hydria is constant at all stages.

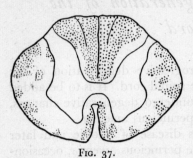

FIG. 37.

THE SITUATION OF THE LESION IN SUBACUTE COMBINED DEGENERATION. Subacute combined degeneration of the cord, showing the situation of the lesions in posterior, lateral, and anterior columns. The dotted areas are those affected.

Symptoms.—Subjectively the mode of onset is fairly constant. The patient begins to complain of sensations of tingling, numbness and pins and needles in the toes, later in the feet and then in the fingers. There may also be sensations of coldness, wetness, or of swelling of the toes and feet, and a feeling when the patient walks in bare feet as though he were treading on cotton wool. Within a very short time of the onset of these symptoms weakness of the legs is noticed. The patient tires rapidly and his legs begin to feel heavy on exertion. Unsteadiness of gait is soon added. The numb fingers become clumsy for fine movements and the patient drops small objects.

If there be anæmia of any severity, breathlessness on exertion, and some œdema of the feet and ankles, and the appearance of the characteristic yellowish pallor are noticed. At some time during the initial stage it is not uncommon for a complaint of sore tongue to be made. In many instances by the time the patient comes under observation his pallor is noticeable. There may be a history of recurrent short attacks of diarrhœa or of gastric discomforts, sometimes accompanied by slight fever, the nervous symptoms increasing after each such episode.

The subsequent course of the illness, its physical signs and its response to treatment depend upon the localization of the greatest intensity of pathological change in the nervous system, and it may be said that there are two clinical types: *a flaccid type*, in which the signs indicate the predominance of change in the peripheral nerves, cord changes being—at least in the early stages—minimal; and *a spastic type*, in which the signs indicate a severe involvement of the lateral columns, dorsal column and peripheral nerve change being less severe. The flaccid type is fortunately the more common; it is the type that responds well to treatment.

(1) THE FLACCID TYPE.—Examination reveals weakness of the legs, which is most marked in the distal segments. There is no consider-

able wasting but the muscles are notably tender to pressure, especially those of the sole and the calf. There is impairment of cutaneous sensibility to touch, but not always to pin-prick or to temperature, over the feet and legs, normal areas of sensibility being reached at or about the level of the knees. Vibration sense is lost at the ankles and often right up to and including the pelvis. This degree of loss is more extensive and profound than can easily be accounted for by peripheral nerve change alone and reveals that in all cases the posterior columns are involved. There is also marked impairment of postural sensibility in the legs as tested by passive movements and as revealed by ataxy of gait and by Rombergism. The knee and ankle jerks are commonly both lost. The plantar responses may be flexor in the early stages, but sooner or later an extensor plantar response develops and thus indicates involvement of the pyramidal tracts in the lateral columns of the cord.

In the arms the signs and the disability are usually much less severe, but are of the order already described. The abdominal reflexes are sometimes retained in the early stage of the malady. It will be seen, then, that this clinical picture is in most respects indistinguishable from that of multiple peripheral neuritis. It is the depth and extent of loss of vibration sense and of postural sensibility that serve to put the observer on the track, and, of course, the associated blood and gastric secretion anomalies.

(2) THE SPASTIC TYPE develops as a spastic paresis, with all the reflex phenomena characteristic of this: increased tendon jerks, clonus, hypertonus. As the weakness progresses flexor spasms make their appearance and ultimately the condition already described as paraplegia-in-flexion ensues. As this approaches, sensory loss becomes more profound and sphincter paralysis and bedsores make their appearance.

It should be emphasized that pictures transitional between these two extremes are sometimes encountered, and all the various states found depend for their features upon the relative severity of the lesion in dorsal columns, lateral columns, and peripheral nerves respectively. That the last-named are always involved may be seen from *the almost constant presence of tenderness of the calf and plantar muscles, a tenderness not encountered in any other disease of the spinal cord* and, therefore, of diagnostic value in subacute combined degeneration. In a certain proportion of cases of the malady, mental symptoms may be present, sometimes early in its course, and in no correlation with the degree of anæmia present. These may range from apathy and mental slowness to hypomanic or even maniacal excitement, or to persecutory ideas with hallucinations.

Diagnosis.—As has already been mentioned, subacute combined degeneration is one of the common progressive nervous diseases of the second half of life, and is, therefore, a malady the doctor should always have in mind when the following sequence of symptoms makes its appearance at the appropriate age period. The patient is usually middle-aged, the story of his increasingly uncomfortable peripheral paræsthesiæ and of his slowly increasing weakness and unsteadiness of gait, the characteristic yellowish pallor of the skin and the pallor of the lips and conjunctivæ, the smooth and shiny tongue, when these are present, together with the physical signs already enumerated, suffice when they are found to allow of diagnosis. It has, however, to be stated that pallor and a shiny tongue are not invariably present and that the neurological signs may on routine examination be indistinguishable from those of multiple peripheral neuritis. In these circumstances such a clinical picture in a middle-aged or elderly subject should lead to an examination of the blood, and if this be not conclusive, to a gastric analysis. From one or both of these, confirmatory evidence will be obtained. In the flaccid type, to which alone these remarks apply, the diagnosis of tabes dorsalis is one to be taken into consideration. In this the characteristic pupillary signs and the absence of any muscular tenderness, the history of disorder of the vesical sphincter and of lightning pains, together with the virtually constant painlessness of the tendo achillis to pressure, serve to make error of diagnosis improbable.

In the spastic type, subacute combined degeneration can be differentiated from other varieties of spastic paraplegia by the presence of muscular tenderness and by the changes in the blood and gastric secretions.

Course and Prognosis.—Before the introduction of liver treatment all cases of subacute combined degeneration ended fatally within three or four years.

Now with adequate treatment, early cases of the flaccid type can be restored to almost normal physical capacity, later cases can be improved and maintained at a reasonable level of capacity, but cases characterized by marked spasticity, despite the most intensive treatment, commonly develop a progressive paraplegia, and this although the blood state can be remarkably improved, and end as cases of paraplegia-in-flexion. It is on account of this differential response to treatment that a distinction between flaccid and spastic types is of importance, and the basis of the difference is almost certainly that in the flaccid cases, at least in their earlier stages, the signs and symptoms are referable to changes in the peripheral nerves; changes that are reversible, while when the cord is severely involved the changes are essentially irreversible and often incapable of being checked. Even in those favourable early cases where a restoration to normal capacity is achieved, the patient commonly continues to notice some tingling of the feet and toes and a complete disappearance of paræsthesiæ is exceptional. In patients over sixty years of age the prognosis is not so good, however thorough treatment may be, as in younger subjects.

Treatment.—This consists primarily and essentially in the administration in adequate and adequately maintained dosage of a liver extract. Massive doses of liver extract should be employed if there is no early improvement in the neurological aspect of the case, and mere changes in the blood picture should not be made the criterion of what is necessary in this respect. The amount and duration of treatment are both greater than are necessary for a restoration of the red cell count to its normal level, and it is generally found that when treatment is in progress no great improvement in the nervous condition occurs until this level is reached and passed. In other words, the amount of treatment sufficient for an uncomplicated pernicious anæmia is not sufficient for the treatment of subacute combined degeneration, and not a few unsatisfactory results are due to ignorance of this important fact of clinical experience. When treatment is begun daily parenteral injection of one or other of the available liver extracts is necessary (2 to 5 c.c. of Campolon, Anahæmin or other comparable product, given intramuscularly and continued for as long as may be necessary at this level of dosage). In addition Blaud's pill or an equivalent in doses of 40 to 60 grains daily should be given. Some observers report good results from the administration of thyroid extract also, in large doses over a short period. All these modes of treatment should be correlated with periodical blood counts. After the first month and in the presence of a satisfactory response of blood and of nervous symptoms daily dosage may give place to maintenance dosage, weekly or fortnightly according to circumstances, a dosage that must be continued indefinitely, if not for life. In cases with severe anæmia that come late under treatment an initial blood transfusion may be necessary. The patient should be kept at rest until recovery is well under way, but when the general condition allows it is as well to give him active exercises for the legs while he yet remains in bed, so that ataxy may be minimized against the time when he resumes walking. Graduated exercise follows later.

The general management of cases with severe paraplegia is discussed in Chapter XXV (page 304).

The anæmia of *tropical sprue* in its more severe grades is frequently accompanied by loss of knee and ankle jerks, sometimes alone and sometimes in association with vibration and postural sensory loss. Although these patients may show extreme generalized muscular wasting there is rarely any degree of true paralysis, and in the writer's experience an extensor plantar response is never seen. In other words, there is no clear evidence of spinal cord lesion.

CHAPTER XV

The Heredo-Familial Ataxies: Friedreich's Disease

UNDER the general title we include a number of syndromes of motor disorder dependent upon degenerative changes in one or more of the following parts of the nervous system: the cerebellum, the brain-stem, and the spinal cord. Heredo-familial factors are usually in evidence. None of the members of the group is common; indeed all but Friedreich's disease are very rare.

Ætiology.—Some form of Mendelian inheritance is commonly present; several siblings may be affected, and the sexes are equally involved. In all the malady makes its appearance during childhood or adolescence. Beyond these simple facts nothing is known of their causation.

Pathology.—There is a primary neurone degeneration with secondary neuroglial proliferation. There may be involvement of retinal, cortico-spinal, cerebellar and spino-cerebellar neurones. Not all are involved in a given type. Thus, in Friedreich's disease the neurones involved are those of the lateral and dorsal columns of the cord, and occasionally those of the retina.

FRIEDREICH'S DISEASE.—This develops during childhood, may affect several siblings and appear in successive generations, progresses slowly, may or may not undergo arrest before disablement is severe, and is characterized pathologically by degeneration in the dorsal columns and of spino-cerebellar and pyramidal neurones in the spinal cord (Fig. 38). There are also sketetal deformities.

Symptoms.—These are insidious in evolution. Appearing usually in childhood, an occasional later case is encountered in which the symptoms appear in early adult life, sometimes after an acute illness of some kind. In such late cases the kyphoscoliosis and the pes cavus, which are the usual deformities, may have been present since childhood, no nervous systems having been noted at this period of life.

Some unsteadiness of gait is usually the initial symptom and it is soon followed by signs of actual weakness of the legs. The hands and arms may slowly develop a relatively slight degree of intention tremor, and often when the patient is observed while sitting in a chair the head will be seen to move in fine mouse-like jerks. A fine nystagmus develops and also a form of dysarthria already described in the case of disseminated sclerosis under the name of scanning speech. All these symptoms gradually increase over a period of several years. They may undergo arrest early, or may progress until the patient can no longer stand or walk and his hands are too unsteady to permit of useful co-ordinated movement. Primary optic atrophy is a rare symptom, not leading to blindness. Examination reveals that these signs are characteristic of a lesion involving the spinocerebellar tracts, the pyramidal tracts, and the fibres underlying postural sensibility in the posterior columns. The nystagmus, scanning speech and tremor of the head have already been mentioned. The arms show an ataxy of cerebellar type. The legs are weak, but not spastic, the knee and ankle jerks are lost, the plantar responses are of extensor type, and the abdominal reflexes are abolished. There is impairment of postural and of vibration sensibility in the legs.

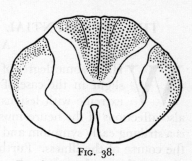

Fig. 38.

THE SITUATION OF THE LESION IN FRIEDREICH'S DISEASE.

Showing the incidence of the lesion in Friedreich's disease.

Diagnosis.—The differential diagnoses from juvenile tabes is made by the absence of the Argyll Robertson pupil, the presence of nystagmus, scanning speech and some intention tremor, of the extensor plantar response and of actual and sometimes severe paresis of the legs. Kyphoscoliosis and pes cavus are not seen in tabes.

Prognosis and Treatment.—No treatment influences the course of this essentially progressive disease. Death ensues from inter-current illness after the patient has been long bedridden.

The forms of progressive and hereditary cerebellar ataxy are very rare and will not be described in detail here. Clinically, they show a progressive cerebellar ataxy, usually without nystagmus.

CHAPTER XVI

Muscular Atrophies

THE DIFFERENTIAL DIAGNOSIS OF MUSCULAR ATROPHY

WHILE some degree of muscular wasting follows motor paralysis, slight in the case of upper motor neurone lesions and often extreme with lesions of the lower motor neurone, there are also affections of the neuro-muscular system in which muscular atrophy is a striking early symptom and remains a prominent feature throughout the course of the illness. Further, in the case of the primary muscular diseases the weakness may be regarded as a sequel of the wasting with which it is associated.

In all we may recognize five main pathological varieties of muscular atrophy, each with its own clinical aspect. (1) Primary Muscular Diseases (Muscular Dystrophy, Myopathy). (2) Peroneal Muscular Atrophy (Neuritic type of muscular atrophy). (3) Motor Neurone Disease (Progressive muscular atrophy). (4) Arthritic Muscular Atrophy. (5) Post-paralytic Muscular Atrophy.

Other pathological processes leading to obvious muscular wasting as an early and prominent feature are cervical rib pressure and syringomyelia.

In any case in which muscular wasting is an early and clinically predominant feature, the following diagnostic generalizations should be borne in mind.

(a) *The presence or absence of heredo-familial incidence.*—This factor is virtually constant in muscular dystrophy and in peroneal muscular atrophy. It is absent in the case of motor neurone disease.

(b) *Age of onset.*—Muscular dystrophy makes its appearance in infancy, childhood, or adolescence, motor neurone disease in the second half of life, and peroneal muscular atrophy and the wasting of cervical rib pressure in early adult life.

(c) *The topography of the wasting.*—It is characteristic of muscular dystrophy that the wasting makes its appearance in the musculature of the limb girdles, that the distal limb muscles are relatively little affected, and that the wasting is not only bilateral but bilaterally equal. In peroneal muscular atrophy the wasting is in the distal segments of the limbs, spares the proximal segments—except for the distal third of the thigh—and is both bilateral and bilaterally equal in degree. In motor neurone disease the wasting almost always appears distally, spreading thence up the limbs to their proximal parts. The wasting starts unilaterally, later becomes bilateral, but is not bilaterally equal since it is greater on the earlier affected side. In arthritic atrophy certain muscles adjacent to the affected joint are involved, with a selective distribution that will later be described.

(*d*) *The presence or absence of fibrillation.*—In muscular dystrophy fibrillation is absent, in peroneal muscular atrophy it is inconstant and never widespread, while in motor neurone disease it is widespread, continuous, and very much in evidence. In arthritic atrophy and in cervical rib pressure it is present while wasting is in progress, but is not a prominent feature.

(*e*) *The presence or absence of muscular tenderness.*—In muscular dystrophy, peroneal muscular atrophy, motor neurone disease and syringomyelia there is no increased muscular tenderness. In arthritic atrophy and in cervical rib pressure the affected muscles are tender to pressure while the wasting process is active.

(*f*) *The presence or absence of other signs of disease in the nervous system.*—In muscular dystrophy and in arthritic atrophy there are no signs of disease of the nervous system, though tendon jerks necessarily disappear from muscles that have lost their contractile tissue. In motor neurone disease and also in peroneal muscular atrophy and syringomyelia there are associated signs of nervous disease.

A further brief reference to fibrillation is necessary. This term is applied to momentary and repeated contractions of small bundles of muscle fibres, occurring spontaneously or following active contraction, or in response to tapping of the muscle. These contractions impart a flickering motion to the muscle and the overlying skin.

It should be borne in mind that localized or widespread fibrillation may be seen in normal health, and may occur continuously or intermittently over long periods of time. It has no untoward significance when it occurs apart from progressive wasting or weakness; that is, as an isolated phenomenon in an otherwise healthy person it is of no practical importance. Its association with muscular and nervous affections is dealt with in this chapter.

The group of primary muscular diseases includes a number that are not commonly comprehended under the title of muscular dystrophy. Most of them are extremely rare, and but one of them, dystrophia myotonica, calls for a brief account. It differs from muscular dystrophy in that the wasting is distal and not proximal in the limbs and is accompanied by a curious condition of delayed relaxation, and also by disorders in certain non-muscular structures.

Peroneal muscular atrophy occupies in some respects a position intermediate to muscular dystrophy and motor neurone disease in that like the former it has an heredo-familial incidence, and like the latter an underlying nervous lesion.

Unhappily, the muscular diseases suffer from a very redundant nomenclature, some of them having as many as three different names. Therefore, to facilitate identification a second name will be given where it seems expedient to do so.

THE PRIMARY MUSCULAR DISEASES

(1) MUSCULAR DYSTROPHY (MYOPATHY)

Ætiology.—This heredo-familial muscular affection is of wholly unknown cause. Males are more frequently affected than females, direct transmission by unaffected females is common, and the types of inheritance differ in different families. The onset is early in life, the clinical types varying in this respect.

Pathology.—The microscopic changes in the muscles are the same in all the clinical variants, and consist in swelling of some muscle fibres with multiplication of the sarcolemmal nuclei. There is an increase in the connective tissue septa and in certain muscles there is a deposition of fat between the hypertrophied fibres. Later also the fibres tend to split longitudinally and to undergo a regressive change into fibrous tissue. Remarkably enough the muscle spindles remain intact in the atrophic muscles.

Symptoms.—(a) GENERAL.—The essential clinical feature in all types is a progressive wasting and paralysis of the muscles of the shoulder and pelvic girdle and of the proximal segments of the limbs. In the final stage the muscles undergo a fibrous change, shorten, and thus lead to the development of skeletal deformities and contractures of the limbs. Certain muscles enlarge owing to the deposition of fat within them. The malady is steadily progressive and ultimately disabling, the different types varying in the rapidity of development and in age of onset. All types have certain striking features in common—winging of the scapula, lordosis, and wasting of pectoralis major—which make them readily recognizable when the patient is inspected.

(b) THE PSEUDOHYPERTROPHIC TYPE is perhaps the most frequently encountered. The subjects are almost exclusively males and all the boys in one generation of a family may be affected. In many instances it is recorded that the child walked late and was never normally nimble, but in others nothing abnormal is seen until between the ages of five and seven years. From this period onwards a slowly growing disability is noted in the child. His gait becomes waddling, he tends to fall easily and frequently, and soon is noticed to have difficulty in getting up again. In course of time he develops a characteristic fashion of doing this. He turns over on to his face, climbs on to hands and knees, then puts both hands on the front of his thighs and working them upwards one by

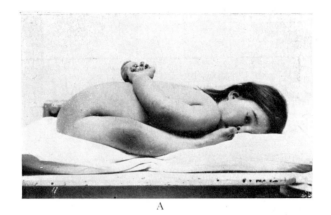

A

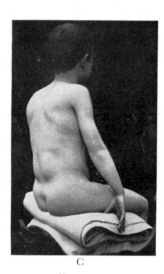

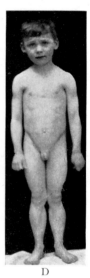

B   C   D

Fig. 39.

FORMS OF MUSCULAR DYSTROPHY.

A.—Amyotonia congenita. A child of 3 years, one of 6 affected siblings in a family of 13 children. (She is now 27 years old, is symptom-free and earns her living at housework, but shows weakness and wasting of the sternomastoids, triceps, trapezii, spinati, pectorals, latissimus dorsi, and deltoids.) The photograph shows the abnormal postures which can be imposed upon the subject, owing to the muscular flaccidity.

B, C, D.—Pseudohypertrophic dystrophy. B, An adolescent case showing enlargement of the calves, and of tensor fasciæ femoris, with wasting of vasti and the adductors of the thigh. C, Showing enlargement of erector spinæ. D, A typical early case with enlargement of calves and thigh muscles, and slight wasting of pectorals and upper arm muscles.

To face page 222.

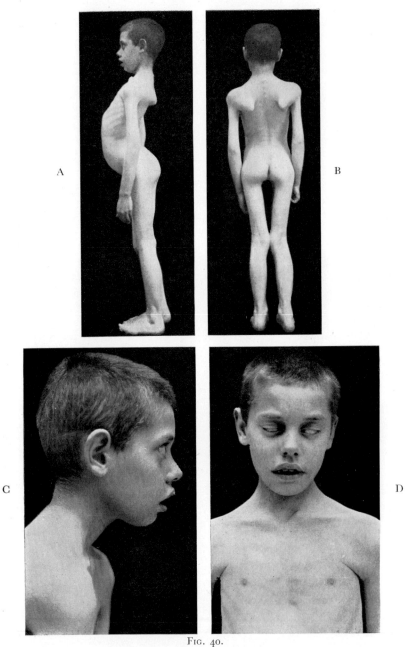

FIG. 40.

FACIO-SCAPULO-HUMERAL FORM OF MUSCULAR DYSTROPHY.

These photographs reveal the characteristic clinical features of the facio-scapulo-humeral variety of dystrophy. In A and B we see the lordosis, winging of the scapulæ, and wasting of the muscles of the proximal segments of all four limbs. C and D show the facies with the thickened and everted lips, and in D the inability of the patient to close the eyes or the lips completely owing to muscular weakness. D also shows the loss of pectoralis major.

To face page 223.

one clambers laboriously on to his feet and finally gains the erect posture.

At or about this stage of the illness the child comes under observation and the following changes are found. There is evident wasting of several muscles in the shoulder region—of the rhomboids, serratus anterior, latissimus dorsi, the spinati, pectoralis major, sometimes of biceps and triceps. The scapulæ are winged. In the lower limbs the thigh muscles, particularly the adductors, are wasted. The flexors of the thigh are not readily visible, but they also are wasted and shortened so that full extension of the thigh is impossible. Hence when standing there is a marked lordosis. Certain muscles are found to be enlarged and to have contours reminiscent of the muscles of the Farnese Hercules. The calves are large and fusiform, the deltoids large and their three portions (anterior, middle, and posterior) tend to stand out as separate masses. Spinati, biceps, and triceps, and the lower portion of erector spinæ, and also the masseters may be enlarged. Some weakness of the facial muscles lends a characteristically angelic quality to the child's smile (Fig. 39 D). At some stage of the illness the tendon jerks tend to diminish and finally they disappear. Ultimately the child becomes bedridden, and often grows extremely fat from inactivity so that the wasting is submerged. The spine develops a marked kyphoscoliosis, the legs become fixed in partial flexion, and the child succumbs to some intercurrent illness before puberty is reached.

(c) THE FACIO-SCAPULO-HUMERAL AND SCAPULO-HUMERAL TYPES have much in common, though the former usually appears at or about the age of ten years, the latter in adolescence or early adult life. Both sexes are affected. There is precisely the same distribution of wasting and paralysis as in the pseudohypertrophic type, though the process is much more gradual and the expectation of life is, therefore, much greater. This is especially the case with the scapulo-humeral variety. The winging of the scapulæ which results from paralysis of serratus anterior and is present in these as in the pseudohypertrophic type, may be the first striking objective sign, and the inability to elevate the arms to which it gives rise may first bring the subject under observation. Later, weakness and wasting of pelvic girdle muscles and lordosis appear. In the facio-scapulo-humeral (Landouzy-Dejerine) type all these signs are present, usually in a more severe and rapidly developing degree, and, in addition, there is profound weakness of all the facial muscles, with pseudohypertrophy of orbicularis oris which gives a characteristic pouting expression to the thick and everted lips. The subject may be unable to close the eyes or to cover the teeth with the lips (Fig. 40).

A slowly progressive wasting of the muscles already enumerated takes place together with an associated weakness. The subjects rarely reach middle life. In both these types traces of enlargement of muscles may be seen, *e.g.* in the deltoids or spinati.

(*d*) A rarer type known as the simple atrophic, or as *amyotonia congenita*, is sometimes seen. It is noticed soon after birth that the child's muscles are unduly soft and flaccid. The limbs can be placed in abnormal positions, the child learns to sit up and to walk very late. Unlike the other forms this is not progressive, and ultimately, despite some muscular wasting and slight contracture the child learns to walk, and may live to lead a life of limited physical activity (Fig. 39 A).

Prognosis.—All cases steadily progress until the subject becomes bedridden. Ultimately, a terminal broncho-pneumonia closes the sequence of events.

Treatment.—Muscular dystrophy is uninfluenced by any known remedy, though favourable claims have been made for the adminis-tration of glycine (10 grams) daily, and more recently for vitamin E. As stated on page 230, carefully controlled observations have failed to substantiate this latter claim. It is best to keep the patient ambulant and to postpone the day of final restriction to bed as long as possible. Massage may slow down the inevitable process of muscular contracture. Electro-therapy has no place in treatment.

(2) DYSTROPHIA MYOTONICA (MYOTONIA ATROPHICA)

An heredo-familial disease characterized by wasting of the distal muscles of the limbs, of sternomastoid and of the facial muscles, by a peculiarly delayed relaxation of certain muscles (myotonia), by testicular atrophy, premature baldness, cataract, and mental deterioration.

Ætiology.—The degenerative process seems to be spread over three generations, appearing as cataract in the first, as pre-senile cataract in the second, and as the fully developed affection in the third. The age of onset is from twenty to thirty years. Males are more often affected than females. The pathological process in the muscles resembles that seen in muscular dystrophy.

Symptoms.—The diagnostic features are weakness and wasting of the facial muscles, the peculiarly mournful set expression of the face, wasting of the sternomastoid muscles which is a constant and unique feature of this malady, moderate wasting of forearm and leg muscles, and delayed relaxation of these and other muscles, *e.g.* the tongue. This delayed relaxation may be demonstrated by tapping the muscle with a percussion hammer, when a local weal appears and slowly subsides. Tapping the tongue produces a local "dimple" which slowly fills up. In normal contractions this delay leads to difficulty in relaxing the grasp and to slowness of movement. Other manifestations include

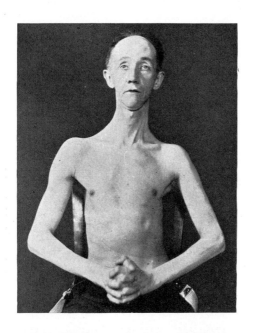

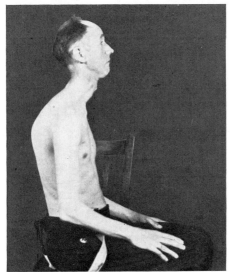

Fig. 41.

Dystrophia Myotonica.

These photographs reveal some of the characteristic features of the malady: namely, the frontal
baldness, the forward curve of the neck owing to
wasting and weakness of the sterno-mastoids, the
prominence of the larynx, the expressionless and
melancholy cast of countenance, and the thin
forearms. Some remaining strands of the left
sterno-mastoid are visible.

To face page 224.

premature baldness, cataract, mental deterioration, and progressive atrophy of the testicles leading ultimately to impotence.

Treatment.—The course of the disease cannot be influenced, but it has been stated that the myotonia may be materially diminished as long as quinine (grs. 10 daily) is administered.

THE PERONEAL TYPE OF MUSCULAR ATROPHY (NEURITIC TYPE)

This relatively uncommon malady resembles muscular dystrophy in that it has an heredo-familial incidence and that muscular wasting is its prominent symptom, and is like motor neurone disease in that these symptoms are due to degenerative changes in the central and peripheral nervous system.

Ætiology.—Nothing is known of its causation. Usually one of the subject's parents is similarly affected, and direct transmission is common though not invariable.

Pathology.—Both motor and sensory neurones are affected. There is atrophy of ventral horn cells and of the dorsal columns of the cord. The ventral (motor) nerve roots are atrophied and there is interstitial neuritis of the peroneal nerves.

Symptoms.—Muscular wasting develops slowly, appearing first in the legs. The muscles are affected in the following sequence: plantar muscles, peronei, calf muscles, and the muscles of the anterior aspect of the thigh in its lower third. The wasting rises like a tide until it reaches the level above mentioned when it ceases to spread. The wasting of the distal part of the thigh imparts to this segment of the limb the general form of an inverted Indian club or champagne bottle. Later in the evolution of the malady the small hand muscles and those of the distal third of the forearm waste. Characteristic of this wasting is the remarkably slight degree of weakness and disability that ensues. The patient walks with foot-drop, but continues to lead an active life for very many years, and the expectation of life is not shortened. All forms of sensation may be impaired within the distribution of the wasting. Pes cavus and hyper-extension of the proximal phalanges develop early.

Treatment.—The slow course of the malady is uninfluenced by treatment. The wearing of a foot-drop support ultimately becomes necessary.

MOTOR NEURONE DISEASE

The essential lesion in this malady is a degeneration of motor neurones, both upper and lower, namely, of the pyramidal fibres, of

P

ventral horn cells, and of cranial motor nerve nuclei. In different cases the relative incidence of degeneration varies. In some the change is maximal in the ventral horn cells of the cervical enlargement of the cord, in others in the cranial nerve nuclei, in yet others the pyramidal fibre sclerosis is severe and adds the appropriate features to the clinical picture. In other words, there are several clinical types of motor neurone disease which give expression to variations in the incidence of the pathological process. For these types various names are in use and are sometimes employed as synonyms for the term motor neurone disease, viz. *progressive muscular atrophy*, *amyotrophic lateral sclerosis*, and *chronic bulbar palsy*.

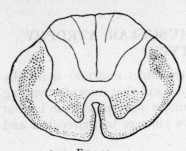

FIG. 42.

THE SITUATION OF THE CORD LESION IN MOTOR NEURONE DISEASE.

Amyotrophic lateral sclerosis, showing the situation of the lesion in the lateral and anterior columns and in the ventral horns. The affected regions are marked by dots.

Ætiology.—Nothing is known of the pathogenesis of this malady. Inheritance plays no part, but as in the case of other maladies of unknown ætiology injury has been invoked as an occasional factor. In the present state of knowledge it is impossible to conceive of a peripheral injury capable of setting up a slowly progressive motor neurone degeneration, and the occasional association of injury and motor neurone disease is accounted for by coincidence more easily than by postulating an obscure and inexplicable relationship of cause and effect. Probably some cases attributed to trauma are not true cases of motor neurone disease, but undiagnosed examples of a lesion to the cervical cord associated with vertebral injury (see page 210). It is a malady of the second half of life and males are more often affected than females. Rarely, a case may be seen in a young adult.

Pathology.—In the spinal cord there is degeneration of descending fibres in ventrolateral columns, especially affecting the pyramidal fibres. There is profound atrophy of motor nerve cells either in the ventral horns of the cervical region of the cord, or in the motor nuclei of the pons and medulla, or in both situations. There is also some pyramidal and Betz cell loss in the motor cortex. The wasted muscles show atrophic changes in the fibres.

It is usual to describe the three following clinical types, but combined and transitional forms also occur, as must be obvious from what has been said of the variable incidence of the pathological process within the motor systems.

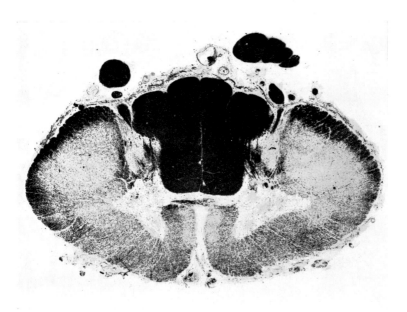

FIG. 43.
AMYOTROPHIC LATERAL SCLEROSIS.
A transverse, Weigert-Pal stained section of the cervical cord. It shows the degeneration in the anterolateral column and especially in the pyramidal tracts. The posterior columns and the direct cerebellar tracts are intact.

To face page 226.

(1) AMYOTROPHIC LATERAL SCLEROSIS

This is perhaps the most frequently encountered clinical variant. The patient is commonly a middle-aged man, often of the labouring class. He complains that he has noticed wasting of one hand, and frequently only a direct question elicits the fact that the hand has also become weak. In an early case, that is, one of less than a year's duration, he may have nothing to say of the opposite hand though inspection may possibly reveal the faint beginnings of wasting there also. Occasionally, if the wasting and weakness be considerable and the hand and arm, therefore, little used there may be an additional complaint of coldness, perhaps even of some tingling in the fingers. Alternatively, if the limb is still in heavy use, this use may be accompanied by some aching in the muscles. Examination reveals wasting involving the small hand muscles—thenar, hypothenar, and interossei—and involving them all in uniform degree. Fibrillation will be seen—most obviously in the first dorsal interosseus muscle—and if not at first then after the muscles have been voluntarily contracted. Further inspection of the limb and shoulders will probably reveal, if not the initial stage of wasting in the forearm, then widespread fibrillation of the limb muscles, of the pectoralis, deltoid, rhomboids, and trapezius. Fibrillation seems to spread widely in advance of wasting and thus always to involve a wider field of the musculature. Even in the opposite and perhaps unwasted arm and hand a degree and extent of fibrillation not less marked may be seen. In short, the combination of uniform wasting of the hand muscles and of widespread fibrillation are highly characteristic of the initial stage of this malady. The tendon jerks in the arms are almost invariably markedly increased, and so also is the mechanical irritability of the entire limb and shoulder girdle musculature. When pectoralis is tapped a large strand of muscle fibres contracts and relaxes rapidly, raising the skin over the contracting fasciculus.

In the lower limbs it is common to find increased tendon-jerks. No other abnormal signs are found, and the paræsthesiæ that are sometimes complained of in the affected extremity have no corresponding objective sensory change.

Some nine or twelve months after the appearance of wasting in one hand the same process develops in its fellow, and in both limbs the wasting then tends to spread steadily up the limb until the shoulder girdle muscles are also affected. The lower part of trapezius wastes and disappears relatively early, the upper portion later and never completely. Latissimus dorsi and serratus anterior are often intact even in the final stages of the malady, so that the winging of the scapulæ so common and so early in muscular dystrophy may not occur at all, though in some cases even these muscles ultimately waste profoundly.

In the majority of instances the process is more marked in one upper limb than in its fellow, that is, in the limb earlier involved.

As this process spreads and deepens, signs of upper motor neurone lesion appear in the legs, the tendon jerks become brisker, ankle clonus and hypertonus may develop, but an extensor plantar response may be strikingly late in development, and the abdominal reflexes disappear even later than the appearance of this reflex and are sometimes retained throughout the illness. Profound weakness of the legs is exceptional and the flexed type of paraplegia is never seen. Occasionally the upper motor neurone element in the disease renders the arms weaker than the degree and extent of wasting can account for. A brisk jaw jerk is not infrequently encountered.

In a few cases the pyramidal fibre degeneration seems to precede the ventral horn cell degeneration, and when this is the case the signs enumerated as present in the legs may for a period of months be present alone, no wasting being visible. It is to this condition that the name of *primary lateral sclerosis* was formerly applied, but most cases so labelled ultimately prove to be amyotrophic lateral sclerosis or some other known affection of the nervous system, and the title corresponds to no special recognized pathological process and should be abandoned.

The combination of progressive and considerable wasting of the muscles, most marked distally, with marked and uniform increase of the arm jerks is, in the absence of sensory and sphincter disturbances, characteristic of this variant of motor neurone disease. It is steadily progressive, though occasional cases of spontaneous arrest lasting for a period of years may be met with. Death commonly ensues within two or three years of onset, but cases of more gradual development occur.

(2) PROGRESSIVE MUSCULAR ATROPHY

Although pathological examination of the spinal cord reveals some degree of sclerosis in the lateral columns, the ventral horn cell degeneration predominates greatly and governs the clinical aspect of the case. The wasting is of the distribution already described, but in this variant it may long remain confined to the small hand and forearm muscles, showing no tendency to spread more widely for many years. Such are the cases that we are apt to think we have arrested by our therapeutic measures. In other cases the spread is rapid and extensive, finally involving the neck muscles so that the head droops and flops passively as the patient sits up or lies down. An extreme degree of muscular wasting may thus come to invade arms, shoulder, and neck. In a few cases this process may begin, not in the upper but in the lower limbs—a state of affairs rarely if ever encountered in amyotrophic lateral sclerosis—or it may appear in the lower limbs later than in the upper. The site of onset and the spread of wasting show little uniformity from case to case when the lower limbs are involved, but fibrillation is as prominent here as in the upper limbs.

Usually the tendon jerks remain at normal—sometimes at heightened—activity. Their disappearance is unusual except in the case of the clinically similar amyotrophic meningo-myelitis of syphilis, which should be suspected when the tendon jerks behave in this way.

(3) CHRONIC BULBAR PALSY

Just as there are two variants of the malady when the limb muscles are concerned—a spastic type (amyotrophic lateral sclerosis) and a purely atrophic (progressive muscular atrophy)—so also there are spastic and atrophic variants of chronic bulbar palsy. In a very few cases the spastic element so far predominates that little wasting may be seen, but instead there is a spasticity of the affected muscles that may lead to a failure to recognize the nature of the lesion. As a rule the condition is what we may call spastic-atrophic, the atrophic element predominating. Usually the patient seeks advice for a slowly increasing difficulty in articulation, shortly followed by difficulty in deglutition. On examination fibrillation will be seen in the muscles in the region of the mouth and chin. The lips are slightly open and saliva trickles from the corners. It may not be possible for the patient to purse the lips or to whistle. The mucous membrane of the tongue is wrinkled and constantly "on the work" over the wasted and fibrillating musculature. The range of movement of the tongue is limited and protrusion beyond the lips may be impossible. On phonation the excursion of the soft palate is diminished. Swallowing is slow and laboured because the weak muscles of the tongue and the floor of the mouth cannot push the food bolus back into the fauces, and pharyngeal deglutition is impaired owing to weakness of the hyoid muscles, the larynx is not fixed and moves up and down, and the nasopharynx is not shut off. For similar reasons articulation becomes grossly disturbed and the voice monotonous. Finally, the patient can make only inarticulate noises, swallowing becomes virtually impossible, and an aspiration pneumonia closes the distressing scene, usually within two years of the time of onset.

When the spastic element is prominent, the face moves as a whole, slowly and in exaggerated degree, and there may be a tendency to what is called spasmodic weeping and laughter of the type found in pseudo-bulbar palsy, with which this variant of chronic bulbar palsy may be confused if the fact of its slowly progressive onset be overlooked. In pseudobulbar palsy the onset is usually sudden after two or more thrombotic attacks (see page 108).

This incidence of the essential pathological process may occur alone or in combination with amyotrophic lateral sclerosis, sometimes one sometimes the other opening the course of events.

Chronic bulbar palsy, whether alone or with amyotrophic lateral sclerosis, usually runs an uninterrupted course to a fatal issue within two years, yet occasional cases may be met in which the process undergoes a temporary arrest for one or more years before again becoming active.

Diagnosis.—The features by which motor neurone disease may be distinguished from the muscular dystrophies, from dystrophia myotonica and from the peroneal type of muscular atrophy, have already been considered. They include the absence of heredo-familial factors, the onset in or after middle life, the topography of the wasting and the presence of persistent and widespread fibrillation, and, finally, in almost all cases the exaggeration of the tendon jerks even when the extensor type of plantar response does not develop.

Sensory loss is absent, there are no skeletal deformities or trophic lesions, and these negative points distinguish motor neurone disease from syringomyelia. In amyotrophic meningo-myelitis of syphilitic origin, the arm jerks, and sometimes also the tendon jerks in the lower limbs, are diminished or absent, though the Argyll Robertson pupil reaction is by no means constantly present. Further, the initial onset of wasting in the hand muscles and its continuous spread proximally up the limb is not so constant as is the case in motor neurone disease. In the syphilitic condition the wasting process may begin proximally, or beginning distally may skip muscles as it spreads upwards. Spontaneous arrest is also more often encountered in syphilitic meningo-myelitis than in motor neurone disease. Finally, the reactions in blood and cerebrospinal fluid will betray the presence of syphilis.

Wasting of limb and trunk muscles with fibrillation may accompany thyrotoxicosis (*chronic thyrotoxic myopathy*) and afford a superficial resemblance to progressive muscular atrophy. The condition responds to treatment of the accompanying thyrotoxicosis.

The differential diagnosis of unilateral wasting of the hand will be considered under the heading of cervical rib.

Treatment.—It has to be confessed that no mode of treatment checks or in any way influences the progress of motor neurone disease, and symptomatic measures alone are available.

It has recently been claimed that vitamin E (tocopherol acetate) in doses of from 3 mgms. thrice daily not only checks the progress of muscular wasting in motor neurone disease, but also leads to rapid improvement. A similar claim has been made for this vitamin in respect of the muscular dystrophies. Carefully controlled observations by numerous observers have conclusively shown these claims to be without foundation, and the attempt to differentiate a special variant of motor neurone disease that does respond to vitamin therapy is equally without evidence.

For cases of bulbar palsy the food must be minced and of a pappy consistence. Massage is no more than a placebo, while to stimulate the weakening and wasting muscles by electrical currents is obviously to "whip a tired horse."

ARTHRITIC MUSCULAR ATROPHY

The wasting of the interosseous muscles and the ulnar adduction of the fingers that accompany arthritis of the metacarpo-phalangeal joints are familiar to every clinician, but less uniformly recognized is the wasting that may accompany arthritis of the knee or shoulder joint. In general we may say that the wasting round an inflamed joint does not affect all muscles equally, but is largely restricted to the extensor muscles proximal to the joint. Thus in the case of the knee, wasting falls almost exclusively upon the vasti muscles. It may become extreme, so that extension at the knee is gravely weakened and the leg tends to "give" when weight is put on it in walking, or when the leg is being extended as the patient walks upstairs. In short, a considerable disability may result. The knee jerk may disappear. While wasting is active the muscle is tender and fibrillates. In the case of the shoulder, deltoid and the spinati are particularly affected, and elevation of the arm to the vertical may be impossible. In the case of the hip joint there may be evident wasting of the glutei. The wasting is always more severe and rapid in development in an acute than in a chronic arthritis.

The treatment of the condition is that of the arthritis if this be active. When it has subsided increasing exercise will promote a certain degree of recovery of strength and of bulk, but some residual weakness and wasting may be permanent.

POST-PARALYTIC MUSCULAR ATROPHY

Reference has been made in the opening paragraph of the chapter to the muscular wasting that ensues upon paralysis from lesions of both upper and lower motor neurones. Muscular wasting is not a feature of lesions of the extrapyramidal system.

In both the acute hemiplegia of vascular lesions and the progressive hemiplegia of intracranial tumour, some wasting of muscles makes its appearance. It is never profound and is most clearly evident in the small hand muscles, where after a severe vascular lesion with complete hemiplegia it may become evident within a week or two. In old residual hemiplegia a slight general wasting of the affected limbs, more particularly the arm, may be seen. In this disuse may play some part.

In acute lower motor neurone paralysis (*e.g.* acute poliomyelitis) the wasting necessarily takes sometime to appear. In totally or profoundly paralysed muscles it becomes evident in the third or fourth week and thereupon progressively increases until, unless some voluntary power is restored, affected muscles may waste until no contractile tissue remains. Fibrous contracture with shortening may then develop unless prevented by treatment.

In hysterical paralysis, prolonged disuse may lead to evident muscular wasting in the affected limb or limbs.

RIB PRESSURE SYNDROMES

Ætiology.—The factors that underlie the abnormal development of ribs at the upper thoracic outlet are multiple. One of them is probably the segmental derivation of the brachial plexus. When this receives a considerable contribution from the fourth cervical nerve root, it is said to be "prefixed," and in these circumstances an accessory cervical rib may grow. Less commonly, the fourth root does not join the plexus, which then receives the whole first and a great part of the second thoracic root, and is said to be "postfixed"; that is, it is set a spinal cord segment caudally. When this is so, the first rib may be imperfectly developed. In either case, other anomalies are frequently found; namely, cervico-thoracic scoliosis, deformation of the vertebræ locally, asymmetry of transverse processes, and even in some cases, syringomyelia has been found. Thus other developmental factors than the derivation of the brachial plexus are probably at work. In short, what is produced is an abnormal upper thoracic outlet. This is asymmetrical, higher and narrower on one side and abnormally tilted. It is in these terms, rather than in terms of the abnormal costal element alone, that we should think of this state of affairs. Given this abnormal outlet, the lower components of the brachial plexus and the subclavian artery are liable to be subjected to pathological stresses as they pass out of the thorax to gain the narrow space between thoracic brim and clavicle. These stresses are aggravated if—as often happens—there is a sagging of the shoulder girdles, such as may be due to atonia of the relevant muscles from illness, fatigue or undue physical strain, and a drooping shoulder girdle may precipitate the appearance of pressure symptoms in the possessor of an abnormal rib at the upper thoracic outlet. It is because the shoulder is set lower in women than in men, that most cases of rib pressure occur in women. Even with a normal thoracic outlet, a sagging shoulder girdle may produce pressure symptoms (the so-called normal first rib pressure syndrome).

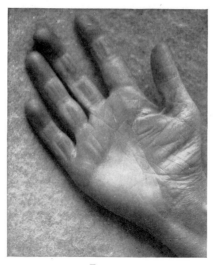

Fig. 44.

The Thenar Wasting in Cervical Rib
Pressure.

The right hand of a man with wasting of
opponens pollicis and the characteristic
appearance of the thenar eminence. A
cervical rib was present.

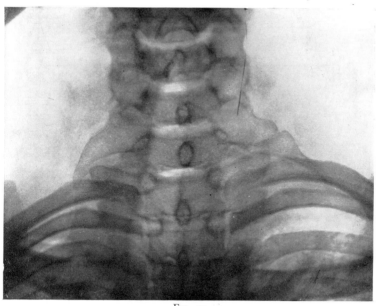

Fig. 45.

Radiogram of Cervical Ribs.

Bilateral cervical ribs. The right rib is non-articulated, sloping and tapering,
and had produced the characteristic clinical symptoms of rib pressure in the
patient, a woman of 30. The left rib is articulated and passes down to the first
thoracic rib. It had produced no symptoms. The radiogram also shows a
drooping of the shoulder on the right side.

To face page 232.

The nerve roots in these circumstances (seventh and eighth cervical and/or the first thoracic) may be subjected to tension and compression, leading to muscular weakness and wasting and to pain and sensory loss. The subclavian artery also, alone or in association with nerve root compression, may also be compressed, angulated and otherwise damaged, with the production of vascular disorders in the upper limb.

Clinically, it is probably indifferent whether the abnormal rib is cervical or rudimentary first thoracic. The latter anomaly is often mistakenly identified as a cervical rib, owing to unsystematic radiography and the failure to determine the vertebral derivation of the abnormal costal element present, but it is the rarer of the two anomalies.

An accessory cervical rib may be no more than an abnormally large transverse process, drooping and pointed, or it may be a short articulated rib ending on an exostosis on the first rib, or passing into a fibrous anterior extension which reaches the manubrium. In other words, a cervical rib may be largely fibrous and may thus be missed in a radiogram. The rudimentary first rib is commonly larger and longer and may fuse anteriorly with the second rib, the anterior part of which is then apt to be abnormally broad and like a first rib in contours (see Fig. 46).

The thorax moves up and down some 23,000 times in the 24-hour period, and the clavicle moves with each movement of the arm, and thus the subclavian artery and the nerve roots are not only subjected to tension as they cross the rib, but also to recurrent compression between clavicle and first rib. This constant movement leads to the formation of fibrous tissue round the subclavian artery when the thoracic outlet is abnormal and the friction between bony and soft tissues abnormally increased, so that the artery may become bound to the abnormal rib, and its wall damaged by the clavicle. Thus, we see the not infrequent development of an aneurysmal dilatation of the third part of the artery, and sometimes the formation of clot within the aneurysm, and, less frequently, the dislodgement of portions of clot with the formation of embolic infarction in the digital arteries. In some cases nervous symptoms alone are present, in others purely vascular, in yet others nervous and vascular symptoms co-exist. Vascular symptoms alone are far commoner than is supposed.

On this complex anatomical background, factors that lead to a sagging of the shoulder girdles may lead to the onset of pressure symptoms: e.g. illness, debility, unaccustomed heavy work with the arms.

A change of occupation may usher in the appearance of symptoms, as, for example, when a young mother begins to carry her first baby on her arm, or a woman takes to heavy housework for the first time. Thus, a young woman accustomed to serving in a baker's shop began to do the bread round, carrying a heavy bread basket on her left arm. Within a few weeks rib pressure symptoms and the characteristic signs developed. A sempstress developed torticollis, could no longer sew and became a charwoman, scrubbing and carrying buckets of water. Cervical rib symptoms developed rapidly. In both these cases radiograms revealed the presence of accessory ribs. Trauma, *e.g.* lifting heavy weights, may lead to the sudden appearance of symptoms.

Symptoms.—There are three possible components in the clinical picture: sensory, motor, and vascular. The last-named component is frequently absent, though there are cases in which it alone is present.

The sequence of events is usually as follows. The patient, following a change in occupation or the assumption of heavier work, begins to complain of aching and shooting pain in the muscles of the forearm and in the hand. This pain may come on during the course of the day's work and often develops with great severity after the patient has gone to bed. During the night she may be kept awake and there are various positions adopted to obtain relief. Some patients like to adduct the arm and to place the forearm and hand across the chest, some find relief from elevating the limb above the shoulder and placing it on the pillow. Others again prefer to let the arm hang downwards over the edge of the bed for some minutes. During the daytime it may be noticed that the carrying of a parcel or the wearing of a heavy coat induces pain. The degree and persistence of pain vary greatly from case to case, and there are sufferers from cervical rib whose attention is first drawn to the condition by the appearance of wasting of the thenar eminence, though these are the exception. Tingling and numbness in the fingers are also commonly and early complained of. Usually these sensations are referred to either radial or ulnar side of the hand rather than to all the fingers equally.

On examination very little may be found. Objective sensory loss is absent or slight and of indefinable distribution, but corresponding approximately sometimes to the median, sometimes to the ulnar, nerve distribution. Tenderness on pressure is, however, virtually constant in opponens pollicis and less frequently in the first dorsal interosseous muscle. When wasting is present its distribution is in most cases characteristic of the condition. The radial half of the thenar eminence is flattened and sometimes hollow, as though scooped out (see Fig. 44). This appearance is due to wasting of opponens pollicis and abductor pollicis. As the pressure continues this selective incidence of wasting remains obvious, but the interossei may also show some degree of wasting, and all the wasted muscles are very tender to pressure. An occasional flicker of fibrillation may be seen in the wasted opponens pollicis. In early cases where obvious wasting is not to be seen, palpation of the two thenar eminences simultaneously may reveal a curious softness of opponens on the affected side.

In other cases the wasting is ulnar in type and involves the interossei and hypothenar muscles. It is in association with this type of wasting that ulnar paræsthesiæ are usually found. It seems probable that when wasting is confined to the thenar muscles named above, the seventh cervical nerve root is the one subjected to pressure, and with the ulnar type of wasting the eighth nerve root.

The vascular symptoms, which may be present alone, are of three orders: (1) coldness, cyanosis, or pallor of the hand. These are aggravated by traction upon the arm, and this may lead to obliteration of the radial pulse at the wrist; (2) the above symptoms with the addition of abnormal pulsation of the subclavian artery above the clavicle, a palpable thrill over the artery and a bruit which is not conducted downwards into the arm, but may be conducted upwards to the skull. This group of symptoms probably indicated a patent aneurysmal dilatation of the artery; (3) coldness, weakness and pallor or cyanosis of the arm and hand, permanent pulselessness at wrist and elbow, and an absence of pulsation, thrill and bruit over the artery in the neck. This betokens clot formation within an aneurysmal sac. In such cases, the sudden appearance of infarcts in the digits may occur—red, swollen, painful areas which become gangrenous.

All these vascular disorders have wrongly been attributed to pressure on sympathetic fibres in the first thoracic root, but for various reasons this hypothesis is untenable, and mechanical interference with the blood flow through the subclavian artery is the operative factor.

Occasionally Horner's syndrome has been present, and is probably due to traction upon the stellate ganglion, or to its involvement in fibrous tissue as it lies against the subclavian artery. On the whole, this group of vascular syndromes is less commonly seen than the syndrome of somatic nerve fibre compression.

Pressure symptoms produced by a normal first rib, and the so-called Scalenus Anticus syndrome

It happens from time to time that patients are encountered in whom there are present symptoms suggestive of pressure upon nerves or artery by an abnormal rib at the upper thoracic outlet, but in whom a skiagram reveals no bony anomaly of this order. The symptoms in these cases are commonly largely subjective: pain, coldness, cyanosis and tingling of the hands, though the more severe nervous and vascular phenomena already described may be met. Here the thoracic outlet is normal, and perhaps the chief operative factor is a sagging of the shoulder girdles, due to causes already enumerated, which leads to an increase in the tension of artery and/or nerves as they cross the first rib on their way into the space between rib and clavicle. We know that the mesial edge of the first rib is sharp and that the lower trunk of the brachial plexus may lie in a deep grove on the rib. Indeed, in the effort to achieve adjustment between nerve trunk and rib, the latter may be bent downwards prior to its ossification. In these circumstances a dropping of the shoulder girdle tends to stretch the structures passing over the rib. Since the first rib slopes downwards from its tubercle, the stretched structures crossing it may tend, when under increased tension, to cross as far forwards as possible: that is immediately behind the tendon of scalenus anticus, which may then indent the artery and add another compressing factor to the nerve trunk. But even when this last factor is present it is clearly only secondary, the primary and essential factors being stretching over the rib when the shoulder girdle drops.

The occurrence of a "normal first rib pressure syndrome" has long been recognized, and in the past was dealt with surgically by resection of part of the rib, but of late years it has become the increasing habit to employ the term "scalenus anticus syndrome" for this state of affairs. The term is unfortunate in that it implies a primacy in the action of scalenus anticus that even the proposers of the term do not claim for it, and it obscures the multiplicity and relative importance of the operative factors. It is true that relief of symptoms is sometimes achieved by section of the tendon of this muscle, but this is scarcely a justification for a terminology that artificially simplifies a complex anatomical situation.

Diagnosis.—The presence of pain in one forearm and hand, behaving as detailed above, and occurring in a woman in the third or fourth decade of life should, even in the absence of objective signs, lead to the search for a possible accessory rib by radiography. In the presence of *wasting of the muscles of one hand* a wider diagnostic problem arises. Characteristic of rib pressure is the selective wasting already described. In motor neurone disease the wasting of the hand muscles is global, or uniform in degree and not selective. Also in this disease the muscles are not tender and there is no history of pain radiating down the limb. It should also be remembered that cervical ribs do not in most cases produce any symptoms, and that there is nothing impossible in the presence in a given person of an asymptomatic cervical rib and motor neurone disease. In short, whatever information be derived from the study of the radiogram, the clinical aspect of the case should be the essential determinant in diagnosis. In syringomyelia the wasting of the upper limbs may be unilateral at onset and may involve small hand muscles first. In these circumstances, the presence of scars of old or recent burns and injuries on the hand, of the characteristic type of sensory loss, of skeletal deformities, of lost arm jerks, and the global character of the wasting distinguishes syringomyelia from rib pressure.

Treatment.—In early cases without wasting, we may as a trial step seek to ascertain whether the relinquishing of heavy work and the employment of massage and active exercises to the shoulder girdle muscles, with a view to elevating the shoulders, will relieve symptoms. Such measures occasionally provide complete relief, but if wasting be present and if the patient's circumstances make a change of occupation impracticable, the surgical removal of the rib or the division of its fibrous prolongation is necessary. This step should not be delayed if wasting is progressing or disabling. In characteristic cases of the syndrome when X-ray examination fails to reveal the presence of any abnormal costal element, the possibility that a normal first rib is exerting pressure on the roots must be considered. When this is thought to be the case, the mid-portion of the rib may be resected.

ACROPARÆSTHESIA

The extremely widespread syndrome that goes by this name is typically found in middle-aged women, particularly in those who are debilitated and forced to unaccustomed manual work. Formerly found chiefly in washerwomen and charwomen, it is now found more widely, owing to wartime conditions which have forced women of all classes to engage in housework, etc. It consists in numbness, tingling and sometimes in severe burning pain in the hands and fingers, accompanied by clumsiness of the hands. These symptoms are most disabling when the patient awakes in the morning, but tend to diminish during the day, returning with severity during the night and disturbing slumber. The onset is gradual, symptoms reaching a maximum in a few weeks or months, and then remaining, with temporal variations, for an indefinite period. The subjects are debilitated, tired and overworked women of middle age or later, or younger women with the additional burdens of pregnancy and the care of infants. On examination, objective signs are extremely scanty, but tenderness of the extensor muscles in the forearm and of thenar and thumb adductors, slight blunting of cutaneous sensibility over the digits and some coldness and cyanosis of the digits are usual. There is no loss of tendon jerks, true paresis, wasting or gross sensory loss. The condition is not a polyneuritis, but in all probability is due to stretching and compression of the lower components of the brachial plexus, and sometimes of the subclavian artery also, as these structures pass across the first rib. This traction and compression are due to drooping of the shoulder girdles. This drooping increases in all women in middle age, but reaches abnormal proportions in states of fatigue and debility when the musculature becomes atonic.

Treatment.—If the ætiology be as here submitted, relief from work and rest and general tonic treatment are indicated. These suffice to afford relief in almost all cases without other measures. Massage to the shoulder girdle muscles is an additional measure that may be useful. It is obvious that to regard the condition as a polyneuritis in the commonly accepted and correct sense of this term is erroneous, and it is not surprising that the administration of vitamin B_1, diathermy, radiant heat, ionization and the like are consistently ineffective.

SYRINGOMYELIA

A chronic and slowly progressive disease of the spinal cord characterized pathologically by cavitation and gliosis in the spinal cord, and clinically by the combination of wasting of the upper limbs, by loss of painful and thermal sensation over several spinal segments and by a variable degree of spastic paresis of the legs. Sometimes the process extends upwards into the medulla (syringobulbia), producing symptons referable to cranial nerves.

Ætiology.—It is probable that syringomyelia arises from the proliferation of rests of embryonic glial cells in the central region of the cord. In this proliferated mass cavitation secondarily occurs. The lesion may be associated with other structural deformities such as spina bifida, cervical rib, or asymmetry of the skull.

The two sexes are affected equally; the malady makes its appearance clinically in adolescence or early adult life. A kyphoscoliosis developing in childhood may precede the characteristic symptoms of the developed disease.

Pathology.—The gliosis and cavitation develop in the neighbourhood of the grey commissure of the cord, and they may lead to an irregular enlargement of this in the cervical segments where the process is most advanced. The vertical extent of the lesion may be considerable, cavitation predominating at some levels and gliosis at others. The cavity may occupy the entire extent of the grey matter of one or more segments and may invade the lateral white columns. Its walls are composed of dense glial tissue, and the surrounding normal structures of the cord are compressed and in varying degree destroyed. In the medulla gliosis predominates and appears as a unilateral streak, with or without a fissure, below the floor of the fourth ventricle.

Symptoms.—The patient usually comes under observation in some such circumstances as the following. He may seek advice for a progressive weakening and wasting of his hands, or of one of them, and when they are examined the sores and scars of new and old injuries and burns are seen on the palm and especially on the fingers. Cigarette burns provide many of these lesions which, the patient will say, are

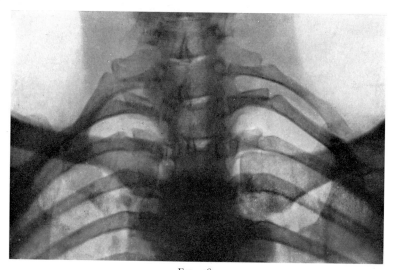

FIG. 46.

RUDIMENTARY FIRST THORACIC RIB ON THE LEFT SIDE.

The rudimentary left first rib ends prematurely upon the upper surface of the second rib, which anterior to this point assumes a broad spatulate form as though the two ribs were fused. There is also some scoliosis of the cervico-thoracic region. The symptoms in this case were predominantly vascular: namely, bruit over the subclavian artery and obliteration of the radial pulse upon traction upon the arm.

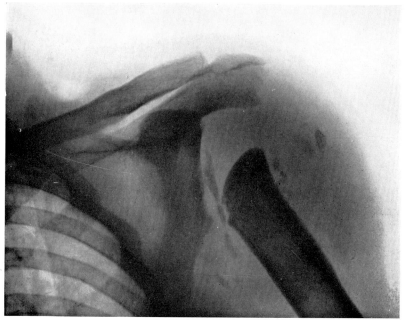

FIG. 47.

OSTEO-ARTHROPATHY OF LEFT SHOULDER JOINT IN A CASE OF SYRINGOMYELIA.

To face page 238.

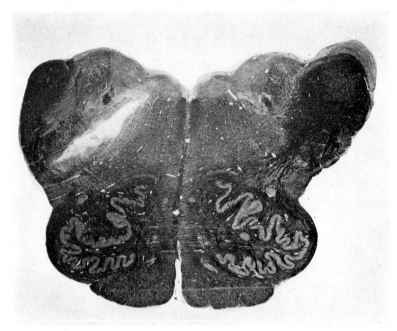

A.

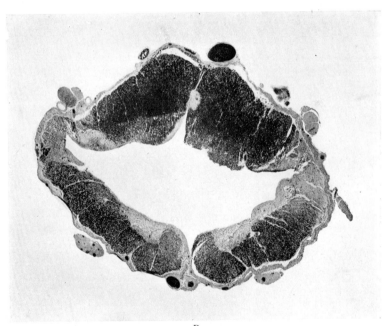

B

Fig. 48.

Syringobulbia and Syringomyelia.

Transverse sections, A of the medulla and B of the cervical region of the spinal cord. A shows the characteristic lateral fissure running forwards and laterally from the region of the floor of the fourth ventricle, and cutting off the restiform body from the central part of the medulla. Such a fissure often destroys the descending root of the fifth nerve, and the nuclei of the vagus-glossopharyngeal complex. B shows extensive cavitation extending laterally in the cervical region of the cord.

almost if not quite painless, so that he does not know of their presence until he sees them. Alternatively, such a patient may be in an occupation not rendering him liable to injury, but on changing his employment for rougher work may notice that painless injuries appear in an unaccountable fashion on his hands; as, for example, in the case of a clerk whom circumstances forced to take to bottle-washing and removing bottles from an autoclave. At once blisters began to appear on his fingers. Examination revealed in addition the early stages of wasting of the small hand muscles. Thus, either motor or sensory signs may first bring the malady to notice.

Systematic examination will then reveal what may be profound wasting of all the small hand muscles, bilateral but not bilaterally

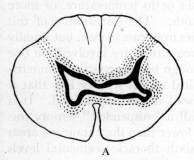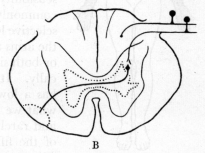

A   B

FIG. 49.

A and B. DIAGRAMS OF THE LESION IN SYRINGOMYELIA.

Two diagrams of transverse sections of the cord. A showing the central cavity surrounded by gliosis and stretching across the midline of the cord. B represents a normal section of the cord in which the lesion depicted in A is marked in dotted lines. The diagram shows how the crossed sensory pathway (pain and temperature sense) is interrupted as it decussates to join the spino-thalamic tract in the opposite half of the cord. The uncrossed sensory pathway on the other hand (postural, tactile, and vibratory sensibility), turns upwards in the posterior columns of the side of entry and thus escapes interruption. In this way the characteristic "dissociated" sensory loss of syringomyelia is produced.

equal in early cases. There may also be wasting of muscles in forearms, upper arms, and shoulder girdle muscles. In some cases the latter muscles are predominantly or exclusively affected, so that no wasting may be visible until the patient is turned round and his back and shoulders inspected. As a rule fibrillation is absent, or if present is minimal in degree and extent.

In cases of longer standing changes in the joints of the upper limbs, or in one of them, identical with those seen in the lower limbs of tabetics (Charcot joint) may be present. The affected joints are swollen by fluid effusion, are abnormally mobile, and may reveal gross crepitation on movement.

The skin of the hands is not normal in texture and appearance as it is in motor neurone disease, but is often cyanosed, and there is a soft, succulent thickening of the subcutaneous tissues which gives the hands a curious, soft and almost boneless quality when they are grasped. Healed and unhealed injuries may be seen on palm and fingers, and some of these may be chronically infected, swollen and granulating. In a few cases recurrent painless whitlows leading to loss of terminal phalanges may be seen.

Examination of sensation reveals the characteristic "dissociated sensory loss." Tactile and postural sensibility are everywhere normal, save perhaps in very long-standing cases where cutaneous sensibility to all forms is lost over the hand and fingers, but there is total loss of sensibility to pain or to temperature, or more commonly to both. The distribution of this selective loss varies from case to case, but usually the arms and forequarters are involved, on one or both sides, though not necessarily symmetrically. It is typical of this sensory loss that it has a lower as well as an upper level. It is what we may call a "suspended" sensory loss and rarely goes lower than the cutaneous areas of the fifth or sixth thoracic segmental levels (Fig. 50). In very long-standing cases it may, however, on one or both sides include all the body below the upper level. This upper level varies from the fourth cervical right up to the limits of the trigeminal nerve distribution, again not necessarily on both sides.

When there is also *syringobulbia* the selective sensory loss may include the fifth nerve area, and there may be unilateral wasting and fibrillation of the tongue, the signs of a sympathetic lesion (drooping lid and small pupil) and nystagmus.

The "suspended" character of the area of sensory loss depends for its production upon the site of interruption of the sensory pathway. It will be remembered that the fibres carrying impulses underlying sensations of pain and temperature end in the posterior horns of grey matter on the side of entry, the pathway being taken up by a second relay of fibres which cross the midline in the region of the grey commissure to turn upwards in the lateral column as the spinothalamic or crossed sensory tract. At their place of crossing

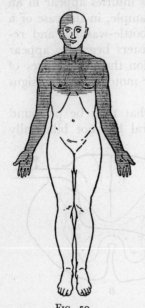

Fig. 50.

Diagram showing the "suspended" Distribution of Sensory Loss in Syringomyelia.

A characteristic distribution of dissociated sensory loss of pin-prick and to thermal stimuli in a case of syringomyelia. On the right side there is total loss to these modes of sensibility over the periphery of the fifth nerve distribution (lesion involving lower part of sensory root of the fifth nerve in the cervical region), and over all the cervical and the upper six thoracic spinal segments. On the left side the sensory root of the fifth nerve has escaped. This diagram illustrates what is called in the text the "suspended" character of the sensory loss.

lies the gliosis and cavitation which form the essential lesion and here the fibres are destroyed. This interruption occurs over a variable number of cervical and thoracic segments, and it is in the cutaneous distribution of these segments that we find loss of painful and thermal sensibility.

The distribution of the muscular atrophy also depends upon compression and destruction of ventral horn cells by the lesion in certain—usually lower cervical—segments, while the later development of spastic weakness of the legs with the appropriate changes in tone and reflexes depends upon compression and sclerosis of the descending pyramidal tracts as they pass through the segments where the lesion is most developed.

Rarely the lesion is prominent in the lumbar enlargement, and in this case we find wasting of the muscles of the legs, with deformities and trophic lesions of the feet and the characteristic sensory loss.

In the matter of skeletal deformities, a marked degree of thoracic kyphoscoliosis and some asymmetry of the skull are the usual findings, and may date from childhood.

Prognosis.—Syringomyelia is a slowly progressive malady, not necessarily shortening life, but ultimately rendering the arms and hands useless, leading to changes in the joints of the upper limb and to some disability of the legs.

Treatment.—Formerly the surgical incision of the cord at the level of maximal involvement (as indicated by the physical signs) and in the midline posteriorly was performed. The serous fluid with which the cavity is filled, and sometimes distended, was thus evacuated, but the cervical region of the cord is a hazardous one to interfere with and the results did not justify the hazard. It is now the custom to give deep X-ray therapy to the cervical region of the cord with a view to the destruction, or shrinkage, of the glial proliferation. It is held that even if this procedure does not lessen the disability it may arrest the downward progress of the malady. Striking claims have been made for this treatment, but no consistent benefit follows it. Treatment is, therefore, mainly symptomatic and palliative and consists in the protection of the hands from injury and the care of injuries when these are sustained. The malady is almost invariably painless.

Q

CHAPTER XVII

Myasthenia Gravis

ALTHOUGH as a muscular affection myasthenia gravis might suitably be considered among the primary muscular diseases, yet wasting is not one of its features and its pathogenesis is peculiar to it. It is, therefore, best treated separately.

Ætiology.—This is unknown, but it has been found that the essential abnormality is a failure of normal conduction of the motor nerve impulse at the neuromuscular junction. The arrival of nerve impulses at this junction normally leads to the liberation there of acetyl-choline which renders the muscle fibres sensitive to the impulse. If this substance be not liberated or if it be prematurely destroyed by the enzyme choline-sterase, contraction does not follow. One or other of these abnormalities is present in myasthenia gravis, and can be temporarily overcome by the injection of physostigmine (or of the synthetic product prostigmin), so that normal contractions follow until the effect of the drug wears off. The malady is more common in women than in men, usually makes its appearance in adolescence or early adult life, and is comparatively rarely found to develop in middle-aged or elderly persons. When it does so, however, it is apt to run a more chronic and benign course than in young persons.

Pathology.—A large persistent thymus gland has been found in very many cases, but whether this is constantly present cannot be certainly stated at present.

Symptoms.—The characteristic symptoms is the extremely rapid development of fatigue and weakness in skeletal muscles when these are in action. The distribution of this disorder of function varies from case to case, and in a given patient from time to time. It may be confined to the muscles moving the eyes, or to muscles supplied by cranial motor nerves, or it may involve almost the entire musculature. Its symptoms are, therefore, transient squint with diplopia and ptosis, facial weakness, weakness of the muscles of articulation, mastication, and deglutition. These symptoms are usually minimal when the patient awakes in the morning and increase during the day. On talking the voice becomes progressively weaker, on chewing the masseters weaken and the jaw drops and may have to be propped up by the patient's hand, on drinking the soft palate weakens and regurgitation of fluid through the nose occurs. Ptosis may increase progressively so that as the day goes on the patient has to tilt his head ever more backwards to see through the narrowing palpebral fissures. The limbs weaken similarly, and when the limb musculature begins to be involved in a case in which only muscles supplied by cranial nerves have hitherto been affected, it is the deltoids which commonly show the first signs of involvement. In severe cases the patient may be bedridden and helpless, and accesses of weakness in the respiratory muscles may imperil his life or end it.

The condition fluctuates widely and spontaneous and permanent recovery is known to occur. Relapses are more common. The tendon jerks remain normal, there is no sensory loss and no impairment of pupillary or of sphincter function. In exceptional cases there may be some muscular wasting with a degree of permanent residual weakness. In elderly patients the weakness may remain restricted to ocular and facial muscles throughout, the trunk and limb muscles retaining normal power. In pregnant subjects the symptoms usually abate, especially during the last three months, and confinement is normal and uncomplicated by myasthenia.

Diagnosis.—The temporal variation in the symptoms and the absence of signs clearly indicative of a lesion of the nervous system, and the dramatic response to injections of physostigmine provide conclusive diagnostic criteria.

Prognosis.—In the individual case this is unpredictable. Complete remissions of many years duration are known to occur, while, on the other hand, a rapidly fatal issue may ensue. These statements are more generally true for young than for elderly subjects, because the chronic case with weakness restricted to relatively few muscles, and these supplied by cranial nerves, is more often seen in an old than a young person.

Treatment.—Prostigmin is the drug of choice, and the technique of its administration has, with experience, become more effective. For most cases the oral administration of pills of prostigmin bromide (15 mgms.) is the method of choice, and the total daily dosage and distribution of doses will depend upon circumstances. Many patients can lead an ambulatory and restricted existence on from 8 to 15 of these pills daily, but it appears that larger doses can be safely used (up to 20 or 25 pills daily). For sudden symptoms of respiratory distress the intramuscular injection may be necessary, and 0·5 mgm. of prostigmin methylsulphate (1 in 2000 soln.) is used for this purpose.

A sheltered existence is obviously necessary for these patients, except during complete remissions.

Good results have recently been claimed to follow the removal of a persistent thymus, but it is not certain that they are always permanent. The operation is one to be especially considered in acute, recent cases in young persons.

CHAPTER XVIII

Multiple Peripheral Neuritis (Polyneuritis)

GENERAL CONSIDERATIONS

UNDER these titles we refer to a bilaterally symmetrical affection of the peripheral nerve trunks to the limbs, involving both motor and sensory fibres. In some instances certain cranial nerves may be affected, and the occasional presence of symptoms of mental disorder indicates that the central nervous system is not immune from the effects of the causative agent.

Pathologically, the striking lesion in long-standing cases that have proved fatal is a parenchymatous degeneration of the long peripheral nerves, affecting most severely the distal portions of the nerves. The heart muscle is also affected.

Ætiology.—Multiple neuritis displays a quite remarkable clinical and pathological uniformity despite the diversity of the poisons apparently able to give rise to it. These poisons range from such an elementary substance as arsenic, through ethyl alcohol to the exotoxins of diphtheria. In these circumstances the question naturally arises as to whether these substances do in fact act *directly* upon the nervous system to produce a single mode of reaction, or whether they may not do so *indirectly* and in virtue of a common disorder of metabolism produced by them, a disorder in the course of which a single toxic metabolite is produced in the body to become in turn the direct neural and myocardial poison. It would be premature to suppose that such an hypothesis necessarily covers every ætiological form of multiple neuritis, yet the clinical and experimental evidence derived from the study of beri-beri, itself a typical form of multiple neuritis, points in this direction.

Beri-beri is probably induced by a toxic product formed in the course of the disordered carbohydrate metabolism that ensues when carbohydrates are taken in large quantities without the vitamin normally found with them in nature, and it is not as biochemists formerly insisted, a simple vitamin starvation-degeneration of the nerves, though vitamin deficiency is a necessary factor in its production. Some as yet uncertainly known component of the vitamin B complex is essential to the carbohydrate metabolism of the nerve cell. In its absence this process is arrested at the stage of pyruvic acid formation, and this substance may accumulate in the cell. Whether it is toxic or not is not known. Yet the essential disturbance of function and the seat of the operative lesion in poly-

244

neuritis is in peripheral nerves, and not in nerve cells. Therefore, there are yet important gaps in the chain of evidence linking B avitaminosis with the development of polyneuritis.

It is thought possible that chronic alcoholism, the cachexia of malignant disease and of chronic tuberculosis may lead to defective absorption of the relevant vitamins, and thus indirectly and by the chain of events already sketched to multiple neuritis.

There are, however, cases of multiple neuritis, some of them severe and even fatal, which in the present state of knowledge cannot easily be harmonized with this hypothesis. Such are acute febrile polyneuritis, and also those cases of rapidly developing multiple neuritis that occur in persons apparently healthy, adequately nourished, and free from all discoverable infections. In such cases it is at present difficult to conceive of an avitaminosis as a factor.

In short, the problems of multiple neuritis are still far from complete solution; the categories of "infective" and "toxic" polyneuritis express this incomplete state of our knowledge, and it is impossible to assign a cause to a considerable proportion of cases.

Pathology.—It is not surprising that in long-standing cases that come to autopsy there should be found visible pathological changes in the peripheral nerves, yet it is certain that disorders of function must precede structural changes capable of microscopic detection. Only thus can we account for the complete or relative absence of visible changes in the nervous system in certain rapidly fatal cases of multiple neuritis (beri-beri, Landry's paralysis), and for the quick recovery in some profoundly paralysed cases. In short, symptoms cannot be closely correlated with microscopically visible changes. In long-standing fatal cases of multiple neuritis degenerative changes of Wallerian type are found in the axis cylinders of the affected nerves, together with some proliferation of the nuclei of the neurilemmal sheath. The nerve cells and fibres of the cerebral cortex may also show a degree of degenerative change, which may perhaps be correlated with the mental symptoms so frequently found in these cases. The heart shows fatty infiltration and myocardial degeneration. In the rapidly fatal cases there may be found acute dilatation of the heart.

Symptoms.—The various ætiological forms of multiple neuritis do not differ essentially in their symptoms or behaviour, but only in rapidity of onset, of development, and of recovery. In some there are special symptoms peculiar to the ætiological variety in question, as, for example, the palatal and accommodation palsies of diphtheritic neuritis, the hyperkeratosis and desquamation of arsenical neuritis, or the œdema of beri-beri. But these specific symptoms are no part of the multiple neuritis, which throughout the entire range of ætiological varieties has a remarkable uniformity.

The essential clinical features of polyneuritis are:

(1) A paralysis of lower motor neurone type with maximal, and sometimes sole, incidence on the limb musculature. The lower limbs are affected earlier and more severely than the upper, and the distal muscles of both more severely than the proximal. There is foot-drop and in severe cases wrist-drop. The muscles are tender to pressure, and the seat of cramps and sometimes of spontaneous pain. In long-standing cases wasting ensues, with the ultimate formation of contractures and deformities when adequate treatment is lacking.

(2) A diminution and later loss of tendon jerks in this sequence, ankle, knee and arm jerks.

(3) An impairment of sensation, varying in depth from case to case, involving all forms of sensibility, and, like the paralysis, maximal over the extremities and diminishing as the base of the limbs is reached. The trunk is rarely involved.

(4) Tachycardia during the active stage of the illness, and in the most severe cases, cardiac dilatation and even fatal syncope. These symptoms are due to direct involvement of the myocardium and are not to be explained, as was formerly done, on the basis of vagus neuritis.

The different ætiological varieties show variations in the relative severity of these symptoms. In the most acute forms, sensory loss is minimal, but the paralysis may spread to involve the trunk musculature and even the facial muscles, and transient sphincter disturbance (retention or incontinence) may develop at the climax of the illness.

It may conduce to brevity if we take three main types as illustrative of polyneuritis: what we may call a fulminating type as seen in the so-called Landry's paralysis and acute febrile ("infective") polyneuritis, the subacute early recovering type seen in diphtheria, and the chronic type as exemplified by alcoholic neuritis.

LANDRY'S PARALYSIS AND ACUTE FEBRILE POLYNEURITIS

It is highly probable that there is no essential distinction between the forms of polyneuritis known by these titles, yet it has to be stated that the term "Landry's paralysis" has in practice become a cover for various forms of acute spreading paralysis, as for example certain cases of ascending poliomyelitis. But since by definition Landry's paralysis is a form of rapidly spreading and often fatal paralysis characterized by the absence of severe or constant changes in the nervous system, so far as these are capable of demonstration by present microscopic methods, poliomyelitis cannot be brought under this heading. The mild and inconstant chromatolytic nerve cell changes reported in fatal cases of Landry's paralysis are, in fact, no more extensive or severe than may be found in any fatal febrile illness and they can scarcely be correlated with the symptoms. In short, it is probable that death has ensued before microscopically visible lesions have had time to develop, a point to which reference has already been made.

In certain acute and severe cases of polyneuritis the cerebrospinal fluid may contain an excess of protein, leading in rare cases to clot formation. Such fluids may be yellow or brownish in colour. Excess of cells is extremely rare. Indeed, in most cases of the malady the fluid is normal.

A brief period of febrile disturbance with headache and malaise, sleeplessness, and gastro-intestinal disorder may precede the appearance of the paralysis, which is of lower motor neurone type, flaccid, with loss of tendon jerks, and develops very rapidly. Commonly the distal parts of the legs are first involved, paræsthesiæ in toes and feet accompanying the development of paralysis, which spreads up the limbs, appears in the arms, may invade the abdominal and back muscles and then the facial muscles. The muscles of respiration do not escape in this rapid ascent, but they are in many cases less severely weakened than the limb and facial muscles, save in those fatal cases where paralysis and asphyxia close the sequence of events. Thus, as also in what is called acute febrile polyneuritis, we may see profound weakness of all four limbs, of the lower abdominal muscles and facial muscles, while the intercostals and other respiratory muscles still maintain an adequate level of activity. Sensory loss is not severe, but in character corresponds to what is seen in other forms of polyneuritis: numbness and tingling in the extremities with some blunting of all forms of sensation in them. Transient retention of urine or incontinence may occur, but quickly passes in surviving cases. The pulse rate may rise to 100 or even 120. Having rapidly reached its maximum, if the patient does not die, the paralysis begins within a few hours or two or three days to diminish, clearing first in the muscles least severely weakened. The recovery process continues rapidly, and only general debility and exhaustion may remain after two or three weeks, though the tendon jerks may take a longer period to reappear. In other words, the pathogenic agent, which must be a poison of some kind, is eliminated or ceases to act before irreversible changes have occurred in the neurones involved.

It is difficult to give a separate description of what has been called acute febrile polyneuritis, for it differs in no essential from what has just been described. Probably the absence of striking ascent of paralysis and a less acute onset are the sole basis of differentiation. It has been said that in acute febrile polyneuritis the muscular paralysis in the limbs is more severe in the proximal than in the distal muscles, but this is not constantly the case, and no clear distinction between Landry's paralysis and acute febrile polyneuritis can be made on grounds so vague. A true lobar pneumonia may complicate the acute stage of the latter, and this together with the febrile prodromata of the illness make it difficult to escape the conclusion that some organismal toxin plays an essential role in causation. A rare accompaniment of these acute cases of polyneuritis is a mild papillœdema, which subsides without producing any measure of optic atrophy or impairment of vision. Only by procrustean exertions can avitaminosis be fitted into the clinical pictures we are considering, and we should for the present be on guard against an artificial simplification of the obscure problems of polyneuritis on these lines, though it remains likely that the further investigations of the mode of action of this factor in producing polyneuritis, which it admittedly may do, will illuminate the general problem of these varying types of polyneuritis.

DIPHTHERITIC PARALYSIS

Involvement of the nervous system may complicate clinically mild infections by the organism of diphtheria as well as severe ones, the former especially if the case be undiagnosed and the patient either remain ambulant or resume physical activity prematurely.

Since diphtheria is mainly a disease of infants, it accounts for the majority of cases of multiple neuritis in this age period.

There are two components in the fully developed clinical picture of diphtheritic paralysis that are not part of the later developing multiple neuritis, but their presence is of value in confirming the diphtheritic origin of the latter. These are the palatal and accommodation paralysis of faucial diphtheria, which commonly make their appearance in the second week of the illness, occasionally even before the membrane in the throat has cleared. The child develops a weak nasal voice, tends to be almost or quite silent when weeping, and regurgitates fluid through the nose. At this stage the sternomastoid muscles may also be extremely weak so that when the nurse's hand is placed behind the child's neck to lift it for feeding purposes, the head flops feebly backwards. Paralysis of accommodation may easily escape notice in an infant, but in adults who are not very ill the blurring of near vision is complained of. When the diphtheritic lesion is unilateral in the fauces, it is noteworthy that the palatal palsy is also unilateral and confined to the side of the infection— a point of interest that will be referred to later.

These symptoms persist for from about ten to twenty days when they quickly clear up. At or about this time a multiple neuritis begins to make its appearance. If the patient be still confined to bed and the nervous system be examined periodically, it may be found that as muscular tenderness develops in the calves the knee and ankle jerks undergo a transient exaggeration which soon gives place to diminution and then to loss, the ankle jerks being the first to go. As this happens, the other symptoms of multiple neuritis make their appearance, tingling and numbness of the extremities with weakness and sensory loss. In the initial illness the heart may have shown signs of involvement, tachycardia, and perhaps some irregularity. The pulse remains rapid—80 to 100 per minute—until the neuritis ceases to progress and begins to clear. The evolution of diphtheritic neuritis is more rapid than that of alcoholic neuritis, it is less apt to be profound and begins under favourable conditions of treatment to clear more quickly without the supervention of wasting or contracture. Even in the mildest cases, however, six months usually pass before normal strength is restored.

In many cases the initial palatal and convergence palsies occur without the addition of a multiple neuritis.

It was just mentioned that a unilateral palatal palsy might be encountered when the faucial lesion was unilateral, a fact suggesting that the toxins may gain access to the nervous system locally from the focus of infection by an ascending neural or perineural lymphatic route. During the war of 1914–1918 the writer observed a large outbreak of cases of cutaneous and wound diphtheria followed by nervous symptoms. In these cases palatal palsy was absent, the initial paralysis being anatomically related to the seat of infection. Thus, a diphtheritic infection of a wound on the hand was followed by an initial weakness of the hand, multiple neuritis ensuing later. Accommodation paralysis was commonly observed in these cases.

It appears, therefore, that the toxins produced in the site of infection ascend along neural channels to the nervous system where they act upon the nervous system locally, giving rise to the initial *local* palsy. In faucial diphtheria this is palatal, in cutaneous diphtheria it is related to the site of infection. Accommodation palsy may occur wherever the local lesion may be, and so also a multiple neuritis may follow. The analogy with tetanus springs to the mind, where there is a local tetanus anatomically related to the site of infection, a specific localization—the trismus—followed by a generalized tetanus. Therefore, in diphtheria it appears that the toxin first gains a local access to the nervous system by the nerves innervating the site of infection, and later by the blood-stream becomes systematized so that—possibly in the way indicated in the introductory remarks—a multiple neuritis may ultimately be produced.

ALCOHOLIC NEURITIS

Usually the onset is insidious, and for weeks or even months before any real disability develops, the patient has been aware of cramps in the calf and plantar muscles at night, of aching in these muscles during use, of ready fatigue of the legs on exertion, and of tingling and numbness in the feet and toes. The upper limbs tend to escape in the initial stages of the illness. These symptoms may persist with little change and may or may not be associated with other indications of chronic alcoholism: looseness of the bowels, morning sickness or nausea, loss of appetite especially for breakfast, some tremor of the hands, and rapidity of the pulse. There may be an enlarged and tender liver. Gradually the legs weaken, subjective sensory symptoms become more prominent. Added to all this there is in some cases an altered mental state that passes by the name of the *polyneuritic psychosis*. The memory is so bad that the names even of familiar objects are forgotten, there may be disorientation as to place and time, and—most typical when present—the patient indulges freely in fictitious reminiscences, describing in detail a daily round of activities that have had no existence and that his disabled condition renders impossible.

If the malady progresses, severe paralysis with wasting and contractures may ensue.

Examination in the initial stage, while the subject is still ambulant and perhaps even engaged in some measure of normal activity, will reveal marked tenderness to pressure of the plantar and calf muscles, the knee jerks may still be present but in all probability the ankle jerks are absent. There is some cutaneous hyperæsthesia over feet and toes, and perhaps a moderate degree of sensory impairment of the same distribution, pain, touch, temperature, vibration, and postural modes of sensibility being all affected.

In later stages there is great loss of power in the limbs, maximal in their distal segments, so that there is foot-drop—with a high-stepping gait when the patient is still ambulant—and less often wrist-drop. Ultimately paralysis may render the patient bedridden. As paralysis progresses the affected muscles waste, and throughout the course of the illness and until recovery is well under way the muscles are spontaneously painful and extremely tender to pressure.

Sensory loss spreads up the limbs in the manner already described. All forms are equally affected, and from the fact that postural sensibility is impaired the ambulant patient is apt to be ataxic and shows Rombergism.

The sphincters are unaffected. In the realm of the cranial nerves the facial nerves are sometimes severely paralysed, the others usually remaining intact.

In severe and inadequately treated cases the wasted and paralysed muscles shorten and contractures and deformities develop. The cutaneous hyperæsthesia so commonly found over the legs below the knees may make the contact of bed-clothes and all handling of the limbs very painful and difficult.

Once the taking of alcohol is controlled and adequate nourishment and complete rest are begun, the downward progress of the illness is checked, and after an interval which varies according to the severity of the condition, recovery slowly begins and progresses to completion unless intractable contractures have been allowed to occur. This process of recovery is a matter of months rather than of weeks. When severe mental symptoms have developed their recovery may lag behind that of the multiple neuritis and in chronic alcoholics some measure of dementia may persist.

A separate account of *arsenical neuritis*, now an extremely rare condition, is unnecessary since it very closely resembles alcoholic neuritis even in the occasional presence of the polyneuritic psychosis. One or more attacks of severe gastro-intestinal irritation will indicate the ingestion of arsenic when large doses have been taken, and these precede the onset of neuritis by a short period of two or more weeks. A possible link between polyneuritis manifestly due to vitamin B deficiency and arsenical neuritis is provided by the recent observation that in arsenical poisoning there is a disturbance of the pyruvate mechanism already mentioned.

OTHER ÆTIOLOGICAL VARIETIES OF MULTIPLE NEURITIS

It is said that certain infections may be followed by a multiple neuritis—*e.g.* typhoid, influenza, malaria, tuberculosis, streptococcal infection—and while this may occasionally be so, it is certainly rare.

Diabetic neuritis is often clinically latent—that is to say, the patient may make no complaints, but examination reveals tenderness of calf and plantar muscles and absence of the ankle jerks. In more severe cases pains in the legs reminiscent of the lightning pains of tabes may be complained of, the knee jerks may also be lost, and the degree of postural sensory loss may produce an ataxic gait and lead to an erroneous diagnosis of tabes dorsalis.

In children there is occasionally observed a form of multiple neuritis known as "*Pink Disease*," in which in addition to the nervous symptoms there is a dusky, reddish swelling of the extremities. In *beri-beri* we are dealing with a multiple neuritis clinically undistinguishable from any other variety of this condition, but often accompanied by a high degree of œdema of the lower limbs and scrotum and by the presence of free fluid in the abdomen. In infantile and in acute beri-beri of adults cardiac symptoms may dominate the clinical picture and may even prove rapidly fatal before neuritis has had time to develop.

Occasionally polyneuritis may occur during pregnancy, either following severe hyperemesis gravidarum with emaciation, or without this complication and during the fifth and sixth months. Not unnaturally deficiency of vitamin B has been invoked as underlying the polyneuritis in the first-named circumstances. The requirement of this vitamin is said to be trebled during pregnancy, and, therefore, although the precise role played by avitaminosis in the polyneuritis remains uncertain, treatment may well take account of this factor. Possibly allied to the polyneuritis of pregnancy and hyperemesis, and to beri-beri in their mechanism of causation are the relatively uncommon cases of polyneuritis that may accompany the malnutrition of gastric carcinoma or ulcer.

Treatment.—In any case recognized as polyneuritis the first essential is complete rest in bed, and the patient should not be mobilized until the pulse rate, which is typically raised while the malady is advancing, has fallen to normal. The liability of cases of diphtheritic neuritis, acute febrile polyneuritis and beri-beri to sudden fatal heart failure is well known, and when death ensues in polyneuritis it is frequently cardiac in origin, though it may, of course, be due to paralysis of the respiratory muscles. In severe cases of febrile polyneuritis grave cardiac dilatation and increasing rapidity and weakness of the pulse may develop rapidly, while ascending and deepening paralysis may involve respiratory muscles. Measures to meet these dangers should be thought out beforehand, so that cardiac stimulants, or a respirator, are at hand when wanted, and the employment of the latter understood by those in charge of the patient. In any case of polyneuritis with increasing paralysis and a pulse rate of 100 or over the patient should be kept completely supine and should not be allowed to sit up for any purpose or should not be raised into a sitting position for nursing purposes. As a cardiac stimulant the following is useful: Atropine sulphate gr. $\frac{1}{200}$, Strychnine sulphate gr. $\frac{1}{100}$, Adrenaline solution 1 in 1000, ℳ5. This is made up to ℳ10 in sterile water, and an injection given four hourly, or as indicated. Fortunately most cases of polyneuritis are not so grave as the preceding lines indicate, but not a few of the exceptionally grave cases are lost through lack of appreciation of their seriousness and of forethought in preparation for a crisis. In particular, nurses in charge of an acute and severe case of polyneuritis should be given explicit instructions for its care.

Even in mild cases of polyneuritis, rest is of paramount importance, and not a few cases of diphtheritic paralysis of apparently slight severity become more severe and long lasting than would otherwise be the case, if the convalescent case of diphtheria is mobilized too soon.

If the limbs be severely paralysed it is necessary to keep them in the position of physiological rest—the legs extended and adducted and the feet at right angles to the leg. A cradle should keep the weight of bedclothes off the limbs. In many cases the muscles are too tender to allow of massage or other local treatment, and gentle passive movements from time to time are all that is necessary.

Active exercises in bed and massage should be reserved for the period of recovery. It has long been the custom to treat polyneuritis by a daily hypodermic injection of strychnine nitrate (gr. $\frac{1}{30}$ daily), or by ♏5 doses of liquor strychnine twice or thrice daily, and in the absence of any more certainly effective remedy this may usefully be employed.

The value of vitamin Bi in polyneuritis has been the subject of immoderate and ill-substantiated claims, and there is now increasing evidence that this component of the B complex may not be related to the nervous system, though it may be to the myocardium. The present writer has found the Bi component (aneurine) wholly inert in poly-neuritis, and he is not alone in this experience. Human illness lacks some of the simplicities of experimental physiology, and the remarkably rapid cures achieved in the so-called polyneuritis of birds have no counterpart in clinical medicine. In chronic cases degenerative changes in peripheral nerves have ensued and take months to recover, but even in acute cases of the "infective" type there is as yet no substantial evidence of a rate of recovery on vitamin therapy greater than that observed in the period prior to the introduction of vitamins. As has been indicated, the role of deficiency is clearest in the case of beri-beri, of alcoholic polyneuritis, and in the polyneuritis of gastric disease and of hyperemesis, and it is, therefore, in these forms of the malady that the use of the entire B complex (in the form of yeast) is most reasonable. When there is marked tachycardia synthetic vitamin B_1 may be given, either by the daily intramuscular injection of 20 to 50 mgms., or by mouth in larger dosage. This should be supplemented by a daily dose of $\frac{1}{2}$ oz. of baker's yeast.

The value of a respirator (box, or Bragg-Paul type) in a case of rapid ascending paralysis is clear, and the prospect of a useful recovery after the patient has been tidied over the crisis is, of course, much greater than in the case of poliomyelitis. Finally, whatever form of medication be adopted, rest in bed until improvement sets in and the pulse rate is normal remains an absolute necessity of treatment. This and a generous diet are the two pillars of treatment and will give good results.

CHAPTER XIX

Lead Poisoning of the Nervous System

LEAD PALSY AND LEAD ENCEPHALOPATHY

LEAD poisoning is an intoxication of the nervous system commonly grouped with polyneuritis, as also are other metallic poisonings of the nervous system, yet both pathologically and clinically they all differ essentially from polyneuritis. Lead exerts its action upon the nerve cells of the brain and spinal cord, upon peripheral motor nerves and upon muscles. This is true also of other and less commonly encountered intoxications of the nervous system, such as carbon monoxide poisoning, carbon disulphide poisoning, etc. Of this group, lead poisoning is perhaps the most frequently met with, and it alone will be described here.

Of the two forms of lead poisoning or "plumbism" in so far as they involve the nervous system, the so-called lead palsy which paralyses certain extensor muscles in the forearm is the most familiar, but a cerebral type, more common perhaps in children than in adults, is also known. In respect of both forms it may be said that they are preceded by visceral symptoms of plumbism—constipation, abdominal pain (lead colic) and anorexia—and in any declared case of lead palsy, or encephalopathy, examination of the blood will reveal characteristic changes (some anæmia, poikilocytosis, punctate basophilia, etc.). The gums may show a "lead line." It follows, therefore, that a complete medical examination, clinical and pathological, is necessary in any case of suspected plumbism involving the nervous system. This is the more important in lead encephalopathy, which, as we have seen, may present features suggestive of intracranial tumour, or of hypertensive encephalopathy.

Ætiology.—Lead poisoning may be industrial or may ensue upon the use of certain lead salts as abortifacients. In the case of children the sucking of lead soldiers, of painted toys, or of other painted objects has been known to induce lead encephalopathy.

Pathology.—In lead encephalopathy the brain is œdematous, and all the elements in the brain are affected, nerve and glia cells alike. In peripheral lead palsy there are degenerative changes in the ventral horn cells and in the peripheral nerve fibres, and also degenerative and necrotic changes in the affected muscles. In children there is a deposit of lead salts beneath the epiphyseal cartilages where its presence is seen in the radiogram as a dark band.

Symptoms.—LEAD ENCEPHALOPATHY.—Prior to the development of cerebral symptoms there is usually a history of impaired health of some weeks' or months' duration, the symptoms being abdominal pain, sickness, loss of appetite, headache, and sometimes increasing pallor. The headache then suddenly becomes intensified, the patient becomes drowsy, vomits frequently and may have generalized epileptiform convulsions, diplopia, and progressive dimness of vision. A state of coma may ensue. Examination reveals intense papillœdema, often indistinguishable from that of intracranial tumour, various ocular palsies in some cases, inconstant changes in the reflexes or even signs of hemiparesis. The blood pressure may be raised or normal, while the pulse rate is usually rapid. Examination will also reveal the other indications of plumbism already enumerated. A blue line on the gums may or may not be present, and lead may be detected in the urine in abnormal amounts. The excretion of lead in the urine continues for some months after the ingestion of lead has ceased.

LEAD PALSY.—This also is preceded by symptoms of chronic plumbism. Wrist-drop is the characteristic symptom, almost always bilateral but not necessarily simultaneous in onset on the two sides, nor of equal severity. There are neither pain nor paræsthesiæ. Examination reveals paralysis of the extensors of the fingers, of the thumb excepting extensor ossis metacarpi pollicis which may escape, and of the wrist extensors. Supinator longus (brachio-radialis) typically escapes. In some severe cases a progressive wasting of the small hand muscles ensues, while in a few instances there may be a rapidly developing weakness and wasting of the muscles of the upper arm as well, so that the entire upper limb becomes wasted and flaccid with an appearance reminiscent of progressive muscular atrophy. Some sufferers from less severe grades of plumbism do not develop either of these characteristic states, but complain of cramps and shooting pains in the limbs.

Diagnosis.—The differential diagnosis of lead encephalopathy has already been discussed on pages 91 and 97. Lead palsy may be distinguished from musculo-spiral paralysis by the integrity in the former of supinator longus (brachio-radialis) and of the two extensors of the thumb mentioned in the preceding paragraph. In hysterical wrist-drop flexion movements at the wrist and digits are also very weak if not lost.

Prognosis.—As has been stated, death may ensue in lead encephalopathy, or survival with a greater or less degree of mental deterioration, defect of vision, and residual paralysis and recurrent convulsions. Complete recovery is rare. In lead palsy, recovery is the rule, save that when the small hand muscles waste or the upper arms become involved considerable weakness and wasting are apt to remain.

Treatment.—In plumbism the lead is widely distributed in the body in a fixed form. Its mobilization and elimination are facilitated by the

administration of ammonium chloride, parathormone, and saline
aperients (sodium and magnesium sulphate). Potassium iodide in doses
of not more than 20 grains daily is also used. When the patient is
severely ill, as in encephalopathy, and the excretion of lead by the urine
is high, the mobilization of lead is not without danger of producing an
acute exacerbation of poisoning. In these circumstances, potassium
iodide and saline aperients are all that should be given. In the case of
peripheral lead palsy the relaxation of the extensors by splinting the
hand in the position midway between flexion and extension at the wrist,
and massage, are indicated.

CHAPTER XX

Common Affections of the Cranial Nerves

THE OLFACTORY NERVE

SYMPTOMS referable to this nerve are rarely of clinical importance, but the following considerations may be stated. The olfactory sense includes the appreciation of flavours as well as of odours. When it is lost the subject retains only gustatory sensibility to sweet, sour, bitter and salt tastes, the savour of his tobacco and of much of his food is lost to him and, therefore, he commonly complains of a loss of taste as well as of smell. Bilateral loss of the sense of smell (anosmia) may be caused in cases of head injury by tearing of the fine olfactory filaments as they pierce the ethmoid plate, while in cases of tumour beneath the frontal pole compression of one olfactory tract or bulb may lead to unilateral anosmia, which is usually associated with primary optic atrophy on the same side, the optic nerve being simultaneously compressed.

THE OPTIC NERVE

The anatomy of the visual pathway and the symptoms referable to interruptions of it at its different parts have already been considered (pages 41-45). The condition of œdema of the optic nerve head, papillœdema, has also been described (page 67).

PRIMARY OPTIC ATROPHY.—The optic nerve may be compressed or severed by fractures which pass through the orbit, or compressed by new growths within the orbit or cranial cavity. It is also subject to degenerative changes, as in tabes dorsalis and dementia paralytica. In all these circumstances what is called primary optic atrophy occurs. Vision fails progressively and blindness ensues. Ophthalmoscopic examination of the atrophic disc shows it to be dead white, with clear-cut edges and a very obvious lamina cribrosa. The retinal vessels remain essentially unchanged. With the onset of blindness the pupil becomes dilated and immobile. The atrophy following papillœdema, known as *post-papillitic or consecutive atrophy*, differs in appearance. The disc edges are fuzzy and indistinct, there is some disturbance of the retinal pigment immediately surrounding the disc, the physiological pit is filled with organized exudate, hiding the lamina cribrosa, and there may be strands of white exudate upon the vessels as they traverse the disc.

RETROBULBAR NEURITIS.—**Ætiology.**—Undoubtedly the commonest cause of acute retrobulbar neuritis is the development in the optic nerve of a focus of disseminated sclerosis. Local infection in the sinuses of the skull is only very exceptionally complicated by retrobulbar neuritis, though it is far too commonly invoked as a factor in the causation of the latter. In disseminated sclerosis both optic nerves may be affected, but never simultaneously, an interval of weeks, months, or even years separating the involvement of the two nerves. The so-called chronic retrobulbar neuritis is in reality a toxic affection of the ganglion cells of the retina caused by various poisons—*e.g.* quinine, methyl alcohol, tobacco ("tobacco amblyopia")—but the symptoms and ophthalmoscopic appearances do not differ from those of true retrobulbar neuritis.

Symptoms.—In acute retrobulbar neuritis vision rapidly becomes blurred in the affected eye. Central vision is not impaired. Blindness does not ensue, but vision may be reduced to perception of light and movement. At the onset there is usually pain on movement of the eye, and pain on pressure on the globe above the cornea. Examination reveals a central or paracentral scotoma for form and colours. Except in rare cases where the lesion is close behind the nerve head, when the optic disc may be swollen and œdematous, ophthalmoscopic examination reveals no abnormality. In the case of disseminated sclerosis visual acuity begins to return in two or three weeks and restoration to normal, or to an acuity almost normal, is the rule. Some weeks later the temporal half of the disc begins to develop some pallor, which persists as a permanent sign of a past retrobulbar neuritis.

In the rare disease known as *neuromyelitis optica*, a severe bilateral retrobulbar neuritis sometimes leading to permanent blindness and primary optic atrophy may be encountered, accompanied or followed by paraplegia (see page 187).

The unilateral development of a retrobulbar neuritis in a young adult is almost invariably a sign of disseminated sclerosis, of which it may be the first indication.

THE THIRD, FOURTH, AND SIXTH NERVES

General Symptoms of Ocular Palsies.—Weakness or paralysis of an external ocular muscle leads to limitation of the movement of the eye, squint and double vision. Two other anomalies follow upon these. They are secondary deviation of the sound eye and error of projection of the image, and are best illustrated by a concrete example. If the right external rectus muscle be paralysed, on conjugate deviation of the eyes to the right the right eye does not move out beyond the middle line. An increased effort is made and the ingoing left eye, therefore, moves too far into the internal canthus—*secondary deviation*. This increased effort corresponds to a greater deviation of the affected eye to the right than is actually taking place, and, therefore, the image is projected farther to the right than the object really is, and if the patient be asked to point to it with a finger he points too far to the right. This is known as *erroneous projection*.

These symptoms necessarily vary in form according to the muscle or muscles paralysed. The following details of these differences may be given in brief.

The third (oculomotor) nerve innervates all the external ocular muscles save the external rectus and superior oblique. It also supplies the levator palpebrae and the ciliary and sphincter muscles within the eye. When it is totally paralysed the upper lid falls (ptosis), the pupil is large and immobile, and the eye diverges (under the unopposed action of external rectus) to the outer canthus. All movement of the eye is lost save abduction and a small range of downward and inward movement. When the lid is lifted there is double vision in all directions save when the affected eye is turned outwards. The two images are crossed—that is, in a left third nerve palsy the false image lies to the right of the true image.

The fourth (trochlear) nerve innervates the superior oblique muscle. There are squint and diplopia only when the gaze is turned below the horizontal. In this case there is an uncrossed diplopia and an internal squint.

The sixth (abducens) nerve innervates the external rectus. When it is paralysed the eye converges and there is an uncrossed diplopia.

These three nerves may be affected singly or in association, an isolated lesion of the fourth being exceptional, and the paralysis may be partial or complete.

Ætiology of Isolated Ocular Palsies.—These may be caused by lesions at any point from the nuclei of origin of the nerves in the brain-stem to their peripheral distribution. These lesions may be purely local, affecting no other nervous mechanisms, they may be part of some general toxic or infective process of the entire nervous system, of a malady with multiple local lesions, or of a systemic degeneration.

The palsies which form part of widespread affections of the nervous system are described under the appropriate headings, and all we need consider here are isolated paralyses of ocular muscles.

ISOLATED OCULAR PALSIES have in the past been regarded as more commonly due to syphilitic meningitis than to any other cause, but it is very doubtful if this view is any longer justified. In elderly persons ocular paralysis involving one or more nerves may appear suddenly, persist for some weeks or months and then clear up. Nothing is certainly known of their ætiology, but it is thought that they may be due to the pressure exerted by an atheromatous internal carotid artery upon the nerves in the region of the cavernous sinus.

As has been described (page 112), an unruptured aneurysm of this artery may be an occasional cause of such local paralyses. In middle-aged and elderly persons a form of neuritis of these nerves may be encountered, involving sometimes a single nerve and sometimes all three in sequence, but on one side only. The onset is sudden with pain in the eye and within the distribution of the ophthalmic division of the trigeminal nerve. The pain may be severe, is aggravated by attempts to move the eye, and persists sometimes for two or three weeks. One nerve after another may be involved until a complete ophthalmoplegia, internal and external, is produced. This usually recovers gradually within a period of from three to six months. Nothing is known of its ætiology, but periostitis of the orbital fissure has been speculatively invoked as a cause. In acute mastoid disease in children, and when the tip of the petrous portion is inflamed, we may see the association of pain of fifth nerve distribution and a sixth nerve palsy.

In a few cases of myasthenia gravis the ocular muscles may alone be affected, at least over a period of time. In this case we see fluctuating squints, diplopia, and usually also ptosis. This chronic localized form of the malady is most often encountered in middle-aged or elderly subjects.

Finally, syphilitic meningitis may produce ocular palsies as its earliest or even its sole symptom.

Treatment.—The isolated ocular palsies of elderly subjects of atheroma require no special treatment save the wearing of an eye-shade to avert the discomforts of double vision, in which the symptom of giddiness may be included. The neuritis of the nerves described above may be so painful as to call for the confinement of the patient to bed and the use of analgesic drugs. The local application of heat may also be useful for relief of pain. In the absence of any known ætiology no specific medication is available, but potassium iodide is usually given.

THE FIFTH NERVE : TRIGEMINAL NEURALGIA

Local lesions involving this nerve rarely give rise to intense pain, and such pain as is present is usually associated with some impairment of sensation within the distribution of the nerve, to a subjective sensation of numbness and—if the ophthalmic division be involved—to diminution or loss of the corneal reflex.

TRIGEMINAL NEURALGIA is a malady of elderly persons and rarely makes its appearance before the age of fifty.

Ætiology.—Nothing whatever is known of this. It is not related to dental sepsis and may make its appearance many years after the patient has been rendered edentulous. On the other hand, the removal of teeth has no influence upon its course. It may occur as a rare complication in disseminated sclerosis.

Symptoms.—These consist essentially in severe paroxysmal pain within the distribution of one or more divisions of the nerve in the complete absence of any signs of impaired function of the nerve.

It is important from the point of view of treatment as of diagnosis to realize that this malady has a characteristic behaviour in time. The paroxysms of pain to be described make their appearance and for a space of time, weeks or months, are frequent and distressing. They then cease and a period of complete freedom from pain, lasting for months or for two or three years, may ensue. The paroxysms then reappear, last somewhat longer this time, only again to cease completely for a considerable time. This sequence of phases of activity and quiescence may continue for several years, but as time passes the pain becomes more intense, the paroxysms continuing for longer periods and the periods of freedom becoming shorter. Finally, a stage is reached when cessation no longer occurs and the patient suffers from paroxysms daily.

The pain makes its first appearance within the distribution of the third or second divisions of the nerve, but never in the first division which, however, is often involved subsequently. It is sudden and shooting in character, a rapid succession of "lightning stabs" of great intensity passing along the course of the affected branches. Each paroxysm consists of an irregular series of these stabs of pain and lasts for some seconds. While it persists the patient stops talking or moving, often presses the palm of the hand to the face, may flush, screw up the face or shed a few tears. The frequency of the paroxysms varies from case to case, and in the individual case from time to time. Pain is usually started by a stimulus of some kind, a puff of cold air, a touch or stroke upon the face, the movements of eating or talking. There are certain "trigger points" on the face from which by light pressure a paroxysm may be "fired off." In the case of the first division the supra-orbital notch, in the case of the second the spot where the nostril meets the cheek, and in that of the third division the mental foramen or the side of the tongue, constitute these points. In severe cases, mastication, opening the mouth, speaking, shaving, washing the affected side of the face are all intolerable, at least for days at a time. The affected half of the tongue may be coated. Between the paroxysms when they are frequent there may be a residual aching pain in the face. The patient often obtains relief from pain during the night.

Examination reveals normal motor and sensory function of the nerve.

Course.—The behaviour of the malady has already been sketched, but it remains to be said that in the very rare cases where it appears in young persons it may clear up permanently before reaching the intensity just described.

Diagnosis.—In practice this should not be difficult if a paroxysm is seen, for the patient's behaviour is quite characteristic. The distribution of pain, its qualities and the absence of any objective signs of involvement of the fifth nerve, or of other parts of the nervous system, all combine to give trigeminal neuralgia a distinct individuality.

Occasionally *frontal sinusitis* produces paroxysms of intense pain in the distribution of the supra-orbital nerve, but these are accompanied by local tenderness to pressure over the sinus, the paroxysms tend to recur at the same time each day, and the second and third divisions of the nerve are unaffected. Nevertheless, sometimes a diagnosis of supra-orbital neuralgia is erroneously made in these circumstances and the underlying sinus lesion overlooked. On the other hand, a complaint of "neuralgia" in the face may be one of the somatic symptoms of a psychoneurosis. In this case it is usually bilateral and does not conform in type, distribution, or in the nature of the precipitating factors to true trigeminal neuralgia, nor does it resemble the pain of local dental or sinus lesions.

The glossopharyngeal nerve is, in rare instances, the seat of a neuralgia comparable with that of the trigeminal nerve and sometimes confused with it. It differs in that the pain is felt deep in the ear and in the throat and that the paroxysms are induced by the movement of swallowing. The pain may be intense.

Treatment.—In the early stages of the malady what we are required to do is to afford relief for what is probably only a matter of weeks until the natural cessation of pain arrives. This can usually be achieved by medication, and the following prescription is useful: R Phenobarbitone sol. gr. $\frac{1}{2}$, Tinct. Gelsem. $\mathfrak{M}$ 15, Phenazone grs. 5, Sod. Bromide grs. 5, Aq. chlorof. ad $\frac{7}{2}$ 6-hourly. When the intensity of the paroxysms is not adequately relieved by such means, and when considerable periods of quiescence have ceased to occur, surgical measures arise for consideration. These consist in alcohol injection into the nerve and section of the sensory root of the Gasserian ganglion. The former when successfully accomplished gives relief for a period of from one to two years. It should be performed only by someone experienced in its use. Surgical division of the sensory root gives permanent relief from pain, but sometimes distressing paræsthesiæ persist, a keratitis may ensue—requiring stitching together of the lids for some months—and the result may thus be less than satisfactory. However, these complications occur only in a minority of cases.

THE FACIAL NERVE

The two common affections of this nerve are facial palsy and facia hemispasm.

FACIAL PALSY: BELL's PALSY.—This is an affection of adult life, and is comparatively rarely seen at an earlier period, apart, of course, from middle ear disease and involvement of the facial nerve in petrous caries.

Bell's palsy has been attributed to exposure to cold and to involvement of the facial nerve in cases of geniculate herpes. It certainly appears true that there is a periodicity in the appearance of fresh cases of Bell's palsy, namely, in the late autumn and early spring. This would suggest a common ætiology for all cases. However, as has been mentioned on page 157 not all cases of facial palsy associated with herpes of the external auditory meatus are accompanied by geniculate herpes, though the available pathological evidence does not exclude the possibility that some such cases may be so associated. The ætiology of Bell's palsy, therefore, remains uncertain, but it is probable that in all cases we are dealing with a neuritis of the facial nerve in its intratemporal course.

Symptoms.—The onset of facial paralysis is usually, though not invariably, preceded by pain below and behind the ear and sometimes by tenderness of the sternomastoid muscle at its point of insertion. Occasionally a large and tender gland may be palpable in the angle between jaw and mastoid. The paralysis is usually sudden in onset and complete at once, but a few cases are seen in which total palsy is not present for from twenty-four to thirty-six hours.

All the muscles of the affected half of the face with the platysma are flaccid and toneless. The face is manifestly asymmetrical even when at rest and the affected half seems to sag. Tears trickle over the margin of the lower eyelid and saliva from the angle of the mouth.

When the patient attempts to close his eye the upper lid descends somewhat owing to reciprocal inhibition of levator palpebrae superioris and the eye rolls up. This upward movement of the eye exceeds the normal upward movement of the eye on the opposite side, and is an over-action strictly comparable with the secondary deviation of the sound eye which we met in the case of ocular palsies (page 258).

The patient cannot whistle or blow out his cheek, fluids tend on drinking to trickle out from the angle of the mouth and solid food to collect within the flaccid and paralysed cheek. Taste is lost over the anterior two-thirds of the tongue if the nerve is affected between the geniculate ganglion and the distal point at which the chorda tympani leaves the nerve. The stapedius muscle is also paralysed, and as a result the patient may complain of increased auditory acuity in the affected ear and of clicking noises.

Course.—Recovery is the rule, and in most cases during the second and third week the marked initial asymmetry of the face at rest diminishes as the still paralysed muscles regain tone. Voluntary movement appears first in the frontalis, then in orbicularis palpebrarum, and last of all in the muscles round the mouth and in platysma. Most cases begin to show voluntary movement within the first three or four weeks and then proceed to complete recovery within about three months. In some instances, however, no visible movement is seen for at least four months, and, in these circumstances, full recovery may not be achieved and the restoration of movement may take over a year to reach its final stage. It is in these cases that during the third week the reaction of degeneration is found in the paralysed muscles. If at this period the muscles still respond to faradism an early and complete recovery may be expected. In elderly persons full recovery is less common than in young adults, and in them and in all slowly recovering cases some contracture of the weak muscles may gradually develop. This tends to minimize asymmetry of the face at rest, but on movement it may be a handicap, for each time the patient chews, the eye screws up and the lids almost meet. In these imperfectly recovered cases isolated movement of the upper or lower part of the face is not regained and the facial muscles contract as a whole.

Sometimes the lower lid sags permanently and tears trickle down the cheek.

So-called Geniculate Herpes. — Recent observations have rendered the status of geniculate herpes doubtful, and the facial palsy that sometimes occurs with herpes occipito-collaris may be a motor neuritis of the facial nerve comparable with that of the third nerve in some cases of ophthalmic herpes. Nevertheless, the clinical picture of facial palsy with herpes deserves description. In a typical case the onset of facial paralysis is preceded by severe neuralgic pain in the external auditory meatus and pinna. There may also be similar pain in the fauces on the affected side and in the tongue. An eruption of herpetic vesicles then appears in the meatus on the adjacent parts of the pinna, sometimes behind the ear, on the pillar of the fauces, and on the anterior two-thirds of the tongue. The pinna may swell considerably and redden, the fauces show several ulcers when the vesicles burst, and look red and swollen. To the observer unfamiliar with this picture it is easy to make a diagnosis of septic throat with secondary infection of the middle ear, and the serous discharge from the burst vesicles in the meatus may be taken for an otorrhœa. When, as a climax, a facial palsy suddenly develops, the idea that the middle ear has been infected obtains an illusory confirmation. Not every case is so striking. Only a few vesicles may be seen in the meatus with no œdema of the pinna, and no vesicles within the mouth. In these circumstances it is the facial palsy that first brings the patient under notice.

Bilateral Bell's palsy is not so uncommon as is generally supposed. When it occurs an interval of four or five days separates the involvement of the two nerves, and the bilateral paralysis of orbicularis oris leads to some difficulty in the formation of labials, so that articulation is not quite normal. *Recurrent* Bell's palsy may also occur, and in the course of a series of attacks both sides of the face may be involved. Occasionally, also, sixth nerve palsies may occur in the course of such a sequence.

Treatment.—In the majority of instances facial palsy makes a complete recovery within three months. For these cases it cannot be said that any treatment is essential, or that the lack of it will prevent a favourable result. The residue of cases which over a period of from one to two years make a degree of recovery short of complete is composed mostly of elderly subjects, and requires more active measures.

In the third week after the onset, if no trace of return can be detected it may be expedient to have the electrical reactions of the paralysed muscles taken. If they respond to faradism an early recovery can be expected. If there be no response to faradism and if the response to galvanism is characteristic of the R.D. it is probable that no voluntary contraction will appear for three or four months and that thereafter improvement will be slow.

With these considerations in mind, and remembering that a Bell's palsy is a disquieting and disfiguring condition for the patient, some treatment becomes a psychological necessity from the outset. For the first week it is wise to keep the patient indoors and away from exposure to cold. The patient, a relative, or—if circumstances make it expedient —a masseur or masseuse should be instructed to rub the face gently with the finger-tips—moistened with ordinary olive oil—for about five minutes morning and evening, paying special attention to the muscles round the eye and the mouth. When, later, the patient begins to go outdoors the face is felt to be uncomfortably stiff after exposure to wind and cold. This discomfort may be relieved by bathing the face with a sponge wrung out of warm water for a few moments. No other measures than these are necessary. When recovery sets in they can usually be dispensed with. In the long-lasting cases where no tone returns to the paralysed muscles after two or three weeks and no voluntary movement in frontalis can be seen, it is wise to use a splint. This consists in a length of silver wire one end of which is curved over the pinna like the sidepiece of a pair of metal spectacles, while the other—covered by a fine piece of rubber tubing—is bent and curved round the corner of the lip. When this is correctly adjusted, movements of the normal half of the face can no longer pull the lips across the midline and thus stretch the paralysed muscles.

This splint need not be worn during sleep.

Gentle massage of the kind already mentioned, which can perfectly well be performed by an amateur, should be continued. In no case of Bell's palsy can it be said that electrical stimulation of the paralysed muscles by galvanism serves any useful purpose. Indeed, if persisted in it may lead to disfiguring contracture of the partly recovered muscles. In brief, the hazard to which the subject of a Bell's palsy is exposed is that of excessive and ill-advised treatment rather than that of neglect. It is common to give potassium iodide and sodium salicylate internally during the early phase of Bell's palsy, and inunction of mercurial ointment over the mastoid region has also been recommended. The influence of these measures upon prognosis cannot be confidently stated.

FACIAL HEMISPASM.—This is an affection of unknown ætiology and pathology usually encountered in middle-aged and elderly persons, more often in women than in men. It consists in the recurrence of irregular clonic muscular twitchings of the facial muscles on one side. In its early stages it usually involves only the muscles of the upper part of the face and is intermittent. In later stages or in more severe cases all the facial muscles, including platysma, are involved, and they may be completely at rest only during sleep (Fig. 51).

Even when the condition has been present for years no weakness of the facial muscles ensues. The spasm is aggravated by voluntary movements of the face and by emotional stimuli. It is painless, but the continual movement of the face and the screwing together of the eyelids in severe cases are uncomfortable and may become exasperating to a degree. It tends to persist indefinitely and rarely ceases permanently (Fig. 51).

Treatment.—The condition is very intractable to all forms of treatment, local and general. Mild sedatives may mitigate the patient's distress but rarely if ever affect the spasm. In the most severe cases, and in these alone, it may be justified—after fully explaining the consequences to the patient—to inject the facial nerve with alcohol, thus paralysing the muscles.

THE EIGHTH NERVE

This nerve has sensory (cochlear) and non-sensory (vestibular) components. The two components have different end organs and different central connections.

Ætiology.—This nerve and its end organs may be involved in many pathological processes. Inflammatory (infective) and degenerative processes may affect the cochlea and labyrinth, and the nerve, together with the fifth and seventh, may be stretched and compressed in the posterior fossa of the skull by an extra-cerebellar growth. Gummatous meningitis is also an occasional cause of eighth nerve disorder.

Symptoms.—*Cochlear division.*—Deafness with or without tinnitus results from lesions of this division. The deafness due to nerve involvement (nerve deafness) may be differentiated from deafness due to middle ear disease by the following tests. Under normal conditions air conduction is more acute than sound conduction through the temporal bone. In nerve deafness this relationship is intact, in middle ear deafness it is reversed. *Rinné's test* is based upon this fact. The foot of a vibrating tuning fork is placed upon the mastoid process until it is no longer heard by the subject. The vibrating prongs are then held close to the pinna. In the normal subject the vibrations are heard again, and in partial nerve deafness also they are still audible. In middle ear disease the

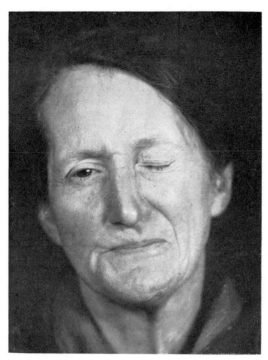

Fig. 51.

Facial Hemispasm involving the Left Half
of the Face.

To face page 266.

vibrating prongs held near the pinna are no longer heard after the base of the fork placed against the mastoid has become inaudible. *Weber's Test.*—The base of a vibrating tuning fork is placed on the vertex of the skull in the middle line. With unilateral nerve deafness the sound is referred to the normal ear, with middle ear deafness to the affected ear. When both ears are normal the sound is referred to the middle line.

In ordinary neurological diagnosis it is perhaps even more important to detect differences in acuity between the two ears.

Slowly progressive lesions involving the eighth nerve are frequently accompanied by tinnitus.

Vestibular division.—Vertigo and certain associated symptoms, *e.g.* ataxy, sickness, result from lesions involving the labyrinth or the vestibular nerve. A complaint of giddiness has always to be investigated as no word is more loosely used by patients. It may be employed to describe sensory ataxy, or feelings of faintness, and it occupies a prominent place in the vocabulary of the psychoneurotic patient when its meaning may be entirely vague. It is necessary, therefore, to ascertain what the patient intends to convey when he speaks of giddiness. The giddiness, or vertigo, due to labyrinthine or vestibular nerve lesions is essentially a subjective sensation of rotation, either of the subject or of surrounding objects. When severe it may be accompanied by vomiting, by gross ataxy of movement so that the patient cannot stand or even sit up, and when the onset is sudden there may even be a momentary blurring or loss of consciousness. Nystagmus is usually present and may cause a sensation of to-and-fro movements of objects.

Ætiology.—A great variety of causes may underlie the appearance of vertigo. Amongst local causes in the ear are blocking of a Eustachian tube, wax in the meatus, inflammatory lesions in the middle ear, lesions involving the vestibular division of the eighth nerve in its intracranial course, and gross lesions of the cerebellum in which the central vestibular connections or the vestibular nerve are involved. It is not a symptom of pure degenerative lesions of the cerebellum. When vertigo is due to an intracranial lesion it is accompanied by other signs of nervous disease.

MÉNIÈRE'S SYNDROME.—This is chiefly encountered between the ages of 30 and 60 and about equally in the two sexes.

Ætiology.—The lesion consists of a dilatation of the endolymphatic system with a concurrent increase of fluid pressure. This in turn leads to a paresis of the nervous mechanism of the labyrinth. This process is peculiar to Ménière's disease, and does not follow suppurative changes. It is essentially bilateral, but one ear is very much more affected than its fellow. There is always some degree of cochlear involvement.

Symptoms.—The syndrome consists in sudden accesses of intense vertigo, occurring at irregular intervals and lasting for variable periods of time ranging from a few minutes to one or more days. The attack may pass off rapidly or may subside into a slight degree of vertigo, which persists for several days. Sudden movements of the head, sneezing, or blowing the nose may precipitate an attack in a susceptible subject, or it may occur with no obvious exciting cause. The sense of rotation may be purely subjective, or there may be a visible tendency to rotate before the patient falls. This fall may be so sudden that the patient cannot guard against it, and consciousness may be transiently lost. Violent sickness ensues in severe attacks and recurs whenever the patient moves. Nystagmus is present at the height of the attack, and diplopia is a rare symptom. Tinnitus may be present.

Between the attacks physical examination reveals no abnormal signs referable to the nervous system, but there is almost always some deafness and a complaint of intermittent tinnitus. The first attacks may, however, antedate the appearance of deafness.

Course and Prognosis.—Frequently the initial attacks are the most severe and the affection tends slowly to improvement. In other cases a progressive deafness sets in and the patient remains liable to recurrent attacks of vertigo until this unilateral deafness is total.

Diagnosis.—Recurrent attacks of intense vertigo associated with a degree of deafness and some tinnitus, in the absence of signs of organic nervous disease characterize Ménière's syndrome.

Treatment.—This is essentially palliative in nature. The following drugs have been used with a measure of success: phenobarbitone, gr. $\frac{1}{2}$ twice daily; or sodium bromide, grs. 10; dilute hydrobromic acid, ℳ 15 to 30, thrice daily; or aspirin, grs. 5, thrice daily. In obstinate cases of frequent attacks, restriction of salt and of fluid intake should be tried. Recently favourable claims have been made for the administration of potassium chloride in doses of from 6 to 10 *grams daily*. In severe and disabling cases where the worst affected ear is deaf, recourse may be had to the operation of labyrinthectomy. Intracranial division of the eighth nerve has also been employed.

THE NINTH, TENTH, AND ELEVENTH NERVES

These nerves are so intimately related in their central connections, and are so frequently affected simultaneously in their contiguous peripheral course, that they are best considered together as the glosso-pharyngeal-vagus-accessorius complex. They contain both motor and sensory fibres. The motor fibres fall into two groups: (1) *a somato-motor* group which innervates the musculature of the pharynx, larynx, palate, sternomastoid, and trapezius. The cells of origin lie in the nucleus ambiguus and its caudal extension. The latter reaches as far as the third cervical segment, where it forms the spinal nucleus of the accessory nerve.

The musculature is represented in this columnar nuclear mass from before backwards in the order named above; (2) *a viscero-motor group* which supplies the involuntary musculature of the alimentary tract and of the air passages, and which arises in the dorsal nucleus of the vagus. The sensory fibres also fall into two groups: *a somato-sensory group*, the fibres of which end centrally in the substantia gelatinosa Rolandi and peripherally supply common sensation to the ear, mouth, pharynx, and the upper part of the respiratory tract; and a larger *viscero-sensory group* which receives afferent fibres from the thoracic and abdominal viscera.

The three nerve trunks leave the skull together by the jugular foramen. The glosso-pharyngeal nerve ends in the posterior third of the tongue, the vagus extends downwards through the neck and thorax to the abdomen, while the spinal accessory (bulbar and spinal portions) sends its bulbar fibres to join the vagus, and its spinal fibres pass to the sternomastoid and trapezius muscles. These three nerves may be involved in focal medullary lesions and by lesions at the base of the skull or in the neck. Various symptom-complexes have been described corresponding to lesions in these different situations.

Lesions in the Medulla Oblongata.—These are not uncommon, and may be the result of focal thrombosis, chronic bulbar palsy, or of syringomyelia with bulbar extension. The symptoms are unilateral paralysis of the soft palate, pharyngeal muscles, and larynx with an associated crossed hemianæsthesia of syringomyelic type affecting pain and thermal sensibility.

Paralysis of the soft palate is also a common symptom in diphtheritic paralysis, and is due to a lesion of the nucleus in the medulla.

Lesions at the Base of the Skull, either of the nature of new growth, fractures, or gunshot wounds, often produce associated ninth tenth, and eleventh nerve palsies. The following syndromes have been described: (1) unilateral paralysis of pharynx, larynx, palate, sterno-mastoid, and trapezius. (2) like the above, with the addition of a hypo-glossal nerve palsy, but in incomplete forms the vocal cord may remain intact.

Lesions in the Neck.—In injuries high in the neck we may see unilateral paralysis of tongue and vocal cord, the palate being intact. The lesion is below the offset of the pharyngeal branches.

The characteristic sign of involvement of the glosso-pharyngeal nerve is sensory loss over the upper part of the pharynx, and loss of taste in the posterior third of the tongue.

The characteristic signs of lesions of the vagus nerve are pharyngeal and laryngeal paralysis. In pharyngeal paralysis the soft palate lies low on the affected side and does not rise on phonation, and there is loss of the pharyngeal reflex on that side. Also, there is the so-called "curtain movement" of the posterior pharyngeal wall, which moves across to the normal side on swallowing. Bilateral pharyngeal paralysis may occur in diphtheritic paralysis.

Total unilateral laryngeal paralysis results from high level lesions of the vagus. The affected vocal cord lies in the cadaveric position. There is weakening of the voice, but no stridor.

Recurrent laryngeal nerve lesions, or lesions of the vagus below the offset of the superior laryngeal branches, produce paralysis of the abductor of the vocal cords. The affected vocal cord lies up against the median plane and does not move on phonation or on respiration. In bilateral abductor paralysis both vocal cords lie approximated in the midline and do not recede during inspiration. There is marked inspiratory stridor and considerable danger of asphyxiation.

Lesions of the Spinal Accessory Nerve.—The bulbar portion joins the vagus at the ganglion of the trunk (inferior ganglion of vagus), and probably provides the majority of the motor fibres which reach the larynx through the vagus. It does not, therefore, need separate consideration. Lesions of the spinal portion produce sternomastoid and trepezius paralysis. It is paralysis of the latter which causes definite disability. The shoulder on the affected side cannot be raised fully. The scapula tends to fall away from the midline and to rotate so that its superior angle lies higher than normal, and protrudes as a hump on the contour of the neck as seen from in front. There is also some winging of the scapula, like that seen in serratus palsy, but most marked when the arm is held extended forwards below the horizontal, whereas the winging of serratus magnus (s. anterior) paralysis is maximal with the arm above the horizontal.

Ætiology of Glosso-pharyngeal-Vagus-Accessorius Lesions.— In the medulla, chronic bulbar palsy, focal thrombosis, tumours, syringobulbia, and diphtheritic toxic lesions may all produce symptoms referable to one or more of these nerves. In their intracranial course, tumours, or syphilitic meningitis, may involve one or more of them. At the base of the skull, injuries or new growth may involve all three in the region of the jugular foramen, while in the neck, injuries, new growths, or aneurysms may compress them. The vagus may be involved in the thorax (recurrent laryngeal paralysis) by aneurysm.

Glosso-pharyngeal Neuralgia.—This comparatively rare condition is in the characteristics of the pain very like trigeminal neuralgia. The patient complains of accesses of severe neuralgic pain in the region of the throat and ear. The paroxysm is commonly excited by the act of swallowing. The patient is usually a middle-aged or elderly man.

Treatment resembles that of trigeminal neuralgia in the matter of medication. In severe and intractable cases division of the glosso-pharyngeal nerve within the skull has been successfully performed.

THE HYPOGLOSSAL NERVE

The twelfth nerve is an exclusively motor nerve which arises in a group of cells on the floor of the fourth ventricle close to the median plane. Its fibres innervate the muscles of the tongue and some of the elevators of the hyoid bone (hyoglossus and geniohyoid).

Ætiology of Lesions.—The nerve nucleus may be involved in medullary lesions, particularly in chronic bulbar paralysis, syringobulbia, tumour, thrombosis, and sometimes in tabes dorsalis. The two nuclei lying close together are generally both affected. The nerve may be affected in its intracranial course by syphilitic meningitis or new growth. Peripherally, it may be involved alone, or, as we have seen with vagus and accessorius, in any disease process deep in the neck.

Symptomatology.—Lesions of the cortico-bulbar (upper motor) neurones at any level higher than the pons may affect the tongue, rendering the organ spastic and small and causing protrusion towards the side of the lesion.

Nuclear or infranuclear lesions lead to unilateral paralysis, the organ when protruded being thrust towards the paralysed side by the unopposed muscles of the normal half, and to wasting and fibrillation. The organ on the affected side is shrunken and wrinkled, and is in constant fibrillation.

CHAPTER XXI

Sciatica and Brachial Neuritis

THE two conditions discussed in this chapter are now less commonly thought of together than has formerly been the case, and this is because new views as to the ætiology and pathology of sciatica have gained ground, and these views have not so far been applied to brachial neuritis. This, it is here submitted, is unfortunate because sciatica and brachial neuritis have striking clinical features in common and it is unlikely that they can commonly have totally differing causes and pathology. The tendency now is to consider sciatica in a vacuum, as it were, but no sound balance of opinion can be looked for in respect of it, except on the general background of what we know of peripheral nerve and nerve root lesions.

Definition.—The problem of sciatica has been needlessly complicated by a deplorable vagueness as to what clinical condition we refer by the term, which has come to mean so many things that it is in danger of meaning nothing save the presence of pain somewhere in the buttock or lower limb. By the term "sciatica" we refer here to a painful malady, of acute or subacute onset, of relatively brief or prolonged course, in which accesses of pain are experienced along the course of the nerve—or part of this course; in which the muscles supplied by the nerve are painful and tender to pressure and to stretching, as well as to the voluntary contraction involved in movement and the active maintenance of posture of the affected limb; in which—in severe cases—there may be some wasting or even weakness in the muscles; in which elevating the extended leg as the patient lies supine, causes pain along the course of the nerve and in the stretched hamstring muscles; in which the ankle jerk may be diminished or lost; and in which there may be a sensation of numbness or objective sensory impairment along the outer side of the foot and leg. These purely neurological signs and symptoms may be accompanied by some rigidity of the lumbar spine, and—when standing—by a tilting upwards of the pelvis on the affected side with a compensatory scoliosis. This statement describes the fully developed clinical picture, but whether all or only some of its components are present depends upon the stage and severity of the cases. It will be seen from the foregoing that sciatica is thus essentially a neurological malady, and not a simple matter of pain in the limb arising from joint, ligamentous, or muscular lesions not directly involving the nerve or its component roots.

Ætiology and Pathology.—There is no general agreement as to the causal factors in sciatica. The old view was that the essential lesion is an inflammation of the nerve sheath—in interstitial neuritis—and observers have described thickening and vascular congestion of the sheath with œdema of the nerve. It must be confessed, however, that since sciatica is a non-fatal malady it has never been possible to establish firmly the reality of this patho-logical process. More recently, rupture of an intervertebral disc, between fourth and fifth lumbar or between fifth lumbar and first sacral vertebrae, with herniation into the spinal canal of the nucleus pulposus of the disc has been increasingly in-voked not only as a cause, but as *the* cause of all cases of sciatica (Fig. 52). Yet others regard lumbar spondylitis or lesions of the sacro-iliac joint as the essential factors. Com-mon to all these hypotheses is the craving of their authors to simplify the problem by invok-ing a single pathology for all

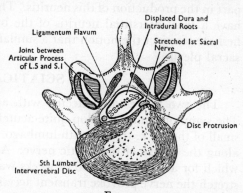

Fig. 52.

A diagrammatic drawing of a section made through a fifth lumbar intervertebral disc in which pro-trusion has occurred on the right. The anterior position of the first sacral nerve on the unaffected side is indicated. The fifth lumbar nerve which would curve laterally around the vertebral pedicle and above the plane of the section has not been represented. (J. O'Conell, *Brit. J. Surg.*)

cases, but nature is not interested in simplicity, certainly not in purely verbal simplifications, and the probability is that while acute single-attack cases may be due to an interstitial neuritis, a proportion—as yet unknown —of chronic and recurrent cases may follow upon herniation of an inter-vertebral disc and the compression of fifth lumbar, first or second sacral roots.

It is virtually impossible to assess the role of lumbar spondylitis, since this condition is very common in middle-aged and elderly men and is often wholly symptom-free, while it is frequently absent in young adults suffering from sciatica. Fibrositis of the lumbosacral muscle sheaths is an even vaguer and less satisfactory explanation, but may account for certain cases of pain referred to the distribution of the nerve. In short, it is likely that single-attack cases of very acute onset and relatively brief duration (four to eight weeks) are due to an interstitial sciatic neuritis, but that chronic or recurrent cases occurring in young adults subject to severe physical stresses, and associated in many instances with a history of strain to the lower back, are predominantly due to rupture of an intervertebral disc. In the present state of knowledge no more dogmatic statement can be made.

As has been said, the symptoms and course of an acute sciatic neuritis

s

bears many resemblances to an acute brachial neuritis, though in the latter objective signs (wasting, reflex, and sensory changes) are less common. Injuries to the cervical spine (see also page 205) may lead to rupture of a cervical disc, but when this occurs the symptom-complex is rarely that of acute brachial neuritis, and this lesion plays no known part in the production of this neuritis. Therefore, the probability that we have a true interstitial neuritis of the brachial plexus should make us hesitate to reject the notion that a similar process may affect the lumbo-sacral plexus.

SCIATICA

The two nerves are affected with approximately equal frequency. The symptoms may develop quite acutely with pain and stiffness in the small of the back, that is, with lumbago, and in a few days pain appears along the course of the sciatic nerve. Another mode of onset is that in which for a variable period of weeks walking or movements tending to stretch the nerve provoke transient accesses of pain along it. Finally, the pain rapidly reaches a climax of intense and disabling severity. When this occurs, any position of the limb in which the nerve is on the stretch becomes acutely painful, the pain radiating from buttock or hip to foot. It is often most intense in the region of the buttock just mesial to the great trochanter, near the posterior iliac spine, at the sciatic notch, in the middle of the back of the thigh, behind the knee, and down the lateral aspect of the leg and on the dorsum of the foot. It is paroxysmal with a residual dull aching pain, the paroxysms being burning and lancinating. The patient is usually least uncomfortable when lying down with the leg slightly flexed at hip and knee and rotated out. When standing the leg is kept flexed at these joints, with the heel just off the ground and the pelvis tilted up on the affected side. A compensatory scoliosis offsets this tilting (Fig. 54).

Tingling sensations are felt over the cutaneous distribution of the sciatic nerve, that is, over the lateral aspect of the leg and dorsum of the foot. All muscles supplied by the nerve are extremely tender when pressed or stretched, and they become flabby. The calf and plantar muscles are exquisitely painful and may be the seat of recurrent cramps.

The tendon jerks are usually all brisk in the initial acute stage, but in severe and in many chronic cases the ankle jerk may be diminished or abolished, and some wasting and weakness of muscles, more especially of the dorsiflexors, may ensue. Fibrillation in the muscles is not uncommon and may persist for years after recovery. If, with the patient lying on his back, the extended leg be lifted by the heel, great pain is felt as soon as the nerve becomes taut, that is, when the leg has been lifted through about 40° above the horizontal. Pressure over the nerve is also painful.

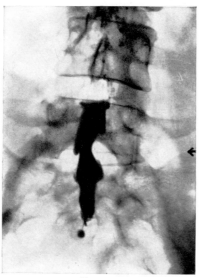

FIG. 53.

RADIOGRAM OF THE LIPIODOL PICTURE IN
HERNIATION OF THE INTERVERTEBRAL DISC.

Herniation of the vertebral disc between the fifth
lumbar and the first sacral vertebræ. Lipiodol has been
injected intrathecally, and the notch in the shadow of
the lipiodol indicates the site of the protrusion of the
herniated disc into the spinal canal. (This radiogram
was kindly given by Mr. J. Pennybacker.)

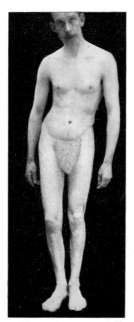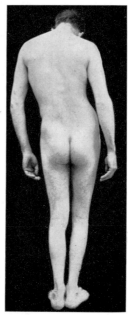

FIG. 54.

THE SCOLIOSIS OF SCIATICA.

Shows the scoliosis of a case of right-sided sciatica.

To face page 274.

The severity and duration of the affection vary widely from case to case, and depend largely upon how soon the patient took to his bed after the onset and how long he was kept there. During the first week the pain may be excruciating in severity, but it then progressively abates, and in uncomplicated and adequately treated cases recovery ensues within six to eight weeks. However, some cases become chronic, chiefly those that remained ambulant in the early stage, and the pain persists, with wide fluctuations in frequency and severity, for many months. On the whole, acute attacks of maximal severity are less subject to recurrence than attacks of subacute or insidious development: a fact that may be due to those differences in ætiology already discussed. Certainly subacute attacks may recur at varying intervals of years for long periods, with intervals of complete or of incomplete freedom from pain.

The clinical picture and course especially associated with rupture of a lumbar or lumbosacral intervertebral disc may be summarized as follows: There is commonly, though not invariably, a history of a strain to the back. The patient is bending to lift a heavy object. This may slip from his grasp, or its weight may suddenly increase if some helper allows it to drop from his grasp. Something is then felt to "give" in the patient's lower back and either an acute "lumbago" follows or he becomes recurrently aware of aching pain and stiffness in this region. Then follows a variable period of what is called "low back pain," and ultimately pain begins to radiate down the back of the thigh and then the lateral aspect of the leg to the ankle. Stooping increases this pain, as also does standing and sometimes sitting on a hard chair. Thereafter the picture is that already described as typical of sciatica. In the early stages nothing may be found other than rigidity of the lumbar spine and the tilting of the pelvis and scoliosis already mentioned (Fig. 54). The muscles supplied by the sciatic nerve are commonly tender to pressure, and straight leg raising is painful. Sooner or later the ankle jerk diminishes or is abolished, and there is some subjective numbness along the outer side of the leg with or without objective impairment of tactile or painful cutaneous sensibility. Some wasting of calf muscles and thinning of the tendo achillis ultimately ensues.

Intrathecal air injections (air myelograms) may reveal the presence of some projection into the thecal space. Lipiodol intrathecally, formerly used for this diagnostic purpose, has been abandoned, as the retention of the substance in the theca may cause root irritation and pain (Fig. 52).

Diagnosis.—Few familiar conditions are more often erroneously diagnosed upon inadequate grounds than chronic sciatica. Osteo-arthritis of the hip is not infrequently so diagnosed. In this there is no noteworthy tenderness of the sciatic nerve or of the muscles supplied by it, and the ankle jerk is never affected, but there is limitation of the range of active and passive movement at the hip. If the heel of the extended leg be struck a smart blow by the observer's palm, there is pain in the region of the hip in arthritis but not in a chronic case of sciatica.

A SYMPTOMATIC SCIATICA due to pressure upon the nerve or its component roots by a vertebral or intrapelvic growth does not really present a close resemblance to the affection just described. The nerve is never so tender to pressure nor are the muscles, relief from pain is more rapid and complete when the patient is put to bed, and the pain has not the intense burning character of true sciatica. Moreover, in the latter the affection is always unilateral; while in cases of pressure, bilateral signs and symptoms are common. Sooner or later progressive paralysis, wasting, and sensory loss in the distribution of the affected nerve roots make their appearance, together with the clinical indications of the underlying growth.

In every chronic case of what appears to be sciatica, a rectal and a radiological examination should be made.

Treatment.—Rest in bed is an imperative necessity in every case of sciatica, whatever its ætiology, and the prognosis as to duration is always best when this step is taken at once. The patient generally finds his own positions of maximum comfort, and fixation of the limb in the adducted and extended position is rarely tolerated in early and severe cases. The leg should be supported fully by pillows in whatever position it lies. Even in cases where the severity of the pain allows the patient to leave his bed for the closet, he should be discouraged from doing so, and if the use of the bedpan is, as it may be, extremely painful or objected to, a compromise may be made by the use of a commode in the bed-room. For the first few days the use of morphia may be necessary to secure sleep and to relieve pain, but as soon as possible aspirin with or without codeine (gr. $\frac{1}{8}$ to gr. $\frac{1}{4}$) and given at regular intervals should be substituted. A barbiturate at night may also be indicated, or a combination of chloral (grs. 10) and sodium bromide (grs. 20). The latter may be given at about seven o'clock in the evening and repeated some three hours later if necessary. In elderly patients it is best to avoid heavier bromide dosage than this. As neither sciatica nor brachial neuritis is primarily an affection of the nervous elements in the nerves or nerve roots concerned, it follows that the employment of vitamin B_1 preparations has no place in treatment. The limb should be kept warm with cotton wool or woollens. The gentle application of a methyl salicylate liniment followed by the application of an ordinary radiant heat lamp may give relief, or an electrically heated pad may be applied. In the acute stage no more active treatment should be given. Massage, movements, or diathermy should be reserved for the convalescent stage or for chronic cases.

The chronic case of sciatica presents one of the most difficult of therapeutic problems, and many remedies at first hailed as universally successful have had their brief day of apparent triumph and have passed, or are passing, into oblivion. They include stretching the nerve under anæsthetic, injecting it with normal saline solution, injecting the sub-cutaneous tissues of the thigh with oxygen, turpentine baths, cupping, "ray" treatment and electro-therapy of various forms. More recently epidural sacral injections of a normal saline solution containing novocain have been employed, while spa treatment and all that this implies in baths and mechano-therapy is still with us. In the individual case not one of these can be confidently relied upon to secure relief, but it must be admitted that their frequent failure is often to be attributed to their use *as a substitute* for the only really essential element in treatment, namely, an adequate period of rest in bed. Rest is monotonous, lacks the im-pressiveness of electro-, mechano-, and "ray" therapy, and may be economically difficult or impossible, yet an adequate period of rest is not seldom far more economical in the long run than a changing over from one method of active treatment to another. Therefore, the ambulant case of chronic sciatica should be first put back to bed and while there massage, radiant heat, diathermy, or other chosen method can be given a reasonable opportunity to prove its value. Other modes of treatment call for brief mention. The highly variable procedures known as "manipulation" of the lumbar spine or sacro-iliac joints have their followers, but it is probable that such success as they achieve is in cases wrongly diagnosed as sciatica. A somewhat comparable statement may be made in respect of the intramuscular injection of novocain into pain-ful spots in muscles. Whatever the value of this in conditions unassoci-ated with any form of lesion of the sciatic nerve, it can be no more than a palliative of very limited scope in sciatica.

The suspected case of herniated intervertebral disc should always be given an adequate period of complete rest in the supine position before surgical intervention is considered. It is certain that many cases of this kind do become symptom-free after conservative treatment alone. It is already too common to encounter patients who have been subjected to laminectomy but have never been rested. A final balance of opinion as to the indications for surgical intervention has not yet been reached. Each case must be considered on its merits: the severity of pain, its duration, tendency to recurrence, the nature of the subject's work and so on. This can be stated, however, that laminectomy for this lesion should be expertly performed if it is not to produce a disability as severe as that it is designed to remedy.

BRACHIAL NEURITIS

As in the case of sciatica this is an affection of adults, and may be acute or subacute in onset. Pain first appears at the root of the neck in the region of the plexus, spreading within a few days downwards into the arm and hand. In incidence and character the pain resembles that of acute sciatica, and there are usually localized sites on the lateral aspect of the limb where it is maximal. The patient cannot lie on the affected side and the hanging position of the limb, or its active elevation, is very painful. During the night pain may reach almost intolerable intensity so that the patient has to get up and walk about. Physical examination may reveal little beyond tenderness of muscles, pain on pressure over the brachial plexus and upon stretching it. The arm jerks are usually brisk, and wasting, weakness, and objective sensory loss are exceptional.

When adequately treated from the outset, the intense pain dies down in a week or so and recovery is complete in from six to eight weeks.

The brachial neuritis that may follow the injection of foreign proteins (tetanus antitoxin, diphtheria, antitoxin, T.A.B., etc.) is a more serious affair, though, fortunately, a rare one. Within from a few days to about two weeks after the injection, and with or without the usual manifestations of "serum sickness," pain develops in the neck, shoulders, and chest. Weakness comes on rapidly in muscles supplied by the upper roots of the plexus, though all muscles in the limb are liable to involvement. The condition is usually bilateral, though not bilaterally symmetrical. Deltoid, serratus anterior, the rhomboids, the spinati, triceps are the muscles most often affected. Wasting soon appears and the disability may be severe. Pain persists for a varying period, sometimes for several weeks. The tendon jerks vary according to the incidence of the paralysis, and one or more of them may be abolished. Sensory loss is minimal and may be absent. There may be an associated paralysis of one or more cranial nerves. Recovery slowly sets in, but is not always complete in all the affected muscles. This variety of brachial neuritis has also been recorded quite apart from protein injections, and it has been suggested that these play no causative role when brachial neuritis follows them, but that the association is always coincidental will not readily be accepted by those who have seen it.

Treatment.—The same general principles of rest, medication, and local treatment as have been mentioned in the case of sciatica apply here. In severe cases it is best to put the patient to bed at once and to rest the affected arm in the most comfortable position on pillows. Its use should be wholly avoided until recovery is manifestly under way. The necessary immobilization of the limb is apt to lead to some fixation of the shoulder joint, and to avoid this the arm should be carefully moved by the nurse for a few moments morning and evening so as to keep this joint mobile. When this measure is neglected it is not rarely found after recovery that there is partial ankylosis of the shoulder.

In the paralytic form associated with serum injections the principles governing the treatment of the paralysis of poliomyelitis apply.

CHAPTER XXII

Affections of the Spinal Nerves

GENERAL OBSERVATIONS ON LESIONS OF PERIPHERAL NERVES

ÆTIOLOGY.—Injury provides the majority of cases of isolated affection of spinal nerves, and the remainder are what is known as toxic in origin, certain spinal nerves seeming to show a proneness to involvement in the latter way. In the case of trauma, a nerve or nerves may be involved in an open wound (as in gunshot wounds), in a closed injury (as in the case of fracture or dislocation), or by compression or traction. The degree of damage thus sustained by the nerve will vary from (1) complete anatomical division of the entire trunk or of the nervous elements within the sheath only; (2) damage sufficient to cause degeneration of the nerve fibres without solution of anatomical continuity; or (3) damage sufficient to produce physiological block; *i.e.* interruption of conduction, without solution of continuity or subsequent degeneration of nerve fibres. It would, however, be an artificial simplification of the situation to erect these three grades of damage into fundamental types of nerve injury, for it is clear that every intermediate grade of injury and every combination of the three grades may be found in a single case; *e.g.* an injury in which the trunk may be partly severed, some fibres degenerated but not anatomically severed, and some physiologically inactivated without visible structural lesion. Nevertheless, some generalization is possible and useful. The two more severe grades of injury are followed by Wallerian degeneration of axis cylinders, the least severe is not, and, therefore, where there is no degeneration recovery may be expected to be most rapid and most perfect. On the other hand, where there is anatomical solution of continuity recovery is longest delayed and least perfect. A Greek nomenclature has recently been coined to specify the three grades of injury, but as this has to be translated back into English before it can convey anything to the average reader, its employment serves but to complicate what without it is a simple grading.

Moreover, clinically considered, nerve injuries fall into a somewhat different grouping according to disturbance of function as follows:—

Complete Interruption of Conduction.—There is paralysis, followed by wasting, of all muscles innervated by the nerve, and the muscles are painless. The reaction of degeneration (see page 31) appears during the third week, and tapping these denervated muscles yields a slow wave-like contraction like that seen when the galvanic current is employed to stimulate them. At first the area of sensory change is maximal for the nerve involved, but the later invasion of the anæsthetic area by sensory fibres from adjacent nerves tends in time to lessen the extent of sensory loss. There is also sudomotor and pilomotor paralysis within the territory of the nerve.

This picture may be associated with anatomical division of the nerve or with degeneration of nerve fibres without anatomical severance. In the latter case, regeneration (*i.e.* restoration of function) appears earlier and proceeds nearer to perfection than when there is severance of the nerve.

Partial Interruption of Conduction.—Paralysis is not complete and wasting absent or not severe. Pressure on or stretching of affected muscles is painful. This seems especially the case with muscles supplied by the median and medial popliteal nerves. In minimal damage, this pain and tenderness may be more prominent than weakness. As in complete interruption the relevant tendon jerks are lost. Electrical testing may show no qualitative change from normal. The area of sensory loss is less than the full distribution of the nerve and the degree of impairment relative only. There is commonly a small focus of analgesia, surrounded by a larger area of tactile loss within which pinprick has a diffuse and peculiarly painful quality.

Partial Interruption of Conduction with Signs of Irritation.—This syndrome is always the result of partial division by a wound, or of the involvement of an intact nerve trunk in cicatricial tissue from an adjacent wound. The greatest degree of irritation is seen in median and internal popliteal nerve lesions. The irritation varies in degree from slight pain and cutaneous hyperæsthesia with muscle tenderness to excruciating burning pain in the affected region and severe trophic lesions. The signs of interruption of conduction may be trivial. The most severe type is that associated with *causalgia*, a form of pain which may be of intense severity, and when long-lasting reduces the sufferer to a pitiable state. This is aggravated by any movement, active or passive, of the part, or by a jarring of the bed on which the patient lies; the pain is mainly superficial. This clinical picture is commonly the result of gunshot wounds which have just glanced the nerve without severing any or many fibres. Motor signs of irritation are contracture, and fibrous infiltration of muscles, muscular spasms, and, rarely, actual hypertrophy of muscle.

Signs of Regeneration are both motor and sensory. On the motor side the pilomotor muscles in the affected cutaneous area regain function and the limb muscles regain tone before voluntary power returns. On the sensory side percussion of the nerve below the lesion elicits a tingling sensation within the skin area which is the seat of sensory loss. All forms of cutaneous sensibility begin to return together, first at the proximal end of the anæsthetic area, but sensations elicited by stimuli here are referred to the distal end of the anæsthetic area ("peripheral reference"). Gradually the area of sensory change lessens in size, beginning to recede at the proximal end. Thermal and painful sensations are apt to be intensified and to be badly localized.

The electrical reactions also begin to return to normal, and trophic lesions to clear up.

LESIONS OF THE BRACHIAL PLEXUS AND OF NERVES DERIVED FROM IT

The brachial plexus is derived from the lower four cervical and the first thoracic spinal nerve roots. These roots are purely morphological in the arrangement of their nerve fibres, whereas the nerve trunks issuing from the plexus distally are physiologically arranged, flexor muscles being supplied by one nerve, extensors by another. The function of the plexus is to effect this rearrangement, and it follows that the topography of the sensory and motor paralyses in plexus lesions will depend upon the situation of the lesion. There are thus three possible types of plexus lesion: radicular lesions involving the roots entering into the plexus, plexus lesions involving the trunks and cords, and distal lesions which correspond to combined lesions of the peripheral nerves.

RADICULAR LESIONS form the majority of cases, and fall into two groups: (1) *upper plexus type*, in which the fifth and sixth cervical roots are concerned; and (2) *lower plexus type*, in which the eighth cervical and first thoracic roots are concerned. (1) The muscles supplied by the fifth and sixth roots and affected in lesions of these roots are the deltoid, biceps, brachialis anticus, supinator longus (brachio-radialis), supra- and infra-spinatus, serratus anterior, rhomboids, clavicular part of pectoralis major and subscapularis. The sensory loss involves the outer aspect of the shoulder and upper limb; biceps and supinator jerks may be lost. (2) The eighth cervical and first thoracic roots supply the flexor muscles in the forearm and the small hand muscles. The sensory change includes the ulnar aspect of forearm and hand. There may be an associated cervical sympathetic paralysis in first thoracic root lesions. Lesions of the trunks and cords of the plexus are not so common as those of the roots, or of the upper trunk formed by the junction of the fifth and sixth cervical roots. Occasionally, also, in gunshot and stab wounds the posterior cord of the plexus may be injured, giving rise to sensory and motor symptoms in the distribution of the circumflex and musculo-spiral (radial) nerves.

Ætiology of Brachial Plexus Lesions.—The majority of plexus lesions are traumatic in origin and arise from the violent forcing of the shoulder and arm into abnormal positions. Thus, traction on the arm, falls on the shoulder, or pressure exerted on the shoulder from above may tear the upper plexus roots either at their points of attachment to the cord or in the intervertebral foramina. In forced adduction of the shoulder the clavicle may be forced backwards, and may compress the plexus against the first rib. The familiar type of birth palsy involves the fifth and sixth roots or the trunk formed by their union, and results from force exerted on the arm when this does not present normally.

Upper plexus lesions form the majority of cases, and the lower plexus type is relatively uncommon, except when associated with a lesion of the upper plexus.

Apart from trauma, the nerve roots entering into the plexus may be involved within the meninges by tumours or by syphilitic or tuberculous inflammatory processes; within the vertebral foramina by arthritic changes, by tuberculous caries or by new growth; in the neck by new growth or by gunshot or stab wounds. The production of plexus injury by cervical or first thoracic ribs is dealt with on page 232.

Symptomatology.—In upper plexus lesions there is both weakness and wasting of the affected muscles, deltoid and biceps being usually the most severely affected and showing a reaction of degeneration. The arm hangs adducted with the forearm pronated. It cannot be abducted nor can the elbow be flexed. The extent and degree of sensory loss are very variable. In slight injuries one or more of the muscles innervated by the damaged roots may escape. In lower plexus lesions there is weakness and wasting of the hand muscles, and oculo-pupillary (cervical sympathetic) symptoms when the first thoracic root is injured near its point of origin from the cord.

Treatment.—The processes of repair which follow severe injuries to the plexus and include fibrosis and matting of the nerve trunks render surgical treatment out of the question in all but exceptional cases. The treatment of paralysed muscles must be carried out on the lines laid down in the section dealing with "Acute Poliomyelitis" (page 150), and pain when present may be treated by radiant heat and suitable drugs.

THE PHRENIC NERVE.—Paralysis of this nerve is uncommon, but when present may be due to lesions of its cells of origin in the third, fourth, and fifth cervical segments of the cord (poliomyelitis, motor neurone disease, compression), to lesions of its roots (vertebral disease, meningitis), or to lesions of the nerve in neck or thorax, where it is occasionally involved in new growths or inflammatory processes. The symptom is paralysis of the diaphragm. When unilateral this may be difficult to detect apart from radioscopic screening. When bilateral there is slight dyspnœa on exertion, and bulging of the abdominal wall on inspiration.

When associated with paralysis of other respiratory muscles, the

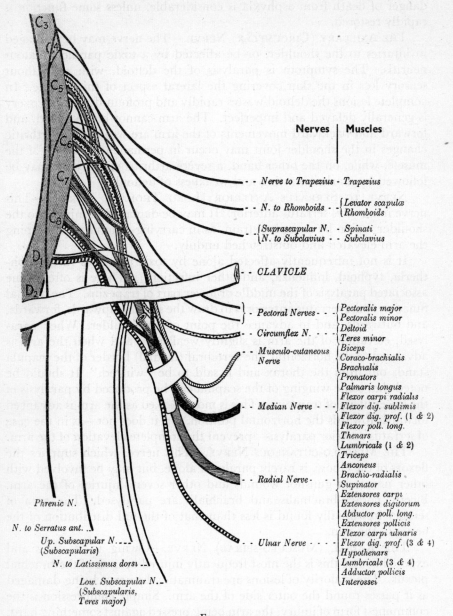

Nerves	Muscles
- - Nerve to Trapezius -	Trapezius
- - N. to Rhomboids - -	{ Levator scapulæ Rhomboids
{ Supraseapular N. - { N. to Subclavius -	Spinati Subclavius
- - CLAVICLE	
} - - Pectoral Nerves - -	Pectoralis major Pectoralis minor
- - Circumflex N. - -	Deltoid Teres minor
- - Musculo-cutaneous Nerve	Biceps Coraco-brachialis Brachialis
- - Median Nerve - -	Pronators Palmaris longus Flexor carpi radialis Flexor dig. sublimis Flexor dig. prof. (1 & 2) Flexor poll. long. Thenars Lumbricals (1 & 2)
- - Radial Nerve -	Triceps Anconeus Brachio-radialis Supinator Extensores carpi Extensores digitorum Abductor poll. long. Extensores pollicis
- - Ulnar Nerve - - -	Flexor carpi ulnaris Flexor dig. prof. (3 & 4) Hypothenars Lumbricals (3 & 4) Adductor pollicis Interossei

Phrenic N.

N. to Serratus ant.

Up. Subscapular N.
(Subscapularis)

N. to Latissimus dorsi

Low. Subscapular N.
(Subscapularis,
Teres major)

FIG. 55.

THE BRACHIAL PLEXUS AND ITS MOTOR INNERVATION.

A diagram of the brachial plexus. The names of the muscles innervated by the plexus are arranged opposite to their corresponding nerves, and the diagram can thus be used to localize lesions of the plexus. (Modified from Meige.)

danger of death from asphyxia is considerable, unless some function is rapidly restored.

THE AXILLARY (CIRCUMFLEX) NERVE.—The nerve may be damaged in injuries to the shoulder, or be affected by a toxic parenchymatous neuritis. The symptom is paralysis of the deltoid, with or without sensory loss in the skin covering the lateral aspect of this muscle. In complete lesions the deltoid wastes rapidly and profoundly, and recovery is generally delayed and imperfect. The arm cannot be abducted, and forward and backward movements of the arm are weakened. Arthritic changes in the shoulder-joint may occur in permanent paralysis of the muscle, while, on the other hand, a severe arthritis of this joint may be followed by marked wasting and weakness of deltoid.

NERVE TO SERRATUS ANTERIOR (LONG THORACIC NERVE).—This nerve innervates serratus anterior. It may be damaged in injuries to the shoulder region by excessive strain, as in carrying weights or in keeping the arm elevated and outstretched unduly.

It is not infrequently affected alone by toxic processes (after diphtheria, typhoid, influenza, and other infections). There is often some associated paralysis of the middle or lower part of trapezius. The normal function of the serratus anterior is to draw the scapula upwards, forwards, and outwards, and to advance the point of the shoulder. When paralysed, elevation of the arm is slightly weakened, and when the arm is advanced to the horizontal, the vertebral (medial) border of the scapula stands out from the thorax and is said to be "winged." It should be noted that some winging of the scapula can be produced by paralysis of the lower fibres of trapezius. This is most marked as the arm is advanced forwards towards the horizontal position, but it does not—as in the case of serratus anterior paralysis—prevent the complete elevation of the arm.

THE MUSCULO-CUTANEOUS NERVE.—This nerve, which supplies the flexors of the elbow, is rarely paralysed alone, but may be involved with other nerves in gunshot wounds and other severe injuries of the arm. Biceps, coraco-brachialis and brachialis are paralysed. The area of sensory loss usually found is less than that of the full distribution of the nerve to the skin.

THE RADIAL (MUSCULO-SPIRAL) NERVE.—Owing to its long and exposed course this is the most frequently injured branch of the brachial plexus. The majority of lesions are traumatic, the nerve being damaged as it passes round the outer side of the arm. Simple compression is the commonest form of injury, the arm being pressed against something hard, or compressed by a tourniquet. It is rare for the nerve of a perfectly healthy subject to sustain damage in this way, the majority of the patients being chronic alcoholics whose peripheral nerves are already poisoned (Saturday night paralysis). Other predisposing factors are debility, chronic plumbism, and recent infections such as typhoid. Other forms of injury are the involvement of the nerve in fracture of the shaft of the humerus, and pressure on the nerve in the axilla by a crutch.

Symptomatology.—This varies according to whether the nerve is damaged distal to the offset of the branch to the triceps or not. In

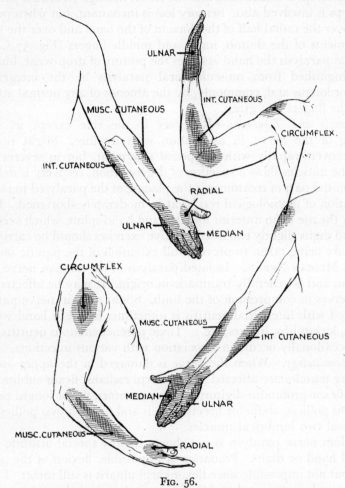

FIG. 56.

AREAS OF SENSORY LOSS FROM NERVE LESIONS IN UPPER LIMB.

The shaded areas represent, not the full cutaneous distribution of
the nerves named, but the areas of sensory change resulting from
lesions of them. The deeply shaded centres indicate total cutaneous
loss, the surrounding areas are those of hypoæsthesia.

the former (and common) case triceps and anconeus escape, and the supinators, extensors of the hand and of the fingers, and the extensors and long abductor of the thumb are paralysed. There is drop-wrist and the wrist and digits cannot be extended, except that the interossei maintain extension of the distal and middle phalanges. The grasp is weakened owing to the flexion at the wrist which accompanies it, and which is due to loss of the synergic fixation of the wrist that is part of the complete movement of grasping. Supination of the forearm is lost, except when the biceps is contracting and the elbow flexing. In crutch paralysis the triceps is involved also. Sensory loss is inconstant, but when present occurs over the radial half of the dorsum of the hand and over the proximal segments of the thumb, index and middle fingers (Fig. 57 C). In hysterical paralysis the hand assumes the posture of drop-wrist, but may be distinguished from musculo-spiral paralysis by the integrity of supinator longus and, commonly, by the absence of any normal attempt to flex the fingers in a grasp.

Prognosis and Treatment.—Recovery is the rule except in severe crushing of the nerve in association with fracture. Slight pressure palsy recovers rapidly without special treatment, but in severer cases where the muscles show a reaction of degeneration, recovery is delayed. The essential part of treatment is the placing of the paralysed muscles in the position of physiological rest, that is, moderately shortened. This is done by the use of an anterior forearm and hand splint, which keeps the wrist and digits slightly extended. Active exercises should be carried out daily, care being taken to prevent full extension of the paretic muscles.

THE MEDIAN NERVE.—Isolated paralysis of the median nerve is not common, and is generally traumatic in origin. It may be affected with other nerves in compression of the limb. Slight median nerve paralysis associated with interstitial neuritis is sometimes found in hand workers (joiners, locksmiths, ironers, etc.). Toxic parenchymatous neuritis of the nerve occasionally occurs in association with various infections.

Symptomatology.—When the nerve is damaged in the upper arm the following muscles are affected: flexor carpi radialis, flexor sublimis and part of flexor profundus digitorum, the pronators, flexor longus pollicis, opponens pollicis, abductor brevis pollicis and flexor brevis pollicis, and the lateral two lumbrical muscles.

Median nerve paralysis is not shown by any special attitude of the affected hand or digits. Pronation is impossible, flexion of the wrist is feeble but not impossible since flexor carpi ulnaris is still intact. Flexion of the thumb, index, and middle fingers is lost, but the ring and little fingers can still be flexed. Some flexion of the first phalanges is possible from the action of the interossei, which are supplied by the ulnar nerve. Opposition of the thumb is lost, and the wasting of opponens produces a hollow on the radial half of the thenar eminence. The full extent of sensory change includes the palm of the hand radial to a line drawn along the long axis of the limb down the middle of the ring fingers, and also the palmar aspect of the digits and thumb (Fig. 57 C and D.) On the dorsum it includes the distal portions of the same digits. In

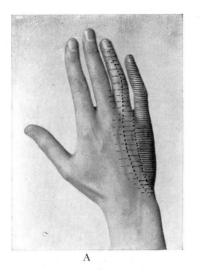

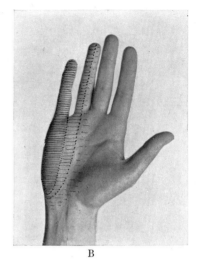

A   B

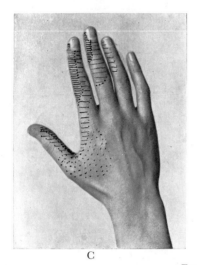

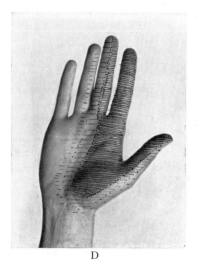

C   D

Fig. 57.

A and B. Sensory Loss in Ulnar Paralysis.   C and D. Sensory Loss in
Median and Radial Nerve Paralysis.

A and B—The dorsal and palmar aspects of the hand showing the extent and
degree of sensory loss after complete division of the ulnar nerve. The most deeply
shaded area shows complete cutaneous anæsthesia, loss of vibration, and postural
sensibility. Surrounding this is a zone of tactile anæsthesia and marked hypoæsthesia to thermal and painful stimuli, with an outer zone of relative hypoæsthesia
to all forms of sensibility merging at its periphery into normal sensibility (lighter
shading).

C and D.—The area and depth of sensory loss following a complete lesion of the
median nerve is shown in the same manner as in A and B. On the dorsum of the
hand the usual distribution of sensory loss from a lesion of the radial nerve is
marked by dots.

To face page 287.

incomplete lesions a less extensive area of altered sensibility may be present. In addition to these objective motor and sensory phenomena, in incomplete lesions of the nerve there may be marked tenderness of the paretic muscles, severe pain in the distribution of the nerve, the so-called "causalgia," and trophic changes in the skin and nails of the affected area. Thus the nails may be rounded and furrowed, and the skin shiny and atrophic.

Prognosis and Treatment.—The prospects of recovery in severe lesions is by no means so good as in the case of the musculo-spiral nerve. In traumatic lesions resection and resuture may be called for.

THE ULNAR NERVE.—This nerve is more commonly injured than the median. Isolated lesions are generally traumatic. The nerve may be crushed in fractures of the internal condyle (medial epicondyle) of the humerus, or may become later involved in callus formation after such a fracture. The paralysis of the nerve in the latter case is gradual and may be long delayed. The nerve may be exposed to repeated minor injuries, as it lies behind the condyle, and develop a neuritis with paralytic symptoms. An isolated toxic neuritis of the nerve occasionally follows some infection.

Symptomatology.—When the ulnar nerve is damaged the following muscles are affected: flexor carpi ulnaris, flexor profundis (two inner bellies), the hypothenar muscles, the interossei, the two inner lumbricals and the adductors of the thumb. Flexion of the wrist is weakened, adduction of the hand is weak, as also is flexion of the ring and little fingers. Flexion of the extended fingers at the metacarpo-phalangeal joint by the interossei is lost, but flexion of the distal phalanges (claw position of the fingers) is retained. It is the paralysis of the interossei which gives rise to the characteristic and severe disability of the hand in ulnar nerve paralysis, for abduction and adduction of the digits is also lost. The paralysis of the adductors of the thumb impairs prehension and this is readily seen if a piece of paper is taken at each end by the finger and thumb of each hand. On the normal side the extended thumb is strongly adducted against the side of the index, while on the affected side, this movement being impossible, the terminal segment of the thumb is strongly flexed and the thumb opposed.

Sensory loss is not invariably present in partial lesions, but when complete it includes the ulnar margin of the hand, the little finger and the ulnar side of the ring finger. Loss to pin-prick is usually confined to the little finger and a narrower zone of the hand than loss for tactile sensibility (Fig. 57, A and B).

In long-standing cases, a partial claw hand is produced (in the little and ring fingers) by the overaction of the opponens of the interossei, and the fingers become hyperextended at the proximal and flexed at the distal joints.

LESIONS OF THE LUMBAR AND SACRAL PLEXUSES

The lumbar and sacral plexuses and the peripheral nerves of the lower limb are much less frequently affected than the plexus and nerves of the upper limb. Isolated paralyses of anterior crural (femoral) or obturator nerves are rare, and while the sciatic nerve is more frequently the seat of disease, it is rarely completely paralysed apart from gunshot wounds.

THE SCIATIC NERVE.—The nerve trunk, or the roots which enter into its formation, may be involved by tumours of the sacrum or in the pelvis, or by a syphilitic radiculitis. The nerve is sometimes the seat of an interstitial neuritis which is the pathological process sometimes responsible for sciatica, a condition which has already been described (page 272). In total paralysis of the nerve there is foot-drop and loss of dorsiflexion, so that when walking the limb has to be lifted high for the toe and foot to clear the ground. There is no muscular power below the knee, and the hamstrings may also be weak when the lesion is high in the thigh. The paralysed muscles waste profoundly, and there is loss of all modes of sensation over the outer and posterior aspect of the lower two-thirds of the leg, over the external malleolus and the tendo achilles. Surrounding this area of total loss is a zone of partial sensory loss. The skin below the knee may be dry and there is hyperkeratosis of the foot and toes. The nails become thick and curved. Trophic lesions may develop within the anæsthetic area and the foot may become red and œdematous. The ankle jerk is lost, but the knee jerk remains intact. Paralysis of this severe order is usually the result of direct injury, as by knife or gunshot wound.

In damage to the nerve from pelvic lesions, tumours or compression exerted by the fœtal head in pregnant women, it is the peroneal division of the nerve which bears the brunt of the damage.

THE PERONEAL NERVE.—Special emphasis should be laid upon the isolated affection of this nerve since it is not uncommon. It may occur in otherwise healthy adults quite apart from discoverable local injury. In these circumstances its ætiology is unknown. Its appearance is often preceded by pain along the outer side of the leg. After this has been present for two or three days a sudden paralysis, usually severe in degree, of all the muscles supplied by the nerve is seen. The foot hangs loosely down in the position of equino-varus. The patient can stand on tiptoe, but he cannot dorsiflex the foot and he cannot run. There is sensory loss of varying degree over the outer aspect of the leg and on the dorsum of the foot to the base of the toes. After some weeks a degree of wasting of the affected muscles makes its appearance, but is rarely profound. Recovery is very slow and frequently incomplete. Among the special circumstances in which this nerve may be paralysed are compression of the nerve trunk by a gaiter or a bandage round the upper end of the fibula where the nerve winds round the bone. In diabetes, and occasionally in typhoid, this nerve may be the seat of a neuritis. Treatment consists in the wearing of a foot-drop support by day and of a night shoe when in bed, so that the foot is constantly kept at right angles to the line of the leg.

THE TIBIAL OR MEDIAL POPLITEAL NERVE.—Apart from gunshot wounds and comparable injuries, isolated paralysis of this division of the sciatic nerve is uncommon. In complete lesions the symptoms are paralysis of the calf and plantar muscles and sensory loss over the sole of the foot and the posterior aspect of the leg in its lower half. The atrophy of the plantar muscles renders the sole hollow, the proximal segment of the toes is hyperextended and the terminal segments flexed. Perforating plantar ulcers may develop when sensory loss is complete.

THE ANTERIOR CRURAL (FEMORAL) NERVE.—Paralysis of this nerve is very rare, and when it occurs is the result of pelvic injuries. The symptoms are paralysis of ilio-psoas, pectineus, sartorius, and quadriceps. There is loss of the knee jerk and weakness of extension of the knee. There may be sensory change on the anterior and medial aspects of the thigh. An uncommon malady is an interstitial neuritis of the lateral cutaneous nerve of the thigh, known as *meralgia paræsthetica*. It occurs in males, and its symptoms are pains, paræsthesia, and slight objective changes in sensibility in the territory of this nerve on the front and lateral aspect of the thigh. The symptoms are brought on by standing or walking.

GENERAL OBSERVATIONS UPON THE TREATMENT OF PERIPHERAL NERVE PARALYSES

The muscles paralysed from a lesion of a peripheral nerve are flaccid and proceed to waste until no contractile tissue is left when they are completely denervated. This wasting is accompanied by fibrillation, and finally the muscle is reduced to a fibrous band which tends gradually to shorten. This process is facilitated if the paralysed muscles are stretched, and it is clear that should innervation ultimately be restored the final result will be imperfect in proportion to the degree to which stretching has been allowed to occur. It follows, then, that the careful splinting of a paralysed muscle is of paramount importance, and should be taken in hand without delay. The principles which govern splinting are as follows:—(1) A paralysed muscle should be splinted in such a position that its origin and insertion are approximated as closely as possible. (2) Prolonged immobilization is contra-indicated unless enforced by accompanying bone or joint injury. In a paralysed limb the joints should be allowed as free a range of movement as is possible without undue stretching of the muscles. (3) Splints should be such as to allow of remedial and occupational activities. The splints should be removed for

T

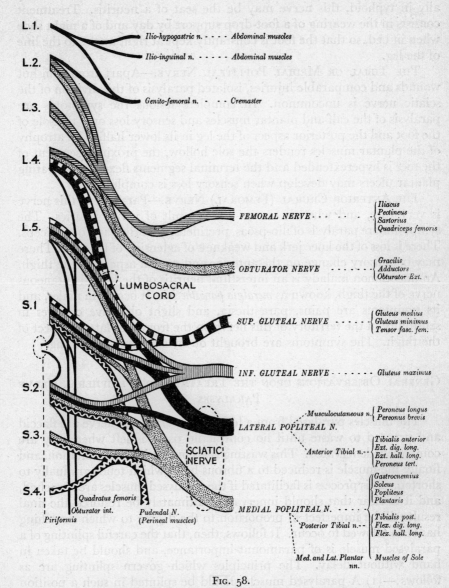

L.1. — Ilio-hypogastric n. - - - - Abdominal muscles

L.2. — Ilio-inguinal n. - - - - - Abdominal muscles

L.3. — Genito-femoral n. - - - - Cremaster

L.4.

L.5.

FEMORAL NERVE - - - - - - - {Iliacus / Pectineus / Sartorius / Quadriceps femoris}

OBTURATOR NERVE - - - - - - {Gracilis / Adductors / Obturator Ext.}

LUMBOSACRAL CORD

S.1.

SUP. GLUTEAL NERVE - - - - - {Gluteus medius / Gluteus minimus / Tensor fasc. fem.}

INF. GLUTEAL NERVE - - - - - - Gluteus maximus

S.2.

Musculocutaneous n. {Peroneus longus / Pereonus brevis}

LATERAL POPLITEAL N.

S.3.

Anterior Tibial n. {Tibialis anterior / Ext. dig. long. / Ext. hall. long. / Peroneus tert.}

SCIATIC NERVE

S.4.

Quadratus femoris
Obturator int.   Pudendal N.
Piriformis   (Perineal muscles)

MEDIAL POPLITEAL N. - - - - {Gastrocnemius / Soleus / Popliteus / Plantaris}

Posterior Tibial n. {Tibialis post. / Flex. dig. long. / Flex. hall. long.}

Med. and Lat. Plantar nn. | Muscles of Sole

FIG. 58.

THE LUMBOSACRAL PLEXUS AND ITS MOTOR INNERVATION.

The right lumbosacral plexus seen from behind. The peripheral and radicular innervation of the muscles is indicated. Sensory supply is not shown.

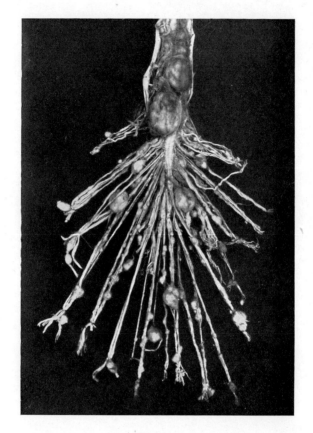

Fig. 59.

THE LOWER END OF THE SPINAL CORD AND THE CAUDA
EQUINA, SHOWING VERY NUMEROUS NEUROFIBROMATA ON
THE SURFACE OF THE CORD AND STUDDING THE ROOTS OF
THE CAUDA.

To face page 291.

two periods of half an hour daily, when the muscles are massaged and all joints passively moved. There can be no doubt that the best results are obtained when experienced orthopædic treatment in an appropriate clinic is available.

NEUROMA

The nerves may be the seat of tumours which are known as neuromata. In the *true neuroma*, or ganglioneuroma, nerve fibres and ganglion cells form part of the structure of the tumour. This rare form of neuroma is found only in connection with the sympathetic nervous system in the thoracic or abdominal cavities. The *false neuroma*, or neurofibroma, is not uncommon. It arises in the connective tissue of the nerve and may be central, separating the nerve fibre bundles or situated at the side of the nerve trunk. It may be the seat of cystic or myxomatous degeneration. Neurofibromata may be single or multiple, and in the latter case the tumours may be confined to a single nerve or nerve plexus, or be widely diffused. In size they vary from tiny nodules to large masses of several inches diameter. They are congenital, of unknown origin, and may be found in epileptic or mentally defective subjects. It is the solitary neurofibroma which is usually responsible for symptoms, and these consist in pain along the course of the nerve, and also, though rarely, in objective sensory and motor symptoms. In *multiple neurofibromatosis* innumerable tumours of soft consistence stud all the peripheral nerves. Occurring on cranial or spinal nerve roots they may produce compression symptoms. Neurofibroma on the auditory nerve forms the so-called *acoustic* tumour, or tumour of the ponto-cerebellar angle.

When multiple neurofibromatosis is associated with cutaneous pigmentation and the presence of multiple sessile and pedunculated tumours on the skin, the condition is known as *von Recklinghausen's Disease* or *Molluscum fibrosum*.

Tubercula dolorosa is the name given to collections of tiny neurofibromata situated on the terminal twigs of cutaneous nerves, and giving rise to considerable tenderness and pain.

All these forms of tumours on nerves tend to be progressive, but do not call for treatment unless pain, or, in the case of tumours within the skull and vertebral canal, signs of compression of adjacent structures occur. In these circumstances the offending tumour may be removed when possible (Fig. 59).

CHAPTER XXIII

Some Common Nervous Affections of Infancy and Childhood

AMONG the many congenital abnormalities, infantile affections and injuries of the nervous system a few are of relatively common occurrence. These include cerebral diplegia, congenital hydrocephalus, infantile hemiplegia, cerebral and peripheral birth palsies and, finally, nocturnal enuresis in children.

CEREBRAL DIPLEGIA

Ætiology.—It was long held that the different clinical forms of diplegia were all related to injuries sustained by the brain during labour and delivery. The pathological evidence indicates that such injury plays no part and that pre-natal factors such as agenesis of certain systems of neurones or their destruction by disease during intra-uterine existence are invariably responsible. The diplegic child is commonly the firstborn of its mother and its birth is as often easy and precipitate as difficult and prolonged. It is very rare for a mother to give birth to more than one diplegic child and her subsequent children are usually normal.

Pathology.—The characteristic naked-eye lesion is atrophy of the cerebral hemispheres, varying in degree and extent in different cases. The affected parts of the hemisphere present shrunken convolutions and gaping sulci. Microscopically, there are atrophy of the parenchymatous elements with secondary neuroglial overgrowth. The pyramidal system is specially prone to be affected.

Symptoms.—The child may be small at birth and have difficulty in sucking. In some cases, however, no early abnormality is noted. In some the child is intensely spastic from birth, but in others attention is first aroused by the child's failure to hold its head up, to sit up and to stand at the proper age periods. Later a failure to talk, or rather a delay in learning to do so, becomes obvious.

In the spastic type there is generalized spasticity most marked in, or perhaps confined to, the legs. The latter are rigidly extended and adducted and the adductor spasm may be so strong that the legs are crossed like the blades of a scissors. When the child is over a year old and is held erect with the feet to the ground this crossing is marked. The feet are plantarflexed and the child cannot get his heels to the ground. Although there is usually considerable voluntary power, the spasticity virtually immobilizes the limbs. When the arms escape, this condition is known as *congenital spastic paraplegia* or *Little's disease*. Such children are frequently normal mentally, but when there is also involvement of the arms a measure of mental defect is usually present.

Another type is that known as *bilateral athetosis*. Here the essential lesion is believed to be in the corpora striata. The entire skeletal musculature is the seat of those writhing movements already described (page 28) under the name of mobile spasm. These render co-ordinated movement impossible. They tend to increase for several years before becoming stationary. The degree of disability that ensues varies from complete helplessness to lesser degrees that permit of some use of all the limbs. Some mental defect is often present. In a few cases the involuntary movements more closely resemble those of chorea. In all cases there may be recurrent epileptic fits.

Treatment.—The cases that offer prospect of useful response to treatment are those of Little's disease where the patient's mental development is normal or approximately so. Remedial exercises and, when necessary, carefully thought out tenotomies or motor nerve sections may greatly increase the patient's mobility.

INFANTILE HEMIPLEGIA
(ACUTE CEREBRAL PALSY OF CHILDHOOD)

Hemiplegia of acute onset is not uncommon in young children during the first five years of life. It is usually primary, that is to say, it develops acutely without preceding illness. It is, however, an occasional sequel of scarlet fever, measles, severe whooping cough, or even mumps. The onset is usually accompanied by severe convulsions which recur in quick succession for some hours, the child subsequently being found to have a hemiplegia. The initial fits are commonly unilateral, may have a focal onset and be accompanied by fever and sickness. A phase of coma may ensue upon the convulsions.

The hemiplegia may be accompanied by sensory loss, or, when right-sided by aphasia, but both these symptoms are short-lived, and the child who survives has a pure motor hemiplegia.

The prognosis depends upon the initial severity of the paralysis, but in the majority of instances, a severe degree of residual hemiparesis remains, and the affected limbs do not grow normally, so that in later life they are shorter and smaller than their fellows.

This hemiparesis is accompanied by a varying degree of spasticity and by the changes in the reflexes characteristic of the hemiplegia of adults, though the abdominal reflexes on the affected side usually return to normal within a few years, and the extensor plantar response may not be well developed.

Another common sequel is a degree of mental defect, varying from the slightest to profound idiocy, and unilateral epileptiform convulsions may appear and recur throughout life.

Perhaps most characteristic of infantile hemiplegia is the development of mobile spasm (athetosis) in the affected limbs. This may increase in severity over a period of years and become profoundly disabling.

Ætiology.—Two views compete for acceptance as to the origin of the condition: one—probably the correct one in the majority of instances —is that the illness is due to arterial thrombosis, or, as Gowers suggests, to thrombosis in cortical veins; the other, that it is due to an encephalitis ("polio-encephalitis") of infective origin. The virus of acute poliomyelitis has been incriminated in this regard, but probably wrongly, and in most cases a vascular lesion is probable.

Pathology.—When the thrombosis is arterial a cavity may be found in the hemisphere of the patient dying in later life, the condition being known as porencephaly. In other cases, there is no gross destruction of cerebral tissue, and Gowers suggested that these may be cases of cortical venous thrombosis.

Treatment.—When athetosis and mental defect, with or without convulsions, are present, nothing can be done to ameliorate the patient's condition, but in milder cases and normal mental development, athetosis being minimal or absent, some improvement may be attained by careful active exercises.

HYDROCEPHALUS : CONGENITAL AND ACQUIRED

Any lesion or developmental abnormality that prevents the outflow of cerebrospinal fluid from the ventricles into the subarachnoid space, or its absorption from the latter into the venous system, will cause it to accumulate within and to distend the ventricles. This distension is known as internal hydrocephalus.

In infants this distension leads to enlargement of the cerebral hemispheres and of the skull.

Ætiology and Pathology.—In about a third of all cases of congenital hydrocephalus there is a developmental defect, usually an atresia or imperfect development of the aqueduct of Sylvius. In other cases the ventricular foramina of exit are blocked by inflammatory exudates, or the space in the opening of the tentorium is similarly occluded. In the remainder a new growth effects a block somewhere in the cerebrospinal fluid system.

In congenital cases the head may be of normal size at birth, enlarging rapidly thereafter, or it may be greatly enlarged at birth, sometimes to such a degree as to render a living delivery impossible. The cerebral hemispheres become reduced to thin-walled cysts and the entire head may be capable of transillumination. The sutures separate and the fontanelles bulge, and from depression of the orbital plates the eyes bulge and look downwards.

Symptoms.—When the head is of normal size at birth it enlarges with great rapidity. This process may be progressive and may end in death, or it may cease relatively early before any gross enlargement or much physical disability or mental defect has developed. In the progressive cases primary optic atrophy and blindness ensue and the child succumbs in the early months. In less severe cases there is survival with a greater or less degree of physical and mental disability. Other congenital abnormalities may also be present: *e.g.* spina bifida, etc. After postbasic meningitis in infancy (or after meningococcal meningitis later in life) inflammatory exudates lead, as already described, to internal hydrocephalus. In the infant there is the same sequence of signs and symptoms as have been enumerated. In older persons there is no visible enlargement of the head.

The head of the hydrocephalic child, whether enlarged or not, may present a "cracked pot" note on percussion.

Treatment.—No success has so far attended surgical efforts to reestablish a free cerebrospinal fluid circulation and hydrocephalus remains an incurable condition.

CEREBRAL BIRTH PALSIES

Intracranial hæmorrhage is not uncommon in the newborn, is found in the majority of stillborn children and in those who die within two weeks of birth. There is no doubt that it plays a major part in the production of cerebral birth palsies, the characteristic expression of which is hemiplegia with or without athetosis.

Ætiology.—Injury to the head during delivery is the essential causative factor, and the varieties of damage done include tearing of the falx associated with moulding of the head and overriding of the parietal bones, and rupture of veins entering the dural sinuses. The hæmorrhage thus caused may be subarachnoid, subdural, or intracerebral. It is probable that the factor mainly operative in producing cerebral birth palsies is not the hæmorrhage itself, but the anoxia which follows the stretching, kinking and compression of blood-vessels which accompany the distortions of the head during labour and delivery. The extreme sensitiveness of nervous tissue to oxygen want has been mentioned (page 93) in the chapter on vascular disease of the brain. These lesions are prone to occur in cases of deformed or contracted pelvis, abnormal presentations, high forceps delivery, and breech presentations.

Pathology.—Areas of cortical atrophy underlie subdural collections of blood, and cysts may form in one hemisphere (porencephaly).

Symptoms.—At birth the child may show a pallid asphyxia with generalized or focal convulsions. The pulse may be slow, or rapid and irregular. The child sucks badly and is feeble, and most cases presenting these symptoms do not long survive. Those who survive and later develop hemiplegia may present no untoward symptoms at birth.

Hemiplegia ensues, severe in some cases, less so in others. The degree of recovery that occurs depends upon the initial severity. When recovery is imperfect the affected limbs do not develop normally and always remain smaller and shorter than their fellows. Sooner or later athetosis develops in the affected limbs in all but the mildest cases. Epilepsy may also make its appearance at some time during childhood.

Treatment.—With severe paralysis and spasticity or athetosis not much improvement can be looked for. In mild cases, active exercises form the essential element in treatment. Massage is of minor importance and electro-therapy is absolutely contra-indicated.

SPINAL BIRTH PALSIES

It has been shown that infants dying during breech presentations have commonly sustained severe damage to the vertebral column and spinal cord, the level of these lesions being the cervical region. In cases that survive the thoracic region is commonly affected and a paraplegia ensues. Such cases are comparatively rare and require the same treatment as the paraplegias of adults.

PERIPHERAL BIRTH PALSIES

Ætiology.—The seat of injury is the brachial plexus, and traction on the arm the common cause. The bringing down of the elevated arm in a breech presentation, or the attempt to bring down the arm in a head presentation may cause rotation of the clavicle which presses upon the component nerves of the plexus. The damage is usually unilateral, but the writer has seen a bilateral brachial plexus palsy caused by movements of the arms carried out to induce respiration in a newborn child.

Symptoms.—The roots damaged are the fifth and sixth cervical, and the muscles paralysed the deltoid, biceps, brachialis anticus, supinator longus, supinator brevis, and infraspinatus. The arm lies with the humerus rotated inwards, the forearm extended, and the hand so pronated that the palm faces forwards. Paralysis of the lower components of the plexus is less common. In this case the muscles of the hand and forearm are paralysed, and the limb is held abducted and slightly elevated at the shoulder. There may be associated bony damage and a cervical sympathetic palsy.

Sensory loss is exceptional in upper plexus paralysis, but lower plexus paralysis is usually more severe and accompanied by sensory loss over the forearm and lateral aspect of the upper arm.

Course and Prognosis.—The plexus lesions of the newborn progress much more favourably than those of adults, and save in the most severe cases recovery is the rule within a few months. Lower plexus lesions and all lesions accompanied by bony damage recover less well.

Treatment.—The principles governing treatment are those obtaining in the case of other peripheral nerve injuries. The paralysed muscles are placed in the position of shortening; that is, with the arm elevated and abducted in the case of upper plexus lesions. This should be done without delay, the muscles being gently massaged and given passive movements of small excursion daily. As soon as possible the limb should be allowed to move actively. Electrical stimulation of the affected muscles cannot be recommended.

ENURESIS IN CHILDREN

It is generally assumed that the problem of nocturnal bedwetting is entirely a psychological one, yet from what has been said of the complex of factors we speak of as ætiology it is inherently unlikely that the matter can be so simple. That there may be a physiological factor, namely, some disorder of the complex process of urinary secretion, is generally ignored, and attention is directed exclusively to the "kind of child" that wets his bed, to his parents, and home. These factors do indeed call for consideration, but until we know more of the clinical and other physiological aspects of bedwetting, we cannot accept explanations based wholly upon psychological hypotheses. These do not come properly into consideration until the physiological problem is understood.

It is said that while some of the subjects are highly-strung, others are phlegmatic and free from all indications of instability or maladaptation to their environments. There is no psychological type more prone to enuresis than another, and the great majority of unstable children do not suffer from this habit. There is no constant relation between enuresis and intelligence. The habit is found throughout the social scale, and irrespective of the hygienic conditions under which the child is reared. In short, the bedwetting child is quite remarkably like other children in all respects save this habit, and the psychological case is not wholly convincing. It may well be that there is more than one category of bedwetting child, one in which physiological and another in which psychological factors predominate, and it must be said that no thoroughgoing study of this problem from all relevant aspects has yet been made. It is a matter of reproach that this should still be so.

The *clinical details* of bedwetting, with which the exponents of the psychogenic hypothesis have never greatly concerned themselves, are as follows: boys are more often affected than girls, and the habit usually ceases at about the age of twelve years. The enuresis commonly occurs within two hours of going to sleep, and a remarkably large quantity of urine is passed when we remember that the child is almost invariably made to empty his bladder immediately before going to bed. It appears that the secretion of urine during this initial period of sleep is abnormally great in these patients, who are usually very deep sleepers. Both these features point to a physiological rather than to a psychological disorder, and indeed it would be astonishing were a purely psychological factor responsible for a somatic disorder of function that characteristically takes place during deep sleep: that is, when psychological activity is probably absent. In this connection it is interesting to recall that the hypothalamus plays an essential part in the regulation of sleep and in the liberation of the so-called "anti-diuretic hormone" by the pars posterior of the pituitary, and also that this hormone has been stated to be ineffective during deep sleep. It is not possible to say how relevant these facts may be to the phenomena of nocturnal enuresis, but they suggest that there is a physiological problem awaiting study before we fly off on the wings of psychological speculation.

A few children show also diurnal enuresis and even fæcal incontinence, and the probability, already mentioned, that there may be more than one ætiological variety of enuresis has never been taken into account. It is possible that a variety in which psychological factors predominate is the one that is said to respond to psychotherapy, while the cases that do not so respond—and they are not few—are predominantly, if not wholly, physiological in origin.

From this statement it will be seen that bedwetting in children, although the subject of much speculation and dogmatic statement, must so far be regarded as imperfectly studied and not understood. The problem is probably far less simple than we have been led to believe.

Treatment.—A preliminary investigation should be made to exclude the presence of organic factors such as spina bifida, or a local lesion of the urinary tract, or abnormality in the urine. The usual devices in the management of the child should be adopted—namely, restriction of fluid intake after tea-time, and the emptying of the bladder immediately before going to bed. When, as is usually the case, the child is a deep sleeper he may be made to micturate again about an hour after going to bed. There is as yet nothing to surpass the old-fashioned mixture containing belladonna and strychnine (tincture of Belladonna ℳ 10 to 15, Liq. Strychnine ℳ 1 to 2, t.d.s.).

Defects in the child's environment in so far as they are capable of improvement should be attended to. Sometimes a short period of hospitalization will give relief, but it has to be confessed that in many instances the habit persists until the usual age of its disappearance arrives, but it would be illogical to conclude that the frequent failure of such routine lines of treatment as are now available, implies that the problem is necessarily psychological.

CHAPTER XXIV

Bromide Intoxication

THIS form of intoxication, not rare though rarely recognized, calls for brief mention. It arises partly because the cumulative effects of continued bromide medication, particularly in elderly persons, are not duly appreciated and partly because the exaggerated notion held by some of the toxic properties of the barbiturates lead them to use large doses of bromide, over long periods of time, in preference.

Ætiology.—Bromides replace the chlorides in the body fluids, and it has been found experimentally in animals that when the replacement reaches a level of 40 per cent, death ensues. This replacement seems to occur more readily in elderly arterio-sclerotic subjects than in young persons, and may in some of the former develop rapidly with the appearance of toxic symptoms. Unfortunately, these symptoms are often attributed to other causes than the bromide and may even lead to an increase in the dosage given. Thus, the restlessness and sleeplessness of the subject of a recent prostatectomy may be treated by regular bromide administration, and when mental confusion is added to the picture more bromide is given to combat it so that the subject becomes demented and drowsy, may develop symptoms suggestive of a cerebral vascular lesion and lapse into stupor and a terminal broncho-pneumonia. Again, it may be deemed unsafe to allow a case of depression or of anxiety neurosis with insomnia to administer phenylbarbitone to himself, he is, therefore, given large doses of bromide in the belief that they are perfectly safe.

Subjects of the following types may be regarded as peculiarly susceptible to bromism: arterio-sclerotics, subjects with anæmia, with organic cardiac disease, or impaired renal efficiency. The older the subject the greater the susceptibility. There is also a wide variation of the toxic threshold in different persons, so that the careful watch for toxic symptoms is advisable.

The normal blood bromide level appears to range from 0·5 to 2 mgms. per 100 c.cms. of serum, and toxic symptoms tend to appear when a level of 225 to 250 mgms. is reached or passed. The threshold, however, is not uniform and in some subjects a level of 150 mgms. may be associated with toxic symptoms.

Symptoms.—In mild cases the patient becomes forgetful, finds difficulty in mental concentration and is apt to be drowsy. In the severe cases any pre-existing mental obfuscation is aggravated. The patient is disoriented and incoherent in speech. His tongue is dry and coated, his speech slurred and his movements unsteady. A certain number of individuals respond by becoming confused and excitable, or even semi-maniacal. From such a degree of bromism recovery takes as long as from seven to fourteen days after the drug is discontinued. In fatal cases the patient lapses into a muttering delirium, is feeble and tremulous, usually incontinent of urine and fæces. He looks ill, wastes, has a dry skin and coated tongue. A terminal pneumonia with coma ends the clinical course.

The incoherence and articulatory defects may lead to a diagnosis of cerebral thrombosis, and the writer has known this to happen in several cases of elderly persons kept on bromide to relieve the insomnia and discomforts following upon operative procedures.

Treatment.—Bromide must be at once discontinued. In severely intoxicated cases large quantities of fluid are given by mouth, and, if necessary, normal saline intravenously. Salt should be given by mouth in solution. If diagnosis be uncertain the blood bromide should be measured. The test cannot be performed except in a properly equipped laboratory, where it can be rapidly and simply carried out. From 2 to 4 c.cms. of serum are required for the test. Finally, in elderly persons, phenobarbitone is a safer and better tolerated drug than bromide for regular medication over any considerable period of time.

CHAPTER XXV

Some General Observations upon the Treatment of Nervous Diseases

I T is widely assumed that organic diseases of the nervous system are more generally incapable of amelioration and cure than are those of other organs and systems. Yet one has only to mention hepatic cirrhosis, the leukæmias, bacterial endocarditis or atheroma to show that the generalization is far from valid. What is true is that a longer period of survival is common with nervous disease than with visceral disease, and this fact and the often grave disability of the sufferer lend an air of hopelessness to the therapeutic problems involved. There is, nevertheless, much truth in the paradox that the more incurable a case of nervous disease the more treatment it requires. If the morale of the sufferer is to be maintained during the long years of his disablement and if he is to be saved from cruel exploitation by charlatans, the greatest patience and judgment are called for in his treatment and general management. Some brief generalizations as to what can be hoped for from the resources at our disposal and what these cannot provide are therefore of importance.

PHYSIOTHERAPY. (Massage and electro-therapy).—In respect of *massage and active remedial exercises* it is necessary to be clear at the outset that in the case of organic nervous disease they have no direct influence upon the pathological process and in that sense they cannot be spoken of as curative. Their purpose is to maintain muscles and joints in as healthy a state of nutrition as possible until normal conditions of innervation and movement are restored, and, in respect of remedial exercises, to help in the re-education of voluntary movements. Thus in a lower motor neurone paralysis of the legs (*e.g.* that of poliomyelitis) the dependent limb tends to become cold and cyanosed and sometimes œdematous. From prolonged immobility atrophic changes occur in muscles and in joints and contracture of muscles and fixation of joints may develop. It is the function of massage and even more of active exercises to improve the local circulation, and to maintain the normal mobility of joints. It is not their function to cure paralysis, and they cannot do so. Active exercises help to aid recovery from wasting and get the best out of such contractile muscle tissue as remains.

In the case of upper motor neurone paralysis, judiciously administered massage may sometimes relieve spasm and abnormal postures and increase freedom of movement in joints. For example, in hemiplegia it is important from the outset to maintain a full mobility of the shoulder joint in which adhesions may form rapidly, especially when the left arm is in question because there is a natural tendency to abandon this arm to its fate and to use the normal right arm and hand whenever a purposive movement is needed. In this type of paralysis active exercises are of great importance when the patient's general health, mental state and expectation of life justify a hope of some useful restoration of function.

The hemiplegic arm and hand tend to become generally flexed, and this tendency must be counteracted from the first by placing the arm alongside the body in an extended position with both wrist and digits also extended. As soon as movement reappears, the subject must be encouraged to use the limb for simple movements. The tendency of the digits to flex may be controlled by placing a large rubber sponge on the palmar aspect and fixing it there by an elastic band passed round it and the hand. Against the resistance thus provided the patient can carry out simple flexion movements of his fingers. Later, he should be persuaded to handle small objects such as dominoes, marbles, or draughtsmen. Sometimes the intermittent wearing of a light splint to keep hand and fingers extended may be advisable. Whenever possible the active use of the hand should be encouraged, for this is of far greater value than any passive manipulation.

In hemiplegia and spastic paraplegia while the patient is still bed-ridden the extended legs should be kept adducted, almost fully extended at the knees and should be prevented from rotating out. The feet should be kept at a right angle to the line of the legs and a cradle placed over the limbs. Gentle passive movements from time to time and later assisted active movements are useful.

It is not possible to make any decisively favourable claims for *electro-therapy* in the treatment of organic nervous disease. In lower motor neurone paralysis there is no convincing evidence that any form of electrical stimulation of muscles averts wasting or accelerates recovery—a hard statement likely to be as unwelcome to doctor as to patient, but nevertheless well substantiated. When used as a substitute for active exercises and passive manipulation, electrical stimulation of paralysed and wasted muscles may be definitely harmful. In facial palsy recovery is commonly achieved with or without treatment, and in slowly recovering cases and especially in elderly persons the galvanic stimulation of the muscles leads to distressing contracture and should on no account be employed.

In upper motor neurone paralysis electrical stimulation increases spasticity and is contra-indicated. A similar objection holds in the case of paralysis agitans, in which both rigidity and tremor are aggravated by electrical stimulation of muscles. In progressive muscular atrophy it tends to exhaust an already failing musculature. In such painful conditions as sciatica or brachial neuritis electrical currents (diathermy, ionization) should be reserved for the chronic stage of intractable cases and not employed in the early and active stage of the malady. It seems clear that ionization can never do more than produce some local warmth since the affected structures are too deeply seated to be reached by the liberated ions. In short, except for its psychological influence electrotherapy is a method of negligible value and one sometimes harmful in the treatment of nervous disease.

Various forms of radio-therapy are now in use, but apart from the use of radiant heat lamps for painful and stiff muscles and joints in association with massage, they have no special place in the treatment of nervous diseases.

THE CARE OF THE PARAPLEGIC PATIENT.—In spinal cord compression, transverse myelitis, or advanced disseminated sclerosis the most important element in the treatment is the nursing care of the patient. He should be nursed on a water or rubber bed over a fracture board. The legs should be in the position of extension and adduction already referred to. The heels should be placed in rings made of wool and bandaging, and the knees and ankles separated by a pad of cotton wool if there be strong adductor spasm. Hot-water bottles should be covered and placed outside the blanket. The undersheet should be kept as free from creases as possible, especially under the buttocks. It may be necessary for part at least of the twenty-four-hour period to have an air ring beneath the buttocks. The weight of the body on this region tends to stop the cutaneous circulation, the skin reddens and, unless the patient be turned slightly on one side from time to time, it chafes, and the epidermis rubs off or necroses.

The pressure points, sacrum, buttocks, trochanters and heels should be washed at least twice daily with soap and warm water, or in the case of a total paraplegia with complete sensory loss, four-hourly. The skin must be carefully dried without undue rubbing, then massaged with spirit or eau-de-Cologne (as long as the surface is intact) and dusted with zinc oxide powder or a powder consisting of starch and zinc oxide. If a hæmorrhagic blister develop over the sacrum it should be carefully snipped and emptied and the skin left in position. Once an area of necrosis develops and separation of a slough begins a boracic or peroxide compress should be applied for a half-hour period twice daily, and the lesion then dressed with a zinc-oxide castor oil paste. Once a separation is complete, further treatment with compresses or with an antiseptic dressing should be employed to clean the ulcer, when paste may again be applied. A chronic, slowly healing ulcer may be given red lotion compresses.

If there be retention of urine, with or without overflow, the bladder should be carefully catheterized thrice daily. Some now prefer to have a suprapubic cystotomy in chronic cases, or to adopt Monro's method of tidal drainage. The last-named requires the willing and skilled attention of a nurse or attendant, and is, therefore, largely restricted to institutional use. But both the latter methods lessen the infection of the bladder and urinary tract that acts so adversely upon all spinal cord lesions.

In patients with incontinence of urine or fæces every effort should be made to prevent or to minimize the wetting of the skin. The precipitancy and slighter incontinence of many cases of spinal cord disease may be helped by the following pill: Ext. Belladonna, gr. $\frac{1}{4}$; Ergotin (Bonjean), gr. i. Ft. Pil. Sig. i. t.d.s.

The flexion spasms of the developing paraplegia-in-flexion are often impossible to prevent since they indicate the increasing dominance of spiral reflexes as higher levels are cut off from the spinal centres by the progress of the lesion. Counter-extension of the limbs is usually contra-indicated as it may aggravate the tendency to flexion and involves much friction of the skin of the moving limbs. Codeine in doses of from gr. $\frac{1}{4}$ to gr. $\frac{1}{2}$ t.d.s. sometimes reduces the force of the spasms. In other cases a combination of soluble phenobarbitone (gr. $\frac{1}{2}$) with tincture of stramonium ($\mathfrak{M}$15) and hyoscine hydrobromide (gr. $\frac{1}{100}$) may be tried.

VITAMIN THERAPY IN ORGANIC NERVOUS DISEASES.—Various references have been made to this subject throughout the text in connection with diseases in which this mode of therapy has been employed, and for which it has been said to be beneficial. In no case, so far, has it been possible, upon a critical view of the evidence, to make any decisively favourable claims. The role that vitamins play in the nutrition of the individual has been defined with differing degrees of precision and completeness according to which member of this group of substances is concerned. Yet, however clear this role may be in the maintenance of normal health, the problems involved in the restoration of health when, through deficiency of one or more vitamins, this has been impaired, appear considerably more complex and obscure. In acute infantile beri-beri, a cardiac illness, it is true that the administration of substances containing the B complex may have dramatic results; while pellagra, a malady not considered in this book, is also known to respond to the B_2 complex. Yet in the case of polyneuritis, in which vitamin B_1 or the B complex as a whole might, upon theoretical grounds, be expected to give clear indications of therapeutic usefulness, the results have been singularly disappointing. Thus, a study of all the cases of alcoholic polyneuritis admitted to a Boston hospital over a period of ten years, has shown no improvement whatever in the recovery rate during the later years of this period in which intensive vitamin therapy has been added to the therapeutic resources previously available. The present writer's experience conforms to the results thus cited. The probability that B_1

U

has no function in relation to the nervous system has already been mentioned on page 253.

These disappointments may be due to defective absorption of the vitamin actually administered, or to the presence of other pathogenic factors not yet discerned. These difficulties may yet be overcome with the advance of knowledge, and in the meantime the administration of the entire vitamin B complex is a reasonable *addition* to the other modes of treatment mentioned in the case of polyneuritis. In the case of sciatica and of brachial neuritis, this treatment is, of course, not rational, and no good comes, or can be expected from it.

In the treatment of motor neurone disease and of the muscular dystrophies, the claims made for vitamins E and B_6 have proved unfounded, and the same may be said for the use of the latter vitamin in paralysis agitans and post-encephalitic Parkinsonism.

In short, despite the sanguine views expressed in the advertising literature upon the vitamins, with its impressive citation of papers from medical journals, the time has not yet come when it can be said that vitamin therapy plays any clearly useful role in neurology, save in the case of Pellagra. An appeal may, therefore, be made for more discrimination in its employment than is at present to be seen.

The problem of saving the subject of an organic nervous disease, which can neither be cured nor materially mitigated, from the host of pseudo-remedies that in the hands of uncritical and unscientific claimants compete for his attention is always difficult, and many patients cannot altogether be saved from exploitation and from the alternation of raised and dashed hopes that so increase the distress of the chronic sufferer. In these circumstances little can be done but to secure as far as possible that financial resources which may be needed for the support of the patient and his dependents and for the provision of comforts are not wasted in the hopeless pursuit of benefits that it is not within human power to obtain. To give a familiar example, it may be much more important for a young housewife threatened with disability, or already partially disabled, by such a malady as disseminated sclerosis to use her resources in the obtaining of additional domestic help, thus securing for herself the rest from exertion that is so essential, than to expend them on some form of physiotherapy or expensive medication from which no candid adviser can promise her anything. Indeed, this consideration should never be absent even in the case of reasonable modes of treatment, and it must often be the doctor's advisory responsibility to see that a due sense of proportion as to the relative importance of the patient's various needs, medical and non-medical, is preserved.

of rest in hospital under a regular routine of life will often cause much improvement. In mild cases tics are often ameliorated when the child is disabused, and even spontaneous movement of the same nature sometimes inevitably helped, e.g. Bromide, 5 gr. (0·3 gm.) in the sodium bromide salt twice or thrice daily.

CHAPTER XXVI

Torticollis and the Tics

A TIC has been defined as "a co-ordinated purposive act, provoked in the first instance by some external cause or by an idea;
repetition leads to its becoming habitual, and finally to its
involuntary reproduction without cause and for no purpose."

The act may be a simple muscle twitch or a complex movement, and
in certain instances there is no such obvious motor act, but a periodical
explosive utterance, or some form of imperative behaviour. These latter
forms are very rare.

It is not certain that spasmodic torticollis has quite the same ætiology
as the other tics, and indeed some maintain that it results from an
organic lesion of the corpus striatum.

SIMPLE TICS : HABIT SPASM

This is an affection of nervous children, most often encountered
between the ages of five and twelve years. The child grimaces, blinks,
twitches its shoulders or shows widespread jerky involuntary movements
somewhat resembling those of rheumatic chorea. At one period blinking
movements predominate, at another some other facial grimace or some
movement of the limbs. Emotion or fatigue tends to increase their
severity. They cease during sleep. They may be present in fluctuating
severity over long periods of time, sometimes for several years, and in
most children they tend to cease at or about the age of twelve. While
they may be precipitated by debilitating factors, the child's temperament is the essential underlying factor in their appearance.

Diagnosis.—The symptoms with which the movements of simple tic
may be confused are those of rheumatic chorea, and the points of
distinction between these two affections have already been fully discussed in the chapter on chorea (page 196).

Treatment.—The child's general health and state of nutrition
require attention, but of equal importance is the securing where possible
of a suitable environment. The patient is not rarely the child of unstable
parents, or the member of a divided or disturbed family circle. The
constant sight of a fidgety or grimacing child acts as an exasperation to a
nervous and possibly overworked, underfed mother, who proceeds to
"nag" the patient and to build up an atmosphere of guilt around his or
her behaviour. If these adverse conditions cannot be corrected a period

of rest in hospital under a regular routine of life will often secure early improvement. In mild cases tics are often best ignored, when they will diminish and cease spontaneously. Mild dosage with sedatives is invariably helpful, *e.g.* Phenobarbitone, gr. $\frac{1}{4}$; or sodium bromide, gr. 5 twice or thrice daily.

SPASMODIC TORTICOLLIS

or wryneck, consists in the recurrence of irregular tonic and clonic spasms of the muscles supporting the head, which is thus forced into abnormal positions, usually of rotation but sometimes of extension.

Ætiology.—Adults only are affected and no age period thereafter is immune. Torticollis may arise without any discoverable exciting factor, but in some cases mental stress and conflict, in others local pain in the neck from spondylitis or fibrositis, may initiate the spasm. It is probable that in the latter group certain inborn qualities of temperamental instability are essential factors. Recently it has been suggested that a local lesion in the corpus striatum may provoke torticollis as a form of "release symptom," and it is true that severe examples of this spasm have been found to follow epidemic encephalitis. Even so, the hypothesis is without any satisfactory basis. Physiologically, torticollis may be regarded as a disorder in the carriage of the head; a complex function peculiar to man, for the head of the quadruped is suspended. It is such recently evolved functions that are so vulnerable to disturbance from factors other than gross focal lesions. It is, in short, impossible to assess the relative role in its causation of physical and psychological factors, and even those who regard the latter as alone operative will be found to show a strange reluctance to assume psychotherapeutic responsibility for a case. Spasmodic torticollis is a comparatively rare affection, a fact which, in view of the widespread incidence of psychoneurosis, may be taken to indicate that its appearance depends upon the rare coincidence in a given subject of the necessary physical and psychological factors.

Symptoms.—The onset is gradual. At first the tendency to rotation is relatively slight, makes itself felt at infrequent intervals, and is easy to control. In time it gains force and will not be denied, the spasms increase in frequency and may, under certain conditions of emotional stimulation, become an almost incessant ordeal, preventing reading, sewing, or writing. Some patients obtain a measure of relief by pressing the hand against the side of the face, and even the contact of the hand in this way may inhibit the tendency to rotation completely for many minutes. Sometimes rotation and lateral flexion of the head are combined so that the occiput is drawn to the shoulder. In other cases the extensors of the neck are primarily involved and then the head is drawn backwards, the eyes and eyebrows being both elevated, the entire synergy of movements indicating that a disturbance of a higher level of physiological function than that subserved by the corpus striatum is in question. In all cases the neck muscles are bilaterally involved, first the sternomastoids, then the trapezii, and finally, in severe cases almost all the neck muscles.

The spasm may be predominantly tonic, or clonic and imposing rapid jerky movements upon the head. After some months of severe spasm the sternomastoids may undergo manifest hypertrophy. Some degree of pain accompanies the spasm, sometimes severe and very wearing to the patient.

Prognosis and Treatment.—The disorder is deep-seated in the sense of being untractable, and the writer has seen a patient with torticollis spasm resume the head movements as soon as she emerged from a coma of three days' duration—an indication of the futility of treatment by sedatives.

Massage combined with remedial exercises and with an initial period of rest in bed may give a measure of relief. The exercises consist in the voluntary performance of movements opposite to those of the spasm, against some resistance. Exercises in which, facing a mirror, the patient holds the head in the normal position for a determined period of seconds and then allows it to turn, are also used. With practice, the period of voluntary fixation of the head is progressively lengthened and some degree of control is achieved. In some cases the fixing of the head and neck in a plaster, celluloid, or metal splint which holds the head erect gives remarkable relief, and normal activities become possible as long as it is worn. But not every case responds to this device. Division of motor nerves or of muscles has in the past been tried without avail.

In mild cases, fluctuations in the severity of the spasm occur spontaneously from time to time, and a period of treatment may initiate such a phase of comparative calm.

CHAPTER XXVII

Occupational Cramps

UNDER this title we refer to a group of disabilities of the hand, characteristically produced by repetitive vocational movements, and consisting of spasm and cramp-like pain in the muscles of the hand and forearm. Perhaps the most familiar of these are writer's and telegraphist's cramps, though both are now less frequent than formerly since the typewriter has replaced the laborious copying of a former generation, and the modern telegraph apparatus is less productive of cramp than the old Morse key. Other forms of cramp have been described after the procedures that give rise to them, as, for example, sempstresses cramp, hammerman's cramp, etc.

With the multiplication of machines and the putting into industrial processes of many thousands of new workers, it would not be surprising if new forms of occupational cramp developed, as in the case of power-operated machines in which the worker pulls levers or turns knobs or handles with great frequency during the working day. Some of the long familiar forms of occupational cramp, *e.g.* writer's cramp, telegraphist's cramp, have been recognized by the State as industrial diseases and have been embodied in the provisions of the Workmen's Compensation Act as notifiable disabilities entitling the sufferer to compensation. The newer forms of cramp referred to above, of which the writer has seen a few examples in factory workers, are not so scheduled at the present time, and thus cannot be dealt with by the certifying factory surgeon who may encounter them.

WRITER'S CRAMP

Ætiology.—There are two acts involved in writing, pen holding and pen moving. The pen is held by the intrinsic muscles of the hand: the interossei and thenar muscles. Pen moving may be done largely by the pen-holding muscles together with the flexors and extensors of the index, middle finger and thumb, the arm remaining fixed. It may be carried out in a free style by movements of the arm as a whole from the shoulder down. In the latter way the muscular effort is spread over a wider field of muscles, and the pen-holding muscles can then maintain a more or less constant tension and length. It is probable that writer's cramp arises in the first group, namely, those who use the pen-holding muscles for pen moving as well. If the subject of writer's cramp be given a piece of chalk and asked to write at face level on a blackboard he is forced to use the entire limb in writing and his "cramp" is less marked and less readily induced; it may even be absent. The use, then, of thenar and interosseous muscles for holding *and moving* involves a heavy burden upon them, and writer's cramp may reasonably be regarded as due to chronic fatigue in over-used muscles.

It may be added that difficulty in writing may arise from a great variety of local causes in the arm, and from organic nervous affections of diverse nature. To a consideration of these we shall later return.

The majority of subjects of writer's cramp are clerks in the third, fourth, and fifth decades of life. The role of a neuropathic constitution in the genesis of the cramp is uncertain and such statements as are made on the subject are wholly speculative.

Symptoms.—The onset is insidious. After continued writing the subject begins to find the pen getting slightly out of control and causing changes in the appearance of his handwriting. The ball of the thumb begins to ache and he finds himself grasping the pen with undue firmness, and driving the nib against the paper with such force that it may either pierce the paper or jerk across it. The thumb and index finger tend to become firmly flexed and to slip up the penholder, and they cannot then be freely extended to perform the upstrokes of letters. Gradually the muscles of the forearm go into spasm and pen movements may become virtually impossible. Pain varies in prominence from case to case. In some it is the main complaint, in others spasm predominates. Variations in the grasp of the pen may give temporary relief, but finally all methods fail to achieve writing. In extreme cases other movements of alternating character may begin to become difficult, such as the use of tooth or shaving brush. But if this spread of disability to other movements is an early symptom, the correct diagnosis is probably not one of writer's cramp.

A comparable "cramp" is seen in telegraphists, but is less frequently seen with modern telegraphic instruments than in the days of the Morse key. Modern instruments have a keyboard the use of which involves the spread of movement over more muscles.

Diagnosis.—Writing is a complex learned act and, therefore, one likely to be interfered with readily if there be any local abnormality of the limb, or any disturbance of innervation from a lesion of the peripheral or central nervous system. Of the local causes we may mention teno-synovitis, arthritis, any painful condition of the muscles, a local neuritis, or muscular paresis. Of central nervous causes we have early paralysis agitans, the slighter degrees of hemiplegia, ataxies of movement due to cerebellar or to sensory disorders. It may confidently be stated that writer's cramp is far more often diagnosed than it is present. The early rigidity of paralysis agitans or of post-encephalitic Parkinsonism if it develop in the right arm is a fruitful source of diagnostic error, for writing is one of the motor functions first impaired. Similar examples might easily be cited. *Therefore, a diagnosis of writer's cramp should not be made until a careful examination of muscles, joints, and tendons has been carried out and until organic disease of the nervous system has been excluded.* Although a process of exclusion is thus essential, true writer's cramp has features of its own: the restriction of the disability to writing, and the action of writing as observed by the examiner. In the case of telegraphist's cramp also these precautions should be most rigorously taken before a diagnosis is made, for in respect of it also errors of diagnosis are not uncommon. Perhaps of all the conditions most often mistaken for writer's or telegraphist's cramp early Parkinsonian rigidity is the most common. The characters of this are described on page 27.

Treatment.—In respect of writer's cramp it is clear that the early inculcation of sound habits of writing—that is, of the most physiological distribution of muscular effort—would probably exclude the later development of this disability. As for curative treatment, it has to be confessed that writer's cramp is a most intractable disability. It develops at **an** age at which the complete recasting of writing habits is difficult if not impossible. Complete abstention from writing is the first essential, and for a period of at least six months. During this time the repeated performance of other small hand movements should be severely restricted; *e.g.* the playing of a musical instrument. Gentle massage is comforting, but whether it or any other form of local treatment can be any more than this is doubtful. Where pain is prominent the splinting of the hand and forearm, as for a Colles' fracture, for a period of a few hours daily, may give relief. Whenever practicable the choice of some other form of occupation than clerical is desirable, for recurrence if the patient returns to his original work is likely, though not inevitable in every case. The use of a typewriter may solve the difficulty in some cases.

In the case of other professional cramps, abstention from the provoking movement is necessary.

CHAPTER XXVIII

The Psychoneuroses

(1) INTRODUCTION

THE great theoretical interest of the psychological problems that underlie the genesis and forms of the psychoneuroses and of psychoneurotic symptoms in sufferers from somatic illness may too easily lead us to forget that the first task of the clinician, face to face with his patient, is one of diagnosis, and that its accomplishment calls for careful clinical examination and an adequate clinical experience. For these, the widest familiarity with psychological hypotheses is no substitute. The following chapter, therefore, concerns itself primarily with diagnosis, and particularly with the differential diagnosis of organic and psychogenic illnesses in which the functions of the nervous system appear the ones predominantly disordered. It is of the first importance to bear in mind that the individual who for any reason, or combination of reasons, develops psychoneurotic symptoms is not thereby immune to any of the range of somatic illnesses to which the human race is liable, and that he is particularly likely to respond to somatic illness by the addition of psychoneurotic symptoms which modify the features and influence the course of this illness. It is, therefore, peculiarly easy to assume, when the patient's past history gives evidence of psychoneurotic trends, or of severe stresses of a mental or emotional order, that his present symptoms are no more than the expression of these trends or stresses, and that he is in fact merely suffering from a psychoneurosis. The error is one too commonly made, and it has its converse in the tendency to attribute all a patient's symptoms and disabilities to some single somatic factor, such as dental sepsis, for example, and to ignore all those factors of personality and environment that may have led to the appearance of a psychoneurosis that is wholly unconnected with the somatic factor. Both these common errors are the fruit of unbalanced and partial thinking, and of an ignoring of the truism that in every case of illness we are dealing with a body informed by a human personality. This notion, which is as old as medicine itself, is pithily expressed by Sterne in his *Life and Opinions of Tristram Shandy* (1759) as follows: "A man's body and his mind, with the utmost reverence to both I speak it, are exactly like a jerkin, and a jerkin's lining; rumple the one, you rumple the other." Here, nearly two hundred years old, we have the clear recognition of the notion embodied in what is now called "psychosomatic medicine."

313

In facing the task of diagnosis, therefore, we have not only to dis-entangle the somatic and psychological components in any given case of illness, or to determine that an illness is primarily and wholly psycho-genic, but we have also to assess the importance of psychological factors in the genesis of somatic illness. So far there is no evidence to suggest that organic disease of the nervous system, apart, possibly, from vascular disease, can be psychologically determined, but in respect of such ill-nesses as peptic ulcer, hypertension, chronic "rheumatism," fibrositis, or thyrotoxicosis, there is some evidence that psychological factors may lead to physiological disorder of function, and through this to structural disease.

It is possible that at present the tendency is to over emphasize this sequence of events, but however this be, it is clear that the clinician in every aspect of medicine must be vigilant not only in making the most careful physical examination of his patients, but he must also take the broadest view of ætiology (see page 8) and bear in mind the wide range of factors that may operate to determine the onset and to influence the behaviour of illnesses of all kinds. Specialism in medicine may be in-evitable, but its peculiar danger is that it leads to excessive concentration upon partial aspects of medical problems, and, therefore, it may be sub-mitted that the assessment of psychological factors in illness is the responsibility not of the psychological specialist only, but of every doctor. Therefore, a chapter on the diagnostic problems raised by the constant interaction of body and mind in all patients, whatever their predominant symptoms and whatever the seat of the significant lesions, is an integral part of every textbook of medicine or of any branch of medicine.

The three common varieties of psychoneuroses are the anxiety neurosis, hysteria, and the so-called "traumatic" neurosis. Less common is the obsessive neurosis, of which, however, brief mention will be made. The diagnostic problem presented by the anxiety neurosis is not so much its differentiation from organic disease as from the depressive psychosis with the milder forms of which it is frequently confused. In hysteria, on the other hand, owing to the predominant part played by somatic symptoms and the superficial resemblance these may show to the symp-toms of organic disease, such diagnostic difficulties as obtain are mainly concerned with the differentiation of hysteria from the latter. The "traumatic" neurosis may present features both of anxiety and of the hysterical reaction.

The psychoneuroses are to be considered as illnesses of the personality and not of the body. They are the expression of abnormal reactions to psychological stress; they are maladaptations of the personality to reality. Yet they are not reactions of the entire personality. This does retain contact with reality, though not perfectly or in all its aspects. On the other hand, in those more profound mental disorders that are the special province of the psychiatrist, the psychoses, the entire personality may be changed, contact with reality and the power to distinguish this from fantasy are lost, as for example when the patient attributes his symptoms to the action of some fantastic external agency.

The different varieties of psychoneurosis show special modes of abnormal reaction to reality. Thus, the anxiety neurosis may be called a reaction by overaction. The patient develops morbid fears and then a number of psychological and physiological reactions expressive of and appropriate to those fears. The somatic symptoms thus consist of reactions resembling the normal physiological responses to fear, but differing from these in their intensity and their persistence. Tremor and tachycardia are examples of physiological reactions produced in this way, not primarily from disorder on the anatomical or physiological levels but psychologically caused. In hysteria, on the other hand, we have a reaction by loss of function; by underaction. This shows itself usually by some striking local loss of bodily function: a paralysis, an anæsthesia or a mutism, or in more profound cases by a splitting of the personality leading to fugues, amnesia, or to double personality.

As has already been stated, the "traumatic" neurosis partakes of the clinical characters of both the above-mentioned forms of psychoneurosis, but it is not traumatic in the strict sense of this word, for in peace time conditions it arises when in addition to trauma there exists the possibility of equating bodily injury with compensation. Injuries sustained in the seclusion of the domestic scene, in the cricket, football, or hunting fields, or at other forms of sport are not followed by traumatic neurosis, which is the sequel solely of road, rail, industrial, and other accidents in respect of which legislation has provided the possibility of monetary compensation. Trauma alone is incapable of causing neurosis.

(2) THE ANXIETY NEUROSIS

This is the most frequently encountered and, fortunately, the most readily amenable to treatment of the psychoneuroses. It is a reaction by the development of morbid fears and anxiety and by mental and somatic symptoms which, originally the outcome of the fears, later become for the patient their apparent cause.

Ætiology.—The subjects of this form of psychoneurosis commonly have a neuropathic inheritance; that is to say, they are the children of unstable parents and not unnaturally they are commonly subjected in childhood and adolescence to that morbid environment that such parents are prone to create round themselves and their families. Thus, both inheritance and environment play a part in the genesis of the anxiety neurosis. The patient is emotionally unstable and given to worrying unduly over all the vicissitudes of life. The final appearance of an anxiety neurosis is but the culmination and exaggeration of tendencies which have always characterized his attitude to circumstances. The precipitating factor is either some overwhelming anxiety which is badly met, or some unresolved conflict between the individual needs—social, sexual, or financial—and the reality with which the subject is faced. When these needs are denied fulfilment in an unstable subject incapable of a satisfactory adjustment an anxiety neurosis may develop.

The development of anxiety and fear is the initial manifestation of the neurosis, but shortly the contemplation by the individual of his difficulties leads to the appearance of emotional reactions, mental and somatic, of the kind normally associated with fear or anxiety. These reactions are exaggerated in intensity, are evoked with undue ease, and have a quality of indefinitely prolonged persistence which distinguishes them from the emotional responses of the normal individual, which are graded in intensity and pass off when the stimulus which evoked them has ceased.

With the appearance of these symptoms the patient proceeds to detach his anxieties from their original external cause and to attach them to the symptoms, which thereupon become for him the overt cause of the anxieties. In this way is achieved the flight from reality into illness which is the essential purpose of the psychoneurosis, and the patient no longer feels any responsibility for his inability to pursue his normal activities or to grapple with his difficulties.

Symptoms.—These are mental and somatic. The mental symptoms include more or less deep anxiety and morbid fears. These in turn induce an inability to concentrate the attention, a defect of memory for current events, irritability in many cases, and loss of sleep. The defects of concentration and of memory readily engender in the patient a fear that he is becoming, or may become, insane; a fear that is in itself a potent source of still further anxiety. Yet there is no mental deterioration, and these symptoms are but the natural sequence of profound anxiety with its distracting influences. Commonly, also, the patient becomes unsociable. He is shy and excessively diffident, and being *au fait* with the jargon of modern psychology, may confess to having "an inferiority complex." This diffidence may be in respect of his mental, moral, social, physical, or occupational endowments.

The somatic symptoms are limited in their range and variety only by the number of bodily structures and functions possessed by the individual. In respect of the nervous system, complaints of pains or of great discomforts in the head are virtually constant. When actual pain is complained of it does not resemble the pain suffered and described by the subjects of organic disease or of migraine, but has bizarre qualities that call for fanciful analogy in their description and is apparently far more disabling than its organically determined counterparts. The discomforts are described variously as sensations of burning, of tingling, of pressure, of compression, of weight, of bursting, etc. All such symptoms are alleged to be aggravated by mental or physical effort or by worry. Pains and paræsthesiæ in the back (or the "spine," to use the term commonly employed by patients, this word lending a sinister import to the complaint) may also be complained of.

On the visceral side there may be tachycardia, palpitations, morbid blushing, excessive sweating, tremor, such gastro-intestinal symptoms as sickness, diarrhœa or constipation, flatulence and sensations of distension. Sexual disabilities in the male include diminution or loss of desire and of potency, in the female dyspareunia, vaginismus or frigidity. While in the male symptoms of this order lead to feelings of great inferiority, they rarely have this effect in the female for whom, commonly, they are purposive and defensive symptoms.

It is characteristic of these somatic symptoms, *firstly* that they are not accompanied by objective evidence of bodily disease. Hence it is that in these cases we so frequently encounter the therapeutic extravagances inherent in an uncritical belief in those most unsubstantial of conceptions, "focal infection" and "auto-intoxication." There are some medical men for whom the notion of psychologically determined ill-health is unattractive or by whom it is imperfectly appreciated, and it is in the hands of these that the exhaustive and expensive search for hypothetical foci of chronic infection in the subjects of the anxiety neurosis is most often undertaken. The easy opportunities which the nose and its accessory sinuses present to the determined seeker after irrelevant bacteria need not be emphasized. It should be borne in mind that with the increasing range of diagnostic procedures, biochemical, bacteriological, radiological and the like, few indeed of us even when we enjoy complete health could hope to escape without the discovery of some imperfection were we so unwise as to submit ourselves to inquisition on these lines. That the subject of an anxiety neurosis has teeth that show signs of wear and tear, nasal catarrh or large tonsils is not necessarily evidence that these blemishes stand in any relation to his symptoms, and to assume that they must do so is a travesty of reasoning that should not have survived the discipline of a scientific education.

Those who work in casualty departments cannot fail to be struck by the frequent presence, in those who seek their aid for minor injuries, of the most extreme and repellent degrees of oral sepsis in subjects who perform the most laborious work and enjoy rude health. It appears, then, not only possible, but even common, to see persons who live in the happiest relations with the hosts of organisms they harbour in sinuses and alimentary tract. This is not to condone such a state of affairs, but simply to stress the absurdity of the obsession that sees in vague shadows in a dental radiogram, in traces of pyorrhœa, or in a sphenoidal sinus that is not sterile, the invariable and constant cause of every variety of psychological disorder from the mildest anxiety neurosis to the gravest psychosis.

Secondly, these somatic symptoms completely engage the patient's attention and become the basis of the most dismal forebodings and anxiety. The patient finds it difficult to talk of anything else than his symptoms, and repeatedly returns to their description and discussion, and to complaints of their profoundly distressing and disabling character. This attitude is in part due to the displacement of the anxiety from its psychological causes to the symptoms, and in part to the fact that it is the essential purpose of the symptoms to be disabling.

In brief, the clinical picture is that of an individual in normal physical health, or of one showing no significant departure from this, who is the prey to anxiety and to morbid fears which he attributes to various mental and somatic symptoms. He is unaware, or but dimly aware, that the latter are in fact but the consequences of his fears and their indirect expression, and that anxiety—with or without mental conflict—is the original and adequate psychological cause of his condition. His anxiety is not necessarily related to long past events and difficulties, and the assumption of some schools of psychological theory that the anxieties and conflicts invariably date from infancy or childhood is inaccurate, nor are they always deeply repressed and completely below the threshold of consciousness or recall. Fortunately for treatment this is not commonly the case. The patient is impressionable in that he responds readily if but transiently, to changes in treatment, but he shows no tendency to spontaneous cure without treatment, and he remains liable throughout life in virtue of his inherent instability to morbid anxieties and to disability arising therefrom, and rarely enjoys prolonged periods of complete freedom from them.

Course and Prognosis.—The majority of cases of anxiety neurosis are relatively mild and amenable to appropriate treatment, subject always to the proviso that in the subject of a neurosis we are not dealing with an individual who is psychologically stable. In many cases a short course of treatment suffices, but in the more severe cases more expert and prolonged psychological treatment may be necessary. In such cases the tendency to relapse should be borne in mind.

Differential Diagnosis of the Anxiety Neurosis : the Depressive Psychosis.—Save in the case already referred to, in which the notion of focal infection is invoked to account for the symptoms of an anxiety neurosis, the most frequent source of error in diagnosis is a failure to differentiate this neurosis from true depression (the depressive psychosis). The prognosis and the treatment of the two conditions differ, and in the latter there is a danger of suicide not present in the anxiety neurosis.

In the depressive psychosis diagnosis may be facilitated if there be a history of previous attacks. These are commonly spoken of by the patient as "nervous breakdown." They may have arisen fairly acutely with no discoverable precipitating factors, or they may be said to have followed a period of prolonged or severe overwork. Their duration is usually one of several months, or even of a year or more, after the lapse of which they have cleared up fairly rapidly leaving the patient normal again and with his full working capacity. Many subjects of the anxiety neurosis attribute their illness to overwork, but usually the plea is without substance. In the case of true depression, however, the statement may at first sight appear to be accurate, for the reason that many subjects of depression have a temperament that fluctuates from an abnormal expansiveness and energy to depression and subnormal energy. This is the so-called "cyclothymic" temperament. This may express itself by periods of restless energy in which the subject overworks, squanders energy, and makes of his leisure a real "toil of pleasure." After some weeks or months of this he then lapses into depression, and not unnaturally his relatives are prone to regard this second phase of the illness as a consequence of the first. Thus the legend of overwork as a cause is born. In many mild depressive subjects, however, these phases of overactivity and expansiveness are never seen.

What we may learn from the past history of such a case is that the patient seems to have recovered more or less spontaneously, and to have enjoyed normal mental and physical health in the intervals between successive attacks. It must be borne in mind, however, that during the course of his illness the patient has received various modes of treatment, probably from a sequence of medical advisers. The form of treatment in use at the moment of recovery and the doctor in the saddle at this fortunate juncture will not unnaturally be credited with the cure. Yet in fact, as a careful assessment of the story will probably reveal, recovery has been quite independent of therapy. Here, as in the case of the retrobulbar neuritis of disseminated sclerosis, treatments that can have no influence upon the course of events score their easy and illusory triumphs, and prominent amongst these modes of treatment are those designed to combat hypothetical focal infections. These features of the depressive psychosis are not present in the anxiety neurosis, in which the patient does not recover "by himself" and rarely enjoys continuous freedom from all symptoms for long periods.

Actually, there are clinical features in the picture of the depressive psychosis which should serve to differentiate it from the anxiety neurosis. The patient's depression is not influenced by changes in his environment and seems to be independent of these. We do not encounter in him those transient improvements so common in the anxiety neurosis from change of surroundings or of medical treatment. The depressive does not respond to factors of this order. He takes no pleasure in anything, nor is he easily moved to active displeasure. He is apathetic emotionally. His mental processes are retarded. He replies slowly and often monosyllabically to questions, and these may have to be repeated more than once to elicit a response. He does not complain volubly of somatic symptoms, but tends to reproach himself for his state and in general to depreciate himself, either as a wrongdoer who has brought his misfortunes on his own head or as an ineffective and useless member of the community. His voice and articulation are monotonous and his movements slow. He is easily exhausted and his physical energy is visibly at a low ebb. Somatic symptoms of much the same order as those complained of by the subject of the anxiety neurosis may be present, but they are not freely volunteered or eagerly complained of, and information concerning them has often to be extracted from the patient. In more severe cases the patient becomes very reticent and presents a picture of congealed misery. He is ready to sit almost motionless all day, has to be pressed to his food, or to any form of activity. He is characteristically inaccessible to discussion and lacks insight into his condition much more profoundly than does the subject of an anxiety neurosis. He tends to regard his state rather as a retribution for his own faults than as an illness, an attitude not encountered in the anxiety neurotic who is only too anxious to interpret his situation in terms of an illness for which he bears no personal responsibility. It will be seen, therefore, that those psychotherapeutic measures which are so essential to and so valuable for the treatment of the anxiety neurosis are both fruitless and even harmful to the depressive, a practical point in treatment that should always be borne in mind.

Finally, a considerable proportion of cases of suicide is recruited from the ranks of the depressives, and a failure to differentiate their illness from the anxiety neurosis necessarily tends to leave them unprotected from this danger, a fact that no reader of accounts of coroners' inquests upon suicides can fail to realize.

Another form of psychosis that may at the outset lead to a diagnosis of anxiety neurosis is *Schizophrenia*. The patient is commonly an adolescent or young adult, whose past history may be one of considerable intellectual ability. The symptomatology of this disorder is protean, and it is when the early symptoms are apathy, intellectual and particularly emotional, inability to keep the attention normally concentrated, and complaints of exhaustion, that a diagnosis of anxiety neurosis is most apt to be made. Sooner or later, however, in the schizophrenic subject some disorder of behaviour will show itself: senseless laughter or chucklings over something the patient does not divulge, a tendency to negativism, shown as an unwillingness to adapt himself to the household regime, accesses of day-dreaming, delusions or hallucinations, and often slowly progressive mental deterioration.

In elderly persons the sudden appearance "out of the blue" of hypochondriacal fears is suggestive of the development of a psychosis. If the patient becomes convinced that he has cancer of the stomach, is reassured and shortly expresses the conviction that he has some other grave bodily disease, and proceeds to repeat this sequence of grim convictions, then grave mental illness may be recognized to be impending.

Among the organic affections to be considered are:

Early paralysis agitans, a malady in which the insidious onset of muscular rigidity may cause disabilities that casual and inadequate examination may fail to reveal. These disabilities and the subjective symptoms that accompany them may give rise to a degree of depression, and it is by no means uncommon for the patient in these circumstances to be regarded as suffering from an anxiety neurosis. The error, however, is one that ordinarily careful physical examination should render impossible.

Early dementia paralytica may first show itself by depression, forgetfulness, and inability to concentrate, and in a middle-aged man the possibility that this malady is developing should be borne in mind. Here, also, physical examination is the chief defence against diagnostic error, but, as has been reiterated in these pages, a careful history-taking is essential. When an individual has reached middle life without showing evidence of past neuroses, and then develops the mental and emotional changes enumerated, the doctor should be chary of making a diagnosis of psychoneurosis until he has excluded organic disease. In such circumstances it is prudent to take the Wassermann reaction of the blood before making a diagnosis.

Treatment.—The anxiety neurosis in its milder forms is extremely widespread, and accounts for a great deal of the chronic ill-health which the doctor is called upon to treat. For very many patients in this situation the advice of the family doctor is all that is available, and, therefore, it should be emphasized that the majority of cases can be adequately dealt with by the family doctor if he will meet the relatively simple requirements of the situation. It is a mistake to suppose that the aid of the psychotherapeutic specialist is always essential, or that the secret of successful treatment resides in the teachings of any particular school of psychological doctrine. In the past, cases of anxiety neurosis have been successfully treated by a wide range of methods, so diverse that many of them have no single point in common save that the patient had confidence in the doctor who employed them.

The general principles that govern treatment may be simply stated. We may begin with the axiom that a psychological illness demands

x

psychological treatment, and that purely physical remedies can never be more than subsidiary. The employment of the latter may, of course, have a suggestive value and they may thus be psychological in their mode of action. Yet if the patient be led to believe, and he will readily accept the view, that his condition is physical in origin and is in fact a bodily illness, such measure of success as physical remedies achieve is limited and transient. Further, when, later on, reasonable psychological treatment is undertaken, the task of persuading the patient to accept a psychological interpretation of his illness will have been rendered infinitely more difficult by the erroneous notions that have previously received the sanction of medical authority. A psychoneurosis is an illness of the personality, not of the body, and treatment should be openly conducted on this understanding.

Careful history-taking and thorough physical examination are an essential and integral part of the treatment of the anxiety neurosis. The patient must be satisfied that he has been allowed to tell his story, and if later he is to accept a psychological interpretation of his illness, the doctor must be in a position to maintain that systematic examination has revealed no bodily disease adequate to account for the symptoms.

In the introductory chapter it was pointed out that history-taking should be a joint undertaking by patient and doctor, and this is nowhere more true than in connection with the psychoneuroses. While the patient may be voluble to a degree concerning certain of his symptoms, there are others he may hesitate to mention, and there are fears that require patient and tactful elicitation if anything is to be heard of them. Further, the history should concern itself not simply with the present illness, but with the entire background of the patient's life. This may reveal evidence of past maladaptations, of somatic illnesses that have not run true to form—that have been unduly prolonged and characterized by symptoms and sequels that suggest the presence of a functional "top-dressing," and of illnesses diagnosed as somatic that were possibly of the nature of psychoneuroses. That engaging figment "chronic appendicitis" is one of the most familiar figures in this galaxy. If it is realized that this painstaking task is part of treatment, the time it may consume will not be grudged, for in the long run treatment properly initiated will prove more rapid in results.

Once it has been decided that an anxiety neurosis is present, the patient is best told the truth about the nature of his illness, namely, that it is the consequence of psychological factors and is not physical in origin or nature. This is not the same as telling him that "there is nothing the matter"; a dangerous half-truth that ignores the fact that the individual possesses a personality as well as a body, and one that may make all attempts at treatment fruitless. To propound a psychological interpretation of his illness to the patient is often a difficult task, for the deeper the purpose this illness serves the more unwilling will the patient be to part with it, and the more he will resent any explanation that seems to place some responsibility for its continuance upon his shoulders. He is apt to accuse the doctor of calling his symptoms "imaginary." The patient history-taking and systematic physical examination that are so imperative in dealing with this category of illness will here stand the doctor in good stead, and will make it possible for him to explain the role of anxiety in the production of symptoms. Some of the more distressing of these may be discussed with the patient in the light of this view, and he should be assured that with adequate treatment he will get well. The temptation to compromise in this psychological interpretation by giving physical remedies to the patient, thus upon a superficial view helping him to accept this view without loss of face, may in fact defeat treatment, since it suggests that the doctor himself is not wholly convinced that physical factors are absent. It is true that such symptoms as sleeplessness may require medication, but the role of this as purely adjuvant should be made clear.

Many subjects do respond in a measure to physical remedies when the fiction of a bodily illness is maintained by the doctor, but the response is incomplete and insecure, and a good final result is rarely obtained by taking the path of least resistance in this way in the case of the anxiety neurosis. In the case of hysteria, on the other hand, whatever may be urged to the contrary, a successful removal of symptoms may often be most rapidly and easily obtained without any attempt to elucidate to the patient the nature and causes of his illness.

In more severe cases of anxiety neurosis, where profound anxiety and marked symptoms develop upon trivial occasion in persons of marked instability, more prolonged and expert psychotherapy may be called for, but, fortunately, the majority of cases are not of this order and are amenable to short courses of treatment at the hands of any sympathetic patient, and careful practitioner.

It has already been stated that this psychological method of approach is both futile and harmful to the subject of a true depressive psychosis, and most of these cases are made worse by psychological inquisitions. They are inaccessible to suggestion or to persuasion. The fact that the patient is a potential suicide indicates that institutional treatment is usually necessary. If he be treated at home he should be under continuous and trained nursing supervision and his life should be one of restricted physical activity. To send such patients away for change of scene or air alone or with a relative is to court disaster. Until his illness undergoes a spontaneous recovery he must be carefully guarded. It is for this reason especially that the depressive psychosis should be differentiated from the anxiety neurosis in which these dangers are not present.

(3) HYSTERIA

The hysterical reaction is essentially one in which the subject responds to her difficulties by the development of a loss of bodily function which completely disables her. While it is true that symptoms of anxiety may be met with in the hysterical subject, in many cases anxiety is conspicuously absent and the patient is emotionally calm and apparently contented. Indeed this emotional tone often wins for the subject of an hysterical illness warm commendations for the fortitude and resignation with which she meets what to a normal person would be disastrous disablement. Thus the anxiety and conflict which lie at the root of this, as at the root of the anxiety neurosis, is said to be converted into a somatic disability and with this conversion conscious anxiety disappears. Undoubtedly a factor in this conversion is the abnormal suggestibility of the hysterical subject. This quality not only determines the appearance of somatic symptoms but also their character, and under treatment plays an important role in their disappearance.

While hysteria is by no means a mode of reaction peculiar to the female sex, in the circumstances of ordinary life adolescent girls and young women provide the majority of cases and tend to the more severe and bizarre forms of somatic disability. Thus dermatitis artefacta, "hysterical fever," and the combination of spasm and paralysis are rarely seen save in women. In men, the so called "traumatic" neurosis may be accompanied by hysterical palsies, spasms and anæsthesias. In the account which follows, this sex incidence of the different somatic manifestations of hysteria will be reflected by the pronouns used.

Ætiology.—What has been said of the inheritance and environment in the case of the anxiety neurosis applies here also. Yet it is probable that the hysterical reaction betrays a more profound instability, for while many might develop excessive anxiety in the face of difficulty, the naïve simplicities and inconsistencies of the hysterical reaction are incompatible with anything approaching the normal in mental stability, or in the power of reasoned contemplation of life and its difficulties. Thus it is that the hysterical reaction is more often seen in the simple-minded, uneducated, and emotionally uncontrolled subjects, while the anxiety neurosis is more characteristic of the intelligent and educated person who has known responsibility. The anxiety reaction may occur at any age period, but the hysterical reaction is most often encountered in the first half of life.

Occasionally, both types of psychoneurosis may develop in sequence in a single individual, and morbid anxiety is also sometimes encountered, though not as a rule, in the subjects of an hysterical illness. This is particularly true of the so-called "traumatic" neurosis.

It is generally assumed that the subject is unaware of the psycho-

logical process by which an anxiety or a conflict is converted into a
physical disability and is wholly convinced of the physical origin of the
latter. This is by no means invariably true, and there can be no doubt
that witting deceit plays a role in the production of the clinical picture
in some hysterics. This is true of such symptoms as dermatitis artefacta,
of "hysterical fever," and of other symptoms which are in a sense self-
inflicted. The rapidity and ingenuity with which the hysteric adapts her
symptoms to circumstances is capable of no other interpretation. Thus
the patient who is prevented from inflicting further cutaneous lesions
upon herself will substitute these by convulsions. If she be prevented
from tampering with the thermometer she will develop a paralysis, and
so on. There is no clear line dividing such cases from the deliberate
simulation of disease. The malingerer is one who with full moral
responsibility for her acts and with full awareness produces bodily
disabilities. She is an actress who knows she is acting. In the hysterical
subject it is probable that neither full responsibility nor full awareness is
always present. The latter certainly tends to diminish, for the hysteric is
often an actress who becomes progressively convinced by her own acting
and may ultimately come to join the audience. Current theories of the
genesis of the psychoneuroses require that the psychological processes
underlying them should be below the threshold of consciousness, and the
clear evidence to the contrary sometimes provided by clinical experience
has been ignored or suppressed in the interests of theory. There can be
little doubt that a capacity for deceit and trickery is inherent in the
hysterical temperament, and this element must always be taken into
account both in diagnosis and in treatment. There is another feature
which differentiates the hysterical from the anxious subject. The latter
may develop and maintain his neurosis alone, as it were, but the hysteric
requires a human background of family or of community with which to
interact. Thus an entire family or household may be influenced by an
hysterical member and come unwittingly to minister to the neurosis and
build it up. To achieve this state of affairs, which profoundly complicates
treatment, is an objective not lost sight of by the hysteric.

Symptoms.—These are mental and somatic. Mental symptoms are
encountered only in the more severe cases where they take the form of
periods of amnesia, of fugues, of somnambulism and, exceptionally only,
of double personality. Much more common are those cases in which
somatic symptoms make up the clinical picture. These consist in local
loss of some bodily function: paralysis, sensory loss, mutism or aphonia,
deafness or blindness. Sometimes hysterical convulsions with or without
associated paralytic manifestations occur. Since these disturbances of the
functions of the nervous system show a superficial resemblance to the
results of organic disease, the principal task in diagnosis is their differentiation from the latter.

These *somatic symptoms of psychological origin* are commonly spoken of as "functional" in contrast to those that arise from primary disorders on the anatomical and physiological level, which we speak of as "organic." The term "functional" has been criticized on many grounds, but it is in general use in the sense here defined; it gives rise to no genuine misunderstanding and may, therefore, be retained as a valuable working term.

Differential Diagnosis of Functional and Organic Somatic Symptoms.—The following general features serve to distinguish somatic symptoms of functional type from those that are organically determined.

THE RELATION OF SYMPTOM TO DISABILITY.—In general we may say that the psychologically normal subject of organic disease is not specially interested in his symptoms or disability, would gladly ignore them, and continues at his normal pursuits as long as it is physically possible to do so. His symptoms, in short, are an obstacle in the way of his obtaining the satisfactions of an active life. Every clinician must be familiar with the patient who continues to struggle to work in the face of increasing disabilities until forced to give up and seek medical advice. His body may be ill, but his personality is not. Wholly different is the patient's reaction to a psychologically determined symptom. He is deeply interested in and preoccupied with it. It forms the main burden of his conversation, and much eloquence may be given to its adequate and reiterated description. It is essentially profoundly disabling, and since the underlying function of a psychological symptom is to afford an escape from a situation which cannot be tolerated it is necessary that it should both appear and be disabling. Thus, we find the hysterical subject disabled by paralysis, anæsthesia, mutism, or muscular spasm.

Therefore, the attitude of the patient to his symptom and the relation of this to the measure of disability it secures for him are factors of diagnostic importance.

In the case of organic disease the total disability may be greatly increased by psychological factors of this kind, and what may be called a "top-dressing" of functional disability may increase the severity and prolong the course of an organically determined illness.

THE DISCREPANCY BETWEEN SYMPTOMS AND ANATOMICAL AND PHYSIOLOGICAL ARRANGEMENTS IN THE BODY.—An essential feature of the somatic symptoms of hysteria is that they do not correspond to disorders produced by, or capable of being produced by, structural lesions or primary physiological disorder, nor is their behaviour compatible with the presence of these. They are, as it were, symptoms that know nothing of anatomy or physiology. They correspond to the patient's notions of his anatomical and physiological arrangements and are clearly influenced in their appearance and disappearance by purely psychological determinants.

(1) *Hysterical Sensory Loss.*—A familiar example of the inconsistency of this loss with known anatomical patterns of sensory innervation are the "glove" and "stocking" anæsthesias. The topography of these correspond to the patient's idea of a bodily unit, her leg, her hand or her arm, and transgress anatomical patterns. They also run counter to physiological arrangements in that the patient loses only those modes of sensation she knows of and understands, not those she knows nothing of —*e.g.* postural sensibility. Thus the patient who at one moment appears to have a total loss of all modes of sensibility in a hand when each mode is separately tested will be seen to perform manipulations with normal address and in a manner clearly indicating that postural sensibility is in fact intact. Again, the subject of hysterical hemianæsthesia will fail to feel the vibrations of a tuning fork placed on the anæsthetic half of the sternum, though these vibrations are transmitted throughout the bone and should, therefore, be perceived from the unaffected half of the sternum.

(2) *Pain of Hysterical Type.*—It has been maintained that this is genuine pain, though the physiological mechanism underlying the appreciation of pain is not involved. Against this view is the fact that the physical concomitants of pain are not usually present, *e.g.* anxiety, sleeplessness, pallor, loss of appetite and weight. These we always find in true physically determined pain when this is persistent and severe. These points have already been considered in the discussion on psychogenic "headache" where the hysterical variety of this mental image of pain was described (page 65). In the anxiety neurosis the patient does not dramatize his situation in this exaggerated fashion, but he is disproportionately disabled by it.

(3) *Hysterical Paralysis.*—In respect of motor paralysis a similar inconsistency is to be found and there are various simple tests for detecting it. Thus, in the case of an hysterical hemiplegia or crural monoplegia the patient appears wholly unable to adduct the affected lower limb when directly asked to do so, yet if she be asked to keep both legs strongly pressed together, both legs adduct strongly since it is impossible forcefully to adduct the normal leg without also adducting its apparently paralysed fellow.

Again, if the patient, lying on her back, be asked to press the heel of the paralysed leg down upon the observer's hand which lies under it, no effort or but a feeble one is made. If now the observer's hand be retained in this position and the patient be asked to elevate the sound leg forcefully, the heel of the formerly paralysed leg will be felt to press down on the observer's hand with a force equal to that of the elevation of the sound limb, because to perform the latter movement strongly against resistance is possible only when the fellow limb is equally strongly pressed in the opposite direction. Again, the hand grasp of a partly paralysed arm in a case of hysterical weakness has characteristic features: the hand is closed round the observer's and held firmly set in a grasp which exerts but the slightest pressure and the sense of power withheld is one that once felt is not easily forgotten. Another feature of hysterical weakness is the tendency to perform a movement opposite to that demanded. Thus if the request be made to the patient to flex the forearm strongly on the arm against resistance a distinct movement of extension may be felt (the so-called "law of antagonistic effort").

In a few cases of hysterical monoplegia the paralysed limb is found to be in intense and sustained spasm. In the case of the leg the limb is extended and adducted with the foot in equinovarus. This spasm which is sustained indefinitely by the patient without apparent voluntary effort may resist all efforts on the part of the observer to overcome it and is of a strength and duration that ordinary voluntary effort could not achieve. Accompanying it we often find cyanosis, coldness, and œdema of the foot and ankle. Apart from spasm these vasomotor changes are not found.

In long-standing hysterical paralysis the affected limbs may show considerable muscular wasting and there may also be contracture with deformity of the hand or foot. These changes are the result of prolonged immobility and are not, as is sometimes assumed, the result of obscure vasomotor disorders peculiar to the hysterical reaction.

Among the various motor disturbances of functional type encountered *tremor* must be included. As seen in the psychoneurosis this is a fine, rapid (six to seven per second) rhythmical to-and-fro movement. It is often confined to the arms. It is finer and more rapid than the tremor of paralysis agitans and is never accompanied by the muscular rigidity that is an invariable concomitant of the latter. It appears when the limbs are extended and may cease when the limb is at rest and supported. Like the long-sustained and intense spasm of hysteria it is incapable of being voluntarily produced and continued. It is rarely sufficiently coarse to cause any disability, though under strong emotional stress it may transiently impair fine movements of the hand. It ceases during sleep.

(4) *The Reflexes in Hysteria.*—We have seen that the sensory and motor disorders of psychological origin commonly depend for their characters upon the patient's notions of her anatomical and physiological arrangements. The patient has *no* notions about either tendon jerks or cutaneous reflexes, nor are these phenomena under any significant measure of voluntary control. In the hysteric, therefore, they show no qualitative change though there may be a uniform increase of the tendon jerks. True clonus of organic type does not occur, the abdominal reflexes remain normal and the plantar responses are of the normal flexor type. In hysterical paraplegia it may be difficult to obtain any trace of plantar response.

(5) *Special Sense Symptoms*.—These show that inconsistency with anatomical and physiological arrangements already described. Thus, there may be peripheral constriction of the visual fields, or unilateral blindness, but not any of the forms of hemianopia that organic lesions may produce. The hysterical subject who complains of the loss of the sense of smell retains the full appreciation of all the flavours, including that of tobacco; in other words, she has not got anosmia, but only what she fancies the loss of the sense of smell to be.

(6) *The characters of the hysterical fit* have already been considered in the chapter on epilepsy (page 124). The fit is sometimes followed by a trance-like state of apparent unconsciousness. It is to be borne in mind that the form sometimes assumed by the automatism that follows a minor epileptic fit may suggest an hysterical attack, and it is not uncommon for a diagnosis of hysteria to be made in these circumstances when the presence of epilepsy is not known. The behaviour of automatism, as has been stated, tends to be repetitive and short in duration, but when doubt exists it is important to see the mode of onset of the attack when, in the case of epilepsy, a transient change in consciousness may be seen to precede the complex behaviour of the following automatism (see page 120).

Amnesia, fugues, and double personality are among the rarer manifestations of hysteria. It may be doubted whether some of the apparent fugues in which the subject disappears from home and is found days later wandering, unkempt, unfed and exhausted, in a remote part of the country are genuine. The subject commonly has an excellent and obvious reason for the flight, such as the discovery by family or employers of some form of irregular conduct, and it is clear that the penalties and retribution this may call for are rendered very difficult of infliction upon the forlorn figure the patient presents when found and restored to his anxious family. In these circumstances the cutting out of the general field of consciousness of the period involved in the fugue is sometimes more apparent than real.

(7) *Other Hysterical Symptoms*.—Among the less common of these may be mentioned *dermatitis artefacta*. This consists of the production by the patient herself of various cutaneous lesions—scratches, abrasions, eruptions, ulcers. The view that such cutaneous lesions as blisters and ecchymoses may arise spontaneously in hysteria, or as a result of suggestion, is not substantiated, and the ingenuity with which cutaneous lesions are produced and the fantastic forms they may take (as in the so-called stigmatization, in which the wounds of the crucifixion are superficially imitated—abrasions on hands, feet, and side) indicate unequivocally their self-inflicted character. The so-called *hysterical fever* is a phenomenon of a like order in that it is produced by manipulations of the thermometer. The readings are usually fantastically high (*e.g.* 110° F.,

this being the top of the thermometer), for graded readings are very difficult to produce. Such "fever" is not accompanied by proportionate changes in pulse and respiration rates, and the simultaneous takings of the temperature in several places—mouth, axilla, rectum—under careful observation will serve to detect the nature of the situation. These dramatic manifestations do not occur as isolated phenomena, but form part of a combination or sequence of hysterical symptoms. They are found almost exclusively in female subjects.

ANOREXIA NERVOSA.—This is in some ways the gravest of the hysterical reactions in that it not rarely ends fatally. The patient is usually a young unmarried woman who has ceased to eat, either because she has come to regard it as wrong to do so, or because she complains that food produces indigestion. A severe degree of emaciation develops and amenorrhœa is an early and constant symptom. Despite the emaciation, a remarkable measure of energy and activity may remain until the later stages of the illness.

In the preceding paragraphs the somatic components of the hysterical symptom-complex that have been described have been referable to the nervous system, but it would be a disastrous error to suppose that the somatic components are always or necessarily of this form.

There is, indeed, no symptom-complex of somatic illness that may not have its hysterical "double." Symptoms referable to almost any of the viscera or to the skeletal structures may dominate the clinical picture, and thus in every field of medicine and surgery the clinician is called upon to differentiate between physically and psychologically determined symptoms. Only by clinical examination and clinical experience can this differentiation be made. What has been said of somatic symptoms of neurological type in hysteria: namely, their incompatibility with organic lesion or their presence without the corresponding indications of organic lesion, applies also to the visceral symptoms. From the fact that in such cases the presenting symptoms are somatic, it follows that they first come under the observation of the general clinician, and not that of the psychologist who in any case is less well placed by the limitation of his experience and interests to recognize them. It is, therefore, important that the doctor should be fully aware of the polymorphic somatic symptomatology of the hysterical neurosis, and should remember that only careful clinical examination suffices for its recognition. This recognition needs to be made as early as possible, since prognosis is best in cases of short duration, and also because much inappropriate treatment may thus be avoided. Such treatment not only fails to relieve, but it makes subsequent treatment of a suitable kind more difficult.

Course and Prognosis.—It is well known that hysterical paralysis may persist for many years, rendering the patient a complete and helpless invalid, or at least protecting her from the burdens and responsibilities of a normal existence. This is particularly apt to be the case when in its initial stages the illness was regarded by the medical adviser then consulted as of organic origin. It is remarkable that for a long period such a diagnosis may be accepted unquestioned by subsequent advisers and, of course, by the patient's family, until no revision of it is acceptable and the time for successful treatment is long past. During all this time the patient has been receiving a satisfactory psychological dividend from her situation in care and attention, in freedom from responsibility, and often in the character she gains for fortitude and edifying resignation to a life of suffering.

In such circumstances an hysterical paralysis may well become incurable and any attempt at cure may evoke a violent and hostile emotional reaction into which the relatives are easily drawn. The writer has seen a case of hysterical hemiplegia with anæsthesia that for eight years had enjoyed a diagnosis of syringomyelia. During this long period she had produced upon her paralysed and analgesic arm a succession of progressively deepening ulcers which, failing to heal, had led to the complete amputation of the arm in three instalments. Thereupon a similar ulcer appeared over, and exposed the shaft of, the clavicle. Neurological examination then revealing the hysterical nature of the illness, the remaining sound arm was encased in plaster to prevent tampering with the ulcer, which promptly healed, no further lesions of the kind developing.

The case is cited to illustrate the severity of the mental abnormality that may underlie the hysterical reaction, the apparent ease with which it may escape medical recognition, and the distressing mutilations to which such a subject may submit herself in respect of lesions which she was knowingly inflicting upon herself.

Fortunately, the underlying mental abnormality is not always so profound, and when dealt with early the hysterical symptoms may readily respond to appropriate treatment, though the subject's personality necessarily remains what it was.

Treatment.—This consists in the removal of hysterical symptoms and the psychological treatment of the mental background upon which they have arisen. As already indicated, the former task is less difficult than the latter, save in such long-standing cases as have been discussed. Whenever the patient's mental capacity, emotional condition, and level of education permit, it is best, after careful history-taking and thorough physical examination, to propound the psychological nature of the illness. This is less often practicable with the hysterical than with the anxiety reaction for reasons which have already been given. When no capacity for the willing reception of the truth exists on the part of the patient, or when the psychological advantage obtained by the illness outweighs the benefits likely to accrue from cure, only dramatic methods with an emotional appeal are likely to be fruitful. These consist, for example, in the application of electrical currents which make the muscles of the paralysed limb contract and thus secure its movement. Once the patient has seen this occur he or she may then be induced to move it voluntarily and by persuasion a complete restoration of function, subject to the measure of disuse atrophy, and joint change present, may be obtained at a single sitting. With more willing and intelligent subjects persuasion alone, coupled with the assurance that no permanent disability is present, may achieve the same result. To employ this method the therapist must not only appear confident, but must possess confidence. The hysterical convulsion often ceases quickly when the patient is left alone and deprived of an audience, and the old-fashioned remedy of a more robust age, namely, a douche of cold water, is usually effective. Vomiting as an hysterical symptom is not serious, and this should be made plain to the patient, who should be kept on a full and ordinary diet despite the recurrent sickness.

The treatment of anorexia nervosa absolutely requires the complete isolation of the patient from every one save her doctor and nurses. Cases of this kind can rarely be safely treated at home. Small and frequent feeds should be given, and much persuasion and patience may be necessary to see that they are actually taken. Psychological investigation is best delayed until the patient's state of nutrition has been improved and she has started to gain weight. Unless these measures are undertaken early and systematically the patient may die, and it is probable that all such cases require expert medical and nursing care. Not a few fatalities are due to delay in starting the necessary measures.

Brief mention may be made of the employment of convulsive therapy for the psychoneuroses described in this chapter. Growing experience seems to indicate that the usefulness of this drastic procedure is confined to the treatment of the depressive psychosis in middle-aged and elderly persons. It does not give consistently good results in hysteria or in schizophrenia, and certainly in the former may act adversely. Prefrontal leucotomy (amputation of the frontal poles) is an irreversible operation, the value and dangers of which we cannot yet assess. It has no place in the treatment of the psychoneuroses, but may prove to have a limited range of usefulness in long-standing and incurable psychoses. Whether the good results claimed for its use in these selected cases will prove permanent it is not yet possible to say.

(4) THE " TRAUMATIC " NEUROSIS

Ætiology.—It has already been stated that this title is a misnomer and that trauma alone cannot be a cause of neurosis.

On the other hand, the factors of inheritance and early environment which go to mould the neurotic temperament and prepare the way for the development of the anxiety and hysterical neuroses appear to play a less consistent role in the genesis of the "traumatic" neurosis, the subject of which may, and often does, reach middle or later life without revealing any indication of this temperament. In this he tends to stand apart from the subject of the anxiety neurosis or of hysteria. If, then, neither trauma by itself nor the neurotic temperament is an essential condition of the development of a "traumatic" neurosis, what is the determining factor?

Cases of this neurosis come within the common experience of most practitioners of medicine, and it can scarcely be denied that the measure of success attained in their treatment falls far short of what is desirable. That this is so is in large part due to factors not within the doctor's control, factors to which subsequent reference is made; but little less important is a widespread unwillingness to face frankly the real issue involved in the production of this neurosis. This issue, as it appears to the writer, may be briefly expounded.

In the circumstances of civilian life if trauma is to be followed by the development of a psychoneurosis it is necessary that the injury, which may be of the most trivial character, should be incurred in circumstances which may render someone liable to pay monetary compensation to the sufferer. In civilian practice the "traumatic" neurosis is a sequel only to road, rail, industrial or other accidents in respect of which legislation has made compensation payable. In war conditions, injury may be followed by neurosis the purpose of which is to remove the sufferer from perilous conditions which he has found himself unable to face or to return to.

In respect of civilian injuries there are several factors which combine to engender neurosis. In the case of injuries sustained at sport and games, tradition requires that the sufferer shall show fortitude, shall minimize his pain, and return with the least possible delay to his game. No sense of grievance is engendered by injuries so sustained and neurosis does not ensue. Unhappily in the case of road, rail, and industrial accidents and injuries there are no such salutary traditions. Circumstances invite the sufferer to make the most of his situation. He is often extremely frightened, and this fright is too readily misnamed "shock" either by the bystanders or by the patient's medical adviser. There can be no defence of this misuse of a technical medical term, but it is extremely common and gives rise in the patient's mind to what may be an exaggerated notion of the severity of his injury. In this way an atmosphere of gloomy apprehension is imparted to the situation and the ground is prepared for the appearance of neurosis. Thereafter the development of a sense of grievance is easy, the notion of compensation dawns in the patient's mind and looms ever larger in his thoughts. Following an injury sustained in the requisite circumstances there may be a period of days or weeks in which no evidence of psychoneurosis is to be seen, but this is a period of incubation, as it were, in which the subject is meditating upon the suffering and the derangement of his life caused by an accident for which he knows someone may possibly be made legally responsible. On the soil thus fertilized by lawyer and doctor a psychoneurosis readily develops. The patient has little inducement to get well, even though he suffers financially while he remains away from work, for if litigation is impending his prospects of compensation are greater if he enters the witness box with his full complement of symptoms than if he does so with no more than a tale of past and now vanished illness to relate. In the case of an industrial accident it may be urged that since the weekly amount payable as compensation is invariably less than the sufferer's normal income, the desire for the former cannot play a primary role in the genesis of neurosis. Yet it must be remembered that financial compensation is all the Workmen's Compensation Act has to offer him, and it becomes a symbol of his desire for redress for his sufferings—as he regards them, and thus is not thought of merely in terms of money value.

The simple fact that he is prepared to accept the financial loss that absence from work involves serves also to demonstrate to himself and to others concerned the reality of his disability. Rationalizations of this kind grow easily in the mind, and lead in these as in other circumstances to a man's acting against his own best interests with varying degrees of conviction. A fear of future ill-health and unemployment is a factor sometimes invoked to account for the persistence of the "traumatic" neurosis, but this can hardly be the case, since the man injured during a game of football may as reasonably have the same fear, yet he does not develop a neurosis. Even when this fear is held by the sufferer it is more often than not a rationalization, born after the development of the neurosis. In short, in these circumstances trauma is but the scapegoat, carrying a responsibility that rests elsewhere, and the "traumatic" neurosis is in fact a nosological impostor.

Symptoms.—These are mental and somatic. Mentally, there is usually a combination of anxiety and a sense of grievance. Complaints of inability to concentrate, of defect of current memory, and of sleeplessness are common. The somatic symptoms depend in a measure on the part of the body which is the seat of the injury, and include complaints of headache, giddiness, tremor, exhaustion, palpitation, tachycardia, etc., with local pains at the seat of injury. For a discussion of the differential diagnosis between the post-concussion syndrome and that of "traumatic" neurosis following head injury see page 202. Hysterical paresis and spasm may be present. In short, the features combine those of the anxiety neurosis and of the hysterical reaction.

Prognosis and Treatment.—"Traumatic" neurosis, especially in middle-aged or elderly subjects, may persist for years and may even be permanently disabling for regular work. Yet when the subject of an accident or injury on road, rail, or in industry is treated wisely and with encouragement from the outset, so that undue fears and a sense of grievance do not develop, the prognosis as to early recovery is sometimes good. However, should the patient unfortunately come, or be persuaded, to regard himself as a symbol of some imagined conflict of interests, and once legal processes are in train and litigation impending, the prognosis inevitably worsens and medical treatment becomes almost if not wholly useless. The dilatory processes by which increasing sums are offered in compensation by one party and refused by the other, the repeated medical and legal consultations to which the sufferer is subjected, and the idleness to which he is condemned, are all potent factors in implanting his psychoneurosis more deeply in his mind. Under such adverse conditions no medical measures can be expected to succeed and the relationship that should obtain between doctor and patient if the former is to help the latter can rarely be achieved.

The remedy for this lamentable state of affairs is not wholly or even mainly in the hands of the doctor, but the latter might do much to avert the development of a psychoneurosis by refraining from alarmist views and prognoses and by maintaining a dispassionate attitude in assessing both disability and prognosis.

Once the legal claims are settled to the satisfaction of the patient at the time of settlement improvement usually sets in. It may do so spontaneously or in response to treatment, more commonly the former, and we encounter the paradox of an illness which, having failed hitherto to respond to rest and a variety of treatments, now proceeds to improve spontaneously and without either. Yet such improvement is not invariably rapid, nor does it necessarily end in complete recovery.

Whenever undertaken, treatment consists in the careful taking of history, systematic physical examination, the general psychotherapeutic method employed in the case of the anxiety neurosis, and when the situation requires the care of whatever degree of physical injury may have been sustained. It may be added that evidence that physical injury has in fact been sustained is not always found either in history or on examination.

The role of the Workmen's Compensation Act in prolonging invalidism after industrial accidents has been stressed by many medical authorities. It makes no provision for the cure and rehabilitation of the injured man, but fixes his attention wholly upon the financial evaluation of his disability and sufferings. The convention of "light work" that so often intervenes between the state of complete disability and the hoped for arrival of full recovery is often most detrimental to recovery, for it commonly consists in unskilled work, or the doing of fatigues, that the skilled workman resents as beneath his occupational status and as not commanding the wage that his former employment brought in. To escape what he feels a humiliation, a withdrawal into complete incapacity for work is a not uncommon sequel, and thus his state is worsened and prolonged by a legal provision that takes no account of human nature. The provision of rehabilitation centres under the control of parties not associated in the sufferer's mind with employers, insurance companies, or workmen's trade organizations, seems an urgent necessity in dealing not only with physical injuries and their direct results, but also with the "traumatic neurosis."

(5) THE OBSESSIVE NEUROSIS

The patient is a victim of a compelling and persistent thought or system of thoughts, which may in some instances lead to compulsive acts, the patient remaining aware of the unreasonable nature of both thought and act. A familiar example is that of the patient who in unreasonable dread of dirt or of contact with infection indulges in constantly repeated hand-washing and in devices designed to avoid touching objects with the bare hand. Other examples are of the individual who has to come downstairs at night after retiring to bed to assure himself that he has locked the door, fastened the windows, or turned out the lights; of the individual into whose mind some distressing or obscene word or phrase persistently comes, with the production of considerable agitation and self-reproach.

The ætiology of this differs in no essential from that of the other varieties of psychoneurosis.

A tendency to obsessive thinking is not uncommon in normal individuals, but it never obtains possession of the patient's attention or dominates his life and activities in the degree encountered in the obsessive neurosis.

The treatment of this form of psychoneurosis is difficult and apt to be prolonged; it cannot be usefully undertaken save by the expert psycho-therapist.

CHAPTER XXIX

A Simple Scheme of Examination of the Nervous System

I. History.—The main symptoms complained of by the patient should be elicited, and if possible the sequence of their appearance. Care may be necessary to distinguish actual symptoms and the interpretations put upon them by the patient. Negative as well as positive items in the story should be taken into account, and these may have to be elicited by more or less direct questions. There can be no element in the student's clinical training of greater or more permanent value to him than the careful and methodical recording of his cases. There is no better discipline in clear thinking and statement, and no better way of fixing in his memory the clinical pictures of disease. The good clinician takes a just pride in his notes, and there is no clearer index of an untidy mind than untidy notes. The student is, therefore, urged not to regard note-taking as drudgery.

Attention should be given to the presence and characters of :—

HEADACHE—its position, its frequency, its duration, the symptoms that may accompany or follow it, and the factors which may seem to provoke or aggravate it.

PAIN—its distribution and character, its frequency and duration, the factors that influence its incidence and severity, and in some cases its response to various modes of treatment.

FITS AND OTHER TRANSIENT DISTURBANCES OF CONSCIOUSNESS—the age of first onset, their frequency and grouping, the usual times of occurrence, premonitory symptoms if any, the presence of cyanosis, of convulsions, of tongue-biting or urinary incontinence, the mode of recovery of consciousness, the mental state ensuing upon this recovery, and any symptoms that may follow. It is also of importance to ascertain in long-standing cases what treatment has hitherto been administered and its results.

VISION—past as well as present visual disturbances should be considered.

It is also necessary to elicit, as far as possible, the precise meaning intended by the patient in the use of such words as "giddiness" and "pain," for these and many other apparently clear terms are used in very diverse senses.

Y 337

II. Mental and Emotional State.—Note the state of consciousness. Is the patient mentally alert, slow, confused, disoriented, or stuporose? Are there hallucinations or delusions. Note the emotional tone. Is the patient depressed or emotionally exalted, is he or she emotionally unstable—prone to facile laughter or to tears? Note the memory for recent and long past events, the association of ideas, and the capacity to give a history.

SPEECH.

Comprehension.—Does the patient understand what is said to him, as tested by his ability to carry out simple or more complex orders, and by his verbal replies? Does he recognize familiar objects, can he read?

Expression.—Can he express himself in words, writing, or gesture? Can he form sentences, has he the normal use of names or does he employ periphrasis? Is he reduced to recurring utterances or single words? Does he recognize his mistakes when these occur? Can he speak or sing when excited? Difficulty in the use and arrangement of words must be distinguished from defects of articulation (dysarthria).

APRAXIA.—Can he, in the absence of paralysis, ataxy or sensory loss, carry out co-ordinated purposive movements at request? Does he appear to understand the use of familiar objects, and when he does, can he handle them appropriately?

III. Special Senses.

VISION.—Acuity for near and distant vision: for slight degrees of visual defect Snellen's types should be used: for more severe defects the ability to count fingers, to detect hand movements, or to recognize the change from light to dark should be recorded. Rough test of visual fields. For the ready recognition of defects in the visual field the method of *confrontation* may be employed. The patient covers one eye with his fingers and fixes the forehead of the observer, who sits opposite to him and about a yard distant, with the uncovered eye. A useful test object is a large white-headed hat pin, or a small square of paper ($\frac{1}{4}$ inch in diameter) fixed between the two prongs of a nib in a penholder. Each quadrant of the field is tested separately by bringing the test object towards the centre of the field of vision from its periphery. In this way the outer limits of the field of vision may be roughly determined. The presence of scotomata may be detected by moving the test object horizontally and vertically across the field.

HEARING.—Subjective—? tinnitus.

Acuity for *air* and for *bone* conduction (watch held near ear, and on mastoid) should be tested (see page 266).

SMELL AND TASTE.—The ability to recognize common aromatic substances presented to each nostril in turn: the ability to recognize salt, sweet, sour and bitter solutions applied to the tongue on either side while this is kept protruded from the mouth.

IV. Cranial Nerves.

III, IV, VI. PUPILS.—Are these normal and equal in size and circular in outline? Do they react normally on illumination (direct and consensual) and on convergence?

EXTERNAL OCULAR MOVEMENTS.—Are these normal in range in all directions, and is deviation well sustained (nystagmus)? Do the ocular axes remain parallel or do squint and double vision develop? Is there any ptosis or retraction of the lids, or any exophthalmos?

V. MOTOR.—Do the masseter and temporal muscles harden and swell equally on the two sides when the jaw is clenched? Is the jaw opened against resistance in the mid-line or does it deviate to one side?

SENSORY.—Note state of corneal reflex and sensibility of skin of face and anterior half of scalp.

VII. Is the face symmetrical at rest and on movement? Are the eyelashes buried to an equal extent on the two sides when the eyes are screwed up, and is the platysma contracted equally well on each side when the angles of the mouth are drawn down? If the face shows any weakness of movement, is this more obvious in the lower half or in respect of voluntary movements made on request rather than of involuntary movements of emotional expression?

VIII. *Vide supra* for hearing tests. Is there any vertigo?

IX, X, XI. Does the palate rise normally and in the mid-line during respiration and phonation? Is there a nasal quality to the voice, or regurgitation of fluids through nose? ? Movement of pharynx, ability to swallow liquids and solids. Pharyngeal reflex. Muscles of larynx, phonation. Trapezius and sternomastoid (cervical part of spinal accessory).

XII. Is there any atrophy or fibrillation of the tongue, and is this protruded straight and well, or deviated to side of palsy?

V. Motor System.—The musculature should be examined limb by limb, then the neck and the trunk muscles. Look for wasting, fibrillation, contractures, changes in the mobility of joints, and for mechanical factors capable of impeding movement that may not be the result of nervous lesions. Note deformities such as pes cavus, kyphoscoliosis, etc. Then note seriatim:—

(a) Changes in muscle tone as tested by passive movement, abnormal postures due to departures of tone from normal. Is hypertonus of pyramidal or of extrapyramidal type? Is "cogwheel" rigidity present?

(b) Voluntary power and range of active movements. Note if any defect of power is due to impairment of movements from central nervous lesion, or to weakness or paralysis of individual muscles. Note any alterations in speed of movement, as in paralysis agitans.

(c) Note the presence and type of any involuntary movements, whether continuous or intermittent, whether occurring during movement or at rest. Are such movements regular (tremor) or irregular (as in chorea)?

(d) Note the co-ordination of movement, and the probable source of any ataxy present. If this is due to impairment of postural sensibility, it will be increased when vision is excluded, and it will include error of projection in the finger-nose test, possibly astereognosis, and in the lower limbs unsteadiness of gait and Rombergism. The extended arms—when the eyes are closed—may fall away from the horizontal, or the fingers may perform involuntary movements like those of athetosis.

(e) Note the gait, whether weak, with dragging of feet or shuffling, whether ataxic, and if so whether aggravated by closing the eyes (Rombergism). Note whether the arms are normally swung in walking (this is early lost in paralysis agitans).

VI. Sensory System.

(a) Subjective disturbances, paræsthesiæ (tingling, numbness, "pins and needles"). Note the distribution of these, their frequency and the circumstances of their appearance. Note the character and distribution of pain, and the influence of posture and of movements upon it.

(b) *Objective.*—Test for loss of sensibility to:—

TOUCH: using cotton wool.

PAIN: using pin-prick for cutaneous pain, and pressure for deep pain.

TEMPERATURE: using tubes of hot and cold water.

SENSE OF POSITION: can patient touch nose with index finger when eyes are closed, or does limb wander and fail to find object? Can he appreciate passive movements of fingers, toes, or larger segments of a limb when eyes are closed? Can he tell position of passively moved limb at any moment in these circumstances? Does ataxy of stance or gait develop when eyes are closed, *e.g.* Rombergism?

VIBRATION SENSE: The foot of a vibrating tuning fork (C°128) is placed over the malleoli and other bony points, and the capacity to detect its vibrations tested.

VII. Reflexes.

TENDON REFLEXES—

    Upper limb—biceps (C. 5 & 6),
                supinator (C. 6),
                triceps (C. 6, 7 & 8).
    Lower limb—knee jerk (L. 2, 3 & 4),
                ankle jerk (S. 1 & 2).

Note whether increased, diminished, or lost, and whether equal on both sides. ? patellar or ankle clonus.

CUTANEOUS REFLEXES—

    Upper abdominal (right and left) (Th. 8 & 9).
    Lower abdominal (right and left) (Th. 10 & 11).
    Cremasteric (right and left) (Th. 12).

PLANTAR REFLEX—

    Flexor or extensor (*i.e.* dorsiflexor).

VIII. Sphincters.

Micturition—hesitancy or retention?
               urgency or incontinence?
               Is there a distended bladder?
Defæcation—incontinence after purgatives?
Sexual power—loss of power, or of desire?

IX. Trophic Changes.

In skin—œdema, atrophy (glossy skin).
Alterations in nails. Bedsores.
In bones and joints (arthropathy).

X. Cerebrospinal Fluid.

Under pressure? Turbidity, pus, altered colour? Coagulum on standing. Presence of blood?
Results of special pathological examination.

VII. **Reflexes.**

—Tendon reflexes—
Upper limb—biceps (C. 5, 6),
supinator, C. 6.
triceps (C. 6, 7 & 8).
Lower limb—knee-jerk (L. 2, 3, 4).
ankle-jerk (S. 1, 2).
Note whether increased, diminished, or lost, and whether equal on both sides... patellar or ankle clonus.

—Cutaneous reflexes—
Upper abdominal (right and left) (Th. 6, 7, 8 & 9)
Lower abdominal (right and left) Th. 10 & 11.
Cremasteric (right and left) (Th. 12).

—Plantar reflex—
Flexor or extensor (i.e. dorsiflexor).

VIII. **Sphincters.**

Micturition—frequency or intermittent.
urgency or incontinence.
Is there a distended bladder?
Defæcation—incontinence after purgatives?
Sexual power—loss of power, or of desire?

IX. **Trophic Changes.**

In skin—œdema, atrophic (glossy skin).
abrasions in nails. Bedsores.
In bones and joints (intra-pelvic?).

X. **Cerebrospinal Fluid.**

Under increase? Turbidity—pus, altered colour? Coagulum on standing. Presence of blood?
Results of special pathological examination.

Index

A

Abdominal reflex, 19
  in disseminated sclerosis, 182
  in motor neurone disease, 228
Abscess, intracranial, 88
  cerebellar, 89
  cerebral, 89
  cerebrospinal fluid in, 90
  diagnosis, 90
  extradural, 90
  pathology, 88
  pyæmic, 89
  extradural, 90
  symptoms, 89
  treatment, 91
Accommodation, paralysis of, 248
Achlorhydria, in subacute combined
  degeneration, 213
Acromegaly, 54, 82
Adenoma, of pituitary, 54, 80
Ætiology, factors in, 8
Afferent Nervous System, 31–36
Agnosia, 50, 52
Agonists, 15
Agraphia, 50–52
Alcohol—
  coma in, 103
  polyneuritis from, 249
Amaurosis, transient, 67
Amblyopia—
  in disseminated sclerosis,181, 262
  quinine, 257
  tobacco, 258
Amnesia—
  hysterical, 325
  retrograde, 199
Amyotonia congenita, 224
Amyotrophic lateral sclerosis (see Motor
  neurone disease)
Anæmia, cerebral, 93, 125
  pernicious, 213
  of sprue, 217
Anæsthesia—
  dissociated, 240
  hysterical, 327
  in tabes, 168
Analgesia—
  in syringomyelia, 240
  in tabes, 168
Anarthria (see Articulation)
Aneurysm, intracranial—
  ætiology, 99, 112
  cerebrospinal fluid in, 113
  diagnosis, 112
  hæmorrhage from, 112
Aneurysm—
  of internal carotid, 112
  prognosis, 112

Aneurysm—
  rupture of, 112
  symptoms of, 112
  treatment, 114
Angioma—
  cerebral, 127
  spinal, 209
Ankle jerk, 19
  in polyneuritis, 246–250
  in sciatica, 272–276
  segmental localization, 19
  in tabes, 168
Anorexia nervosa, 330
Anosmia, 77
Antagonists, 15
Anxiety neurosis, 315–323
Aphasia, 51–53
  in migraine, 134
Apoplexy—
  ætiology, 5, 98
  differential diagnosis, 102
  prognosis, 104
  residual paralyses of, 105
  symptoms, 5, 98
  treatment, 111
Arachnoiditis, 205, 209
Argyll Robertson pupil, 163, 169
Arthritis, muscular wasting in, 231
Articulation, disorders of, 48
  in cerebellar lesions, 30
  in chronic bulbar palsy, 229
  in dementia paralytica, 176
  in disseminated sclerosis, 183
  in pseudobulbar palsy, 109
Aspirin poisoning, 103
Associated movements (see Movements)
Astereognosis, 37
Astrocytes (see Neuroglia)
Astrocytoma, 71, 73
Ataxy—
  cerebellar, 29
  Friedreich's, 218–219
  hereditary, 218
  in medullary thrombosis, 106
  in tabes, 169, 172
  in vestibular lesions, 267, 268
Atheroma, cerebral, 98–100
Athetosis, 28
  bilateral, 296
  in infantile hemiplegia, 296
Athetosis, pathology, 296
  as a release symptom, 6, 27
Atonia, 16
  in cerebellar lesions, 29
Atrophy, disuse, 231, 328
  of iris, 169
  muscular—
    arthritic, 231
    in cervical rib, 234

PRINTED BY J. AND J. GRAY, EDINBURGH